Social Work and Health Care in an Aging Society

Education, Policy, Practice, and Research

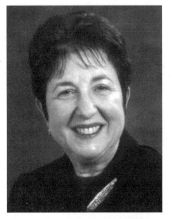 **Barbara J. Berkman, DSW,** is the Helen Rehr/Ruth Fizdale Professor of Health and Mental Health at Columbia University School of Social Work (CUSSW) and Adjunct Professor, Department of Community and Preventive Medicine, Mount Sinai School of Medicine in New York City. Dr. Berkman has directed 23 federally and foundation supported research projects focusing on issues in geriatric care, and is currently Director of the John A. Hartford Foundation's Geriatric Social Work Faculty Scholars Program. She is a former President of the Institute for the Advancement of Social Work Research (IASWR) and is a Fellow of the Gerontological Society of America and of the New York Academy of Medicine.

Linda Krogh Harootyan, MSW, is the Deputy Director for the Gerontological Society of America (GSA) and serves as the Project Officer for the $10 million Hartford Geriatric Social Work Faculty Scholars and Doctoral Fellows Programs. She initiated and secured funding to launch a major initiative within the organization to address minority issues in aging. Ms. Harootyan was a coauthor of *The Common Stake: The Interdependence of Generations* and has edited or directed production of a wide range of publications. Since 1980 she has been a representative to the Leadership Council of Aging Organizations, a Washington, DC-based coalition of more than 40 aging organizations, and currently serves as the Membership Chair. Ms. Harootyan received her Masters in Social Work from San Diego State University.

Social Work and Health Care in an Aging Society

Education, Policy, Practice, and Research

Barbara Berkman, DSW, Editor
Linda Harootyan, MSW, Associate Editor

 Springer Publishing Company

Copyright © 2003 by Springer Publishing Company, Inc.

Springer Publishing Company, Inc.
536 Broadway
New York, NY 10012-3955

Acquisitions Editor: Sheri W. Sussman
Production Editor: Jeanne W. Libby
Cover design by Joanne E. Honigman

03 04 05 06 07/5 4 3 2 1

Library of Congress Cataloging-in-Publication Data

Social work and health care in an aging society : education, policy, practice, and research / Barbara Berkman, Linda Harootyan, editors
    p. cm.
    Chapters are based on the research of the first 10 scholars in the Hartford Geriatric Social Work Faculty Scholars Program, administered by the Gerontological Society of America.
    Includes bibliographical references and index.
    ISBN 0-8261-1543-8
    1. Social work with the aged—United States. 2. Aged—Services for—United States. 3. Medical social work—United States.
4. Aged—Medical care—United States. 5. Aged—Mental health services—United States. 6. Social work education—United States. 7. Aged—Government policy—United States. I. Berkman, Barbara. II. Harootyan, Linda K.
    HV1451.S632 2003
    362.6'0973—dc21   2003042815

Printed in the United States of America by Maple-Vail Book Manufacturing Group.

We dedicate this book with love to Barbara's parents, Sally and Manuel Fox, who always inspire their children and grandchildren to contribute to society in the best ways possible; and in memory of Alice and Leo Harootyan, who showed their family how to age with dignity and grace.

11/03

CONTENTS

CONTRIBUTORS

Margaret E. Adamek, MSW, PhD
Indiana University

Portia Adams, MSW
Washington University of St. Louis

Nancy Capobianco Boyer, MSW, PhD
Boston University

Denise Burnette, MSSW, PhD
Columbia University

Letha A. Chadiha, MSW, PhD
University of Michigan

Daniel S. Gardner, MSW
Columbia University

Scott Miyake Geron, PhD
Boston University

Melanie Gironda, MSW, PhD
University of California at Los Angeles

Marci Guevara, MSW
University of Utah

Irene A. Gutheil, DSW
Fordham University

Suk-Young Kang, MSW
Columbia University

Stacy Kolomer, PhD
University of Georgia

Nancy P. Kropf, MSW, PhD
University of Georgia

Ji Seon Lee, MSSW, PhD
Fordham University

Faith C. Little, MSW
Boston University

James Lubben, DSW, MPH
University of California at Los
Angeles

Peter Maramaldi, PhD, MPH
University of Utah

Philip McCallion, MSW, PhD
State University of New York at
Albany

Matthias J. Naleppa, MSW,
PhD
Virginia Commonwealth
University

Gregory J. Paveza, MSW, DPH
University of South Florida

Cynthia Cannon Poindexter,
MSW, PhD
Fordham University

Stephanie A. Robert, MSW,
PhD
University of Wisconsin

Jeanette Semke, MSW, PhD
University of Washington

Carla VandeWeerd, BSW
University of South Florida

Scott Wilks, MSW
University of Georgia

Bradley D. Zodikoff, MSW
Columbia University

ACKNOWLEDGMENTS

We want to express our deepest gratitude to Laura Robbins, Senior Project Officer, and Corinne Rieder, Executive Director of the John A. Hartford Foundation, without whose intellectual and steadfast support this book never would have been written.

We would like to thank Sarah D'Ambruoso, Program Coordinator of the Hartford Geriatric Social Work Faculty Scholars Program, who worked closely with each of the authors on every phase of bringing this book to fruition; and our special thanks are given to Jennifer Campi, Beth Ciha, and Candace Heinlein for their superior editorial skills.

And we gratefully acknowledge our fellow contributors, each of whom has made significant contributions to social work in gerontology and health care, in education, policy, practice, and research.

Chapter 1

INTRODUCTION

Barbara Berkman and Linda Krogh Harootyan

Over the past 10 years, Americans have read many times about the dramatic changes in health care delivery that have been stimulated by advances in technology and by new approaches to the financing of health care. They also have read about the significant and equally dramatic changes in the demographics of the older population. The statistics, which highlight the increasing proportion of the population who will be older than 65 years and the increasing diversity of the older population, are now familiar to all Americans.

People are living longer because of advances in public health, health care technology, and service delivery. In 1990, 4% of the population (3 million people) in America was aged 65 or older, compared with 13% (35 million) in 2000 (U.S. Bureau of the Census, 2000a). At the end of the decade, in 2011, the baby boom population will begin to turn 65 years old, and by 2050, 20% of the total U.S. population will be aged 65 years and older (U.S. Bureau of the Census, 2000c). The fastest growing segment of the older population in the United States is the group aged 85 years and older, which is expected to grow from 4 million in 2000 to 19 million by 2050. By 2050, about one third of the elderly population will be composed of Blacks, Hispanics, Asians, and other minority groups (U.S. Bureau of the Census, 2000b).

The increasing need for biopsychosocial services to support the independent functioning of older adults and the needs of their caregivers means that more social work assistance will be required to address their health care needs effectively (Browne, Smith, & Ewalt, 1996). Social work professionals with training in aging are even more essential in health care to address the social, functional, psychological, and environmental needs of older people and their families.

This raises the question of whether today's social work education will focus on yesterday's health care practice or whether social work educators will develop educational programs for future designs of practice. Today, social work educators can conclude that within social work, interest in the older person and health care is undergoing a revival. However, the gaps between research, practice, policy, and education must be closed. Regardless of their specialty, social workers need knowledge about aging, yet social work education does not consistently provide this knowledge outside of aging specializations. Only 10% of all social work students take a course on aging (Damon-Rodriguez & Lubben, 1997), although almost all of them will be working with older adults and their families. With little or no knowledge about aging, social workers graduate ill-prepared to meet the needs of the clients and communities they serve.

THE CHANGING WORLD OF HEALTH AND MENTAL HEALTH

Americans live in a changing political, economic, and social world that is aging. Each of these domains presents complex issues for health care and social work. It is understandable that educators, for the sake of clarity, frequently have found it pedagogically efficient to break these domains apart and focus on one dimension at a time, for example, separating health from aging, or policy from psychosocial practice. In this context, social work is a dramatically changing construct in the dramatically changing world of health and mental health. Changes in patient care and in the financing and structure of health care systems are creating new roles and challenges for social workers. Thus, educators cannot use a single factorial model in instructing their students. The biopsychosocial frame is not sufficient without addressing economic, political, social, cultural, and environmental factors.

Today, there are significant changes in outcomes of patient care that are stimulated by technological advances in biomedicine and pharmacology. People are living longer with complex chronic physical and mental health conditions (Berkman, Silverstone, Simmons, Howe, & Volland, 2000). The leading causes of morbidity and mortality are almost all related to chronic diseases, resulting in episodes of illness over a lifetime of chronic complex processes (Paulson, 1994). These elderly people often have significant activity impairments and quality-of-life issues. They will represent an increasing percentage of persons who are served by social workers. Social workers who will be valued in health care will be those who have the necessary knowledge and skills to work effectively with older people and their families.

Americans are witnessing dramatic changes in the financing of health care delivery. The corporatization of health care delivery systems in the United States is having a profound impact on health care professionals who work with older adults. Currently, health care is skillful in its ability to provide high-quality, technologically advanced acute care, but the ability to meet chronic care needs is limited because the service and financing systems are complex and fragmented into many minisystems. There is an overlapping, confusing array of service providers—ranging from the federal government to state and local governments, the proprietary sector, the voluntary sector, and the family. Under managed care particularly, there is movement toward more community-based services. There is the decentralization of expensive diagnostic services to out-of-hospital sites and increasing use of ambulatory procedures and services that were once done only on an inpatient basis.

These changes further complicate the ability of elderly patients and their families to access and use the multiple systems of care effectively. It is not surprising that with the fragmentation of service delivery even the most competent elders and their families have difficulty deciphering the eligibility requirements of different programs. They and their families require special knowledgeable interventions from social workers in order to access and use social and health care systems effectively. Health care is beginning to respond to the increasing need for continuity of care through the creation of community-based networks that link service providers to a continuum of health care that includes long-term care, rehabilitation, home care, and community social services. Thus, there is new opportunity for social workers to serve the aging population through the continuum of care based on predetermined vulnerable points in a chronic illness.

It is important to note that the political environment of health care practice is constantly in flux. Social work practice is affected by changing political priorities, the push and pull of various constituencies, the introduction of new ideas and technologies, and the advent of new policies around health crises, such as HIV/AIDS. The bulk of health care services are financed by monies from the public domain. Policy decisions are made that determine the availability of services, length of service, and type of services provided to patients. Social workers need to have a voice in developing appropriate policies that meet the needs of their clients. These issues also must be incorporated into social work education if social work professionals are to meet the demands of health care practice with competence.

This is also a time of social changes in the expectations for family responsibility. Families are increasingly expected to be responsible for home care needs. With the number of beneficiaries of the Medicare Home Health Program rising significantly, there has been a simultaneous increase in the pressure placed on families (U.S. Special Committee on Aging, 1996). Recent national surveys suggest that one in four households was involved in helping to care for a family member who is aged 50 years or older. More than 9 million people in the United States are informal caregivers (Berkman & Volland, 1997). At the same time, there has been a reduction in the number of family members available to provide care (Scofield, 1995) because of geographic distances and increased workforce participation.

Older persons are not only receiving care, they also are providing it. Half of all people caring for elderly family members are themselves older than age 60, and there are 2.5 million families in the United States that are maintained by a grandparent (Lipsitz & Rosenberg, 2002). However, families may not have the physical, psychological, or financial resources needed to provide such care. The capacity of families to adapt to the patient's health or mental health condition has led to a renewed focus on training social workers for intergenerational family practice.

Another significant social change that is impacting health care and social work is that patients and their families are increasingly seeking more active participation in health care decision-making as they are faced with more complex clinical choices. The complexity of medical decision-making includes issues around providing or withholding treatment, organ donations, and complex or risky surgical and other innovative medical procedures. As individuals and their families become more responsible for decision making, it is obvious that they will need additional education and support from social workers around psychosocial issues in adjusting and responding to illness and necessary role changes. Increased cultural diversity among the elderly population who confront serious physical and mental health problems is another major demographic trend that is impacting health care services and social work practice. There are vast cultural differences in factors that affect the health care of patients in terms of health care utilization and patterns of relationships with providers and family members. Social workers can be leaders among health professionals in understanding and interpreting the importance of culture on health care service delivery.

SOCIAL WORK IN HEALTH CARE

After 100 years of social work in health care, social workers are visible in every facet of service delivery, working as providers in new models of health and mental health practice. Unfortunately, many of these models of care are based on a system in which health and mental health services operate as separate fragmented entities, isolated from social support services, which raises increased concerns about accessibility, efficiency, and comprehensiveness (Berkman & Maramaldi, 2001). As more social health services are provided in neighborhood agencies (senior centers, community centers, housing projects, and churches), there are increased opportunities to develop integrated, linked service-delivery systems (Mellor, 1996). For example, elderly patients with chronic-care needs require rehabilitation and a range of supportive services from home care to meal preparation, counseling to adult day care, respite care, and acute and long-term care. Social workers must be prepared to intervene along the continuum of service delivery.

As case managers and counselors to vulnerable patients and their families, social workers can be crucial to maintaining older individuals in their communities and reducing the cost of health services. However, interventions must be designed that focus on prevention and health promotion, early diagnosis of psychosocial problems, and treatment and rehabilitation along the continuum of service delivery. Consumer and staff education and consultation concerning health coverage and the impact of new technologies are increasingly needed. Case management and care coordination models must be demonstrated. Inherent in these changing roles for social work is the need for new important skills: alternative intervention strategies, such as short-term intensive therapies; screening and identification of psychosocial problems using standardized reliable and valid measures; biopsychosocial assessments that are timely; and the ability to develop critical-path treatment models (Volland, Berkman, Stein, & Vaghy, 2000).

The acute-care model, long the focus of geriatric social work in hospitals, is no longer sufficient to meet the needs of the chronically ill older population who need continuity of care and not just episodic interventions. Social work's biopsychosocial and multidisciplinary approach to care positions social workers to have a principal role within emerging linked health delivery systems. However, as payers increasingly expect the use of critical-path models and outcomes research to promote interventions of a particular type or length, social workers must be able to evaluate the outcome of their practice and use evaluative data in case planning. It is virtually impossible with existing knowledge to determine the effects on client outcomes of most social work interventions, such as family treatment, much less to know whether the effect is preferable to the outcome that may have resulted from other services (such as peer groups) or no services. Thus, it is imperative to conduct research on the outcomes of social work services.

THE GENESIS OF THIS BOOK

Too frequently, social work education has separated the issues of aging from health and mental health issues. This has been evident in the development of specializations and concentrations in aging as separate from health, mental health, and disability. Reality shows practitioners that the vulnerable, chronically ill elderly patient—traditionally the major focus of social work services—presents complex intersecting physical, mental, and social environment problems associated with aging. It is time to bring the concepts of aging and health care together in social work educational programs, social-work policy considerations, social work practice, and social work research. This book is based on the premise that aging and health care are significantly intertwined.

In 1998, the John A. Hartford Foundation began an initiative to improve the capacity of social work educators to train practitioners who would work in geriatric health care to improve the lives of older adults and their families. One of the first projects funded under this agenda was the Hartford Geriatric Social Work Faculty Scholars Program, which is administered by the Gerontological Society of America. The program's goal is to increase the number of faculty in schools of social work who are leaders and scholars in geriatric health care. One of the main objectives of the program is to contribute new knowledge of the contributions of gerontological social work to health care outcomes by supporting the Scholars in community-based research. The first 10 Scholars were selected in 1999 after a highly competitive process that focused on their potential as scholars and leaders in research, teaching, policy, and professional activities.

The chapters in this book are based on the research of the first 10 Hartford Scholars and other scholars who were significantly involved in the beginning phase of the Hartford program. These leaders in gerontological social work have focused their research career trajectories on the improvement of the health and well-being of older adults and their caregivers. Therefore, each chapter is focused on an area of significance in gerontological health-care social work. Each author has placed the importance of his or her area of gerontological research within the broader context of the health and well-being of older adults and their families and has clarified the added value brought by social work practice to each of these areas.

The unique challenge of social work in integrating aging and health care is that social workers do not have the luxury of limiting the number of variables to which health care professionals must relate. If the goal of social work is to support the social functioning of individual and family, it must not offer a narrow basis for practice. Care must be taken that practitioners do not fall into a dogmatic single-factor causality mode of thinking, which too frequently has directed the practices of both biomedically based and psychodynamically based practitioners. And although social work has placed greater emphasis in past years on the psychological and interpersonal elements of social functioning, it is evident to those who practice in geriatric health care that in conceptualizing the content areas necessary in curricula, educators must encompass a blend of cultural, social, psychological, environmental, and biological dimensions of social functioning, with policy issues addressed in each domain.

In framing their chapters, the authors recognize that the issues of health and aging are multidimensional. They address the political, social, and economic issues that drive social work health and aging policies, which in turn impact the accessibility of health care and the social and economic well-being of older adults and their families. In addition, because social work's dynamic role in practice must be based on evidence captured through research, the authors examine the evidence-based knowledge available in their specific area by reviewing prior research, presenting their own current research, and delineating the needs for further research. As these scholars also are faculty members in schools of social work, they make suggestions for integrating this knowledge into the curriculum of master's degree educational programs in social work.

The dramatic changing events—political, social, economical, and technological—in an aging world must not be lost to social workers in health care, who must keep their knowledge base current. Thus, this book represents an effort to present significant issues related to the health, mental health, and well-being of older adults and their significant caregivers. We use a multidimensional approach in which the chapters address critical problems that exemplify the intersect between the biopsychosocial and political domains. Each chapter begins with an introduction to the area of knowledge addressed and its importance to social work, to health care, and to the practice and policy arenas. These chapters are not meant to be all-inclusive of gerontological health-care knowledge, but are focused on some of the issues that are in the forefront of gerontological social work in health care practice in the emerging health care world. Thus, the trends in health-care service delivery are evident throughout. Furthermore, the book attempts to emphasize that research, as the means to acquiring evidence-based knowledge, is an integral part of social-work health care practice and is the frame for directing policy concerns. The reality is that there are many deficiencies in the provision of geriatric social and health care services. Elimination of these deficiencies is a critical concern to all health care professionals. Social work research must be motivated by the desire to clarify social work principles of practice and by the professional concern for questions, such as What are the knowledge and skills needed to improve the health and well-being of social work clients?

Social-work gerontological health-care practice has significantly moved out of the acute care arena and is primarily focused on the long-term care needs of those with chronic illness. In chapters 2 and 3, Margaret Adamek and Jeanette Semke address the older adult with health and mental health long-term care needs. Dr. Adamek's chapter focuses on geriatric depression in institutional long-term care. Depression is the most common mental health disorder in late life, but is not a normal part of aging. Dr. Adamek notes that despite our recognition that mental and physical health are inextricably linked, the emphasis on medical intervention in long-term institutional care continues to overshadow attention to psychosocial needs. She raises the concern that America's current reimbursement policies in long-term care promote a unilateral approach. Dr. Semke focuses on older adults with dementia in community-based long-term care. She clearly identifies the challenges faced in the coordination of community-based social and health services to meet the needs of older persons who are experiencing comorbid health and mental health problems. In addressing policy implications, she voices concern that the move away from institutional care toward community residential care may have preceded the development of more socially oriented models of care that are needed to maximize the health and well-being of older persons.

The vulnerable chronically ill patient, traditionally the major focus of social work services, presents complex interacting medical and psychosocial problems. They and their families require special interventions from community-based social workers to access and utilize social and health care services effectively. Chapters 4 and 5 focus on older adults with community-based service needs. In chapter 4, Ji Seon Lee and Irene Gutheil address social work in home health care. While home health care is a medically oriented service, psychosocial services are often needed and are essential to positive patient outcome. Dr. Lee and Dr. Gutheil clearly elucidate the threats and the challenges to providing psychosocial services posed by the new prospective payment system (PPS). In chapter 5, Matthias Naleppa reviews geriatric case-management as a critical component in the continuum of care, addressing the value of task-centered brief treatment as an intervention modality for case management. He examines case-management services and how its direction has been shaped by social and economic policy. The chapter details the testing of the intervention process and is an excellent example of research for evidence-based practice.

The view that illness is a chronic process raises the question of whether an acute episode can be prevented, placing much more importance on consumers in determining their health care needs and outcomes (Berkman, 1996). The focus of care becomes primary care, with an emphasis on disease prevention and health promotion (Paulson,

1994). The growing empowerment of older adults who wish to participate in decision making about their own health care and treatment is
shifting the decision-making role away from the physician and to the
patient. In chapters 6 and 7, Denise Burnette and Suk-Young Kang
and Letha Chadiha and Portia Adams approach this issue from two
perspectives. Dr. Burnette and Mr. Kang emphasize the importance
of patient self-health care as a critical adjunct to professional care in
the continuum of care for chronic health conditions. They focus on
older African Americans who are particularly disadvantaged in terms
of chronic conditions and disabilities. Dr. Chadiha and Ms. Adams
address the challenges faced by older Black women and their physical
health status, health care, and economic well-being. They recommend
empowerment strategies to enable older African American women to
improve their health and economic well-being.

   Three chapters (8 through 10) focus on caregiving issues when older
adults assume caregiving responsibilities. In chapter 8, Nancy Kropf
and Scott Wilks address the issue of grandparents raising grandchildren. Current intervention approaches to help grandparents with their
health care needs and social functioning are highlighted and there is
presented an innovative intervention for custodian grandparents who
may typically be outside of existing service networks. In chapter 9,
Philip McCallion and Stacey Kolomer focus on older caregivers of
adults with intellectual disabilities. They emphasize that innovative
responses to the needs of caregivers are required if persons with
developmental disabilities are to remain in the community with quality
of life. And in chapter 10, Cynthia Cannon Poindexter and Nancy
Capobianco Boyer highlight older relatives who are taking care of
grandchildren whose parents have HIV disease. They emphasize that
these caregivers can be remarkably strong and resourceful, but that
social workers must still recognize their need for services that are now
lacking. In chapter 11, Gregory Paveza and Carla VandeWeerd address
the important area of elder care, but with a focus on the underserved
issue of mistreatment of elders by caregivers. They emphasize that
this critical issue is largely underdeveloped in educational offerings,
in research, and in national policies.

   The final section of the book focuses on trends that cut across every
problem area addressed in gerontological health-care social work,
biopsychosocial assessments, and consumer-directed outcome measures. Social work in health care should provide a carefully balanced
perspective that takes into account the person in his or her environ-

ment and helps social workers assess the needs of an individual from a multidimensional point of view. Biopsychosocial assessments play an increasingly important role in health planning and clinical practice. The authors in this section deal with significant assessment and measurement issues. Particular recognition is given to the increased importance of consumer involvement in the development of assessment measures and the evaluation of outcome of services (Berkman, 1996; Shortell, Gillies, & Devers, 1995; Volland, 1996). In chapter 12, Scott Miyake Geron and Faith Little lay the foundation by addressing the importance of geriatric assessment, the characteristics of useful measures of practice, emerging areas of assessment research, and the growth of consumer-directed care and consumer-centered outcomes.

Another major demographic trend that is having an impact on social work assessment and service delivery outcomes is the increased social and ethnic diversity of the older population. Health care professionals must be especially cognizant of the cultural diversity among elders who confront serious physical and mental health problems. In chapter 13, Peter Maramaldi and Marci Guevara emphasize the importance of cultural considerations when developing, implementing, and evaluating geriatric health care delivery systems.

Social support, social ties, social networks, and social isolation and loneliness are important assessment variables in geriatrics. They are frequently used in practice, research, and policy, but not necessarily with enough specificity. In chapter 14, James Lubben and Melanie Gironda help us distinguish and understand these constructs as they focus on the centrality of social ties to the health and well-being of older adults and the use of standardized means of measurement.

A major trend affecting all health care practice and professionals is that evaluating the outcomes of health interventions is becoming increasingly necessary (Corcoran & Gingerich, 1994; Rogut, 1995). In this emerging health-care environment, social workers will be expected to demonstrate effectiveness through an evaluative process based on clinical practice guidelines (Lawlor & Raube, 1995; Shueman & Troy, 1994). In chapter 15, Stephanie Robert focuses on the need for, and issues in, evaluation of quality-of-life outcomes in long-term home-care programs from the consumer's perspective, emphasizing the important role for social workers.

The final chapter in the book is written by Daniel Gardner and Bradley Zodikoff, two highly experienced gerontological health care social workers. They acknowledge that health care is changing dramatically and address questions as to whether gerontological social work in health care will meet the new challenge posed by community-based care for complex health and mental health situations. Gerontological social work is now expanding its focus of concern and articulating a new vision for the profession. More than 20 years ago, Elaine Brody, a social work gerontologist, urged social work education to lead rather than lag (Brody, 1970). We believe that the work of the scholars in this book represents a beginning leadership effort.

REFERENCES

Berkman, B. (1996). The emerging health care world: Implications for social work practice and education. *Social Work, 41,* 541–551.

Berkman, B., & Maramaldi, P. (2001). Health, mental health, and disabilities. In R. Feldman & S. Kamerman (Eds.), *The Columbia University School of Social Work: A centennial celebration* (pp. 246–264). New York: Columbia University Press.

Berkman, B., Silverstone, B., Simmons, W. J., Howe, J., & Volland, P. (2000). Social work gerontological practice: The need for faculty development in the new millennium. *Journal of Gerontological Social Work, 34*(1), 5–23.

Berkman, B., & Volland, P. (1997). Health care practice overview. In *Encyclopedia of social work* (19th ed., 1997 Suppl., pp. 143–149). Washington, DC: National Association of Social Workers Press.

Brody, E. (1970). Serving the aged: Educational needs as viewed by practice. *Social Work, 15,* 42–51.

Browne, C. V., Smith, M., & Ewalt, P. L. (1996). Advancing social work practice in health care settings: A collaborative partnership for continuing education. *Health and Social Work, 21,* 267–276.

Corcoran, K., & Gingerich, W. J. (1994). Practice evaluation in the context of managed care: Case-recording methods for quality assurance reviews. *Research on Social Work Practice, 4,* 326–337.

Damon-Rodriguez, J., & Lubben, J. (1997). The 1995 WHCOA: An agenda for social work education and training. In C. Saltz (Ed.), *Social work response to the 1995 White House Conference on Aging: From issues to actions* (pp. 65–77). New York: Haworth.

Katz, I. R., & Parmelee, P. A. (1997). Overview. In R. L. Rubenstein & M. Powell Lawton (Eds.), *Depression in long-term and residential care: Advances in research and treatment* (pp. 1–25). New York: Springer Publishing.

Lawlor, E. F., & Raube, K. (1995). Social interventions and outcomes in medical effectiveness research. *Social Service Review, 69,* 383–403.

Lipsitz, L. A., & Rosenberg, R. (Eds.). (2002). *Harvard Cooperative Program on Aging Newsletter, 31,* 2.

Mellor, M. J. (1996). Special populations among older persons. *Journal of Gerontological Social Work, 25*(1/2), 1–10.

Paulson, L. G. (1994). Chronic illness: Implications of a new paradigm for health care. *Joint Commission Journal on Quality Improvement, 20*(1), 33–39.

Rogut, L. (1995). *Meeting patients' needs: Quality care in a changing environment.* New York: United Hospital Fund Paper Series.

Scofield, E. C. (1995). A model for preventive psychosocial care for people with HIV disease. *Health and Social Work, 20,* 102–109.

Shortell, S. M., Gillies, R. R., & Devers, K. J. (1995). Reinventing the American hospital. *Milbank Quarterly, 73,* 131–160.

Shueman, S. A., & Troy, W. G. (1994). The use of practice guidelines in behavioral health programs. In S. A. Shueman, W. G. Troy, & S. L. Mayhugh (Eds.), *Managed behavioral health care: An industry perspective* (pp. 149–166). Springfield, IL: Charles C Thomas.

U.S. Bureau of the Census. (2000a). *Census 2000 summary file 1 (SF 1).* Washington, DC: Author.

U.S. Bureau of the Census. (2000b). *Population projections of the United States by age, sex, race, Hispanic origin, and nativity: 1999–2000.* Washington, DC: Author.

U.S. Bureau of the Census. (2000c). *Projections of the total resident population by 5-year age groups, race, and Hispanic origin with special age categories: Middle series, 2050 to 2070 (NP-T4-G).* Washington, DC: Author.

U.S. Special Committee on Aging. (1996). *GAO report to the Chairman.* Washington, DC: Author.

Volland, P. J. (1996). Social work practice in health care: Looking to the future with a different lens. *Social Work in Health Care, 23*(4), 35–51.

Volland, P., Berkman, B., Stein, G., & Vaghy, A. (2000). *Social work education for practice in health care: Final report.* New York: New York Academy of Medicine.

Chapter 2

LATE-LIFE DEPRESSION IN NURSING HOME RESIDENTS: SOCIAL WORK OPPORTUNITIES TO PREVENT, EDUCATE, AND ALLEVIATE

Margaret E. Adamek

> No pill or regime known, or likely, could transform the latter years
> of life as fully as could a change in our vision of age and a militancy
> in attaining that.
> —Alex Comfort (1976)

Depression is the most common affective disorder in late life. The highest rates of late-life depression are found in long-term-care (LTC) settings where an estimated 30% to 50% of residents experience some level of depression (Katz & Parmelee, 1997). While currently a small proportion (5%) of the older adult population lives in nursing homes (about 1.5 million people), the proportion of the population who are older is increasing dramatically, particularly with the aging of the baby boom cohort. Thus, it is anticipated that the number of LTC residents will triple by 2040 (Katz & Parmelee, 1997). Considering both the anticipated growth in the LTC residential population and estimates of the proportion that experience depressive symptoms, and in the absence of significant changes in approaches to identification, treatment, and prevention of late-life depression, there will be an estimated 2.25 million LTC residents living with depression by 2040.

Despite documentation of the high prevalence of depression among LTC residents, it is estimated that only 10% of their needs for mental health services are being met (Burns & Taube, 1990). Too often, depression among older adults, particularly LTC residents, is viewed as a normal part of aging and hence is disregarded. As G. D. Cohen (1997) stated, "failure to attend adequately to issues of mental health and aging in long-term-care settings continues to be a pervasive, major public health problem" (p. 211). Untreated depression in late life is of such magnitude that the National Institute of Mental Health identified depression among older adults as a major public health problem (National Institutes of Health Consensus Development Panel on the Diagnosis and Treatment of Depression in Late Life [NIH Consensus Panel], 1992). Unreported, undiagnosed, and untreated depression results in serious consequences in terms of decreased quality of life and increased morbidity, mortality, and health care costs (Buckwalter & Piven, 1999). Late-life depression is particularly costly because of its role in producing excess disability (U.S. Surgeon General, 1999). This issue promises to persist as the growth of the older population, especially the oldest-old, leads to a continuing need for both institutional and community-based long-term care.

SIGNIFICANCE TO GERONTOLOGY, HEALTH CARE, AND HEALTH PROFESSIONALS

Estimates of the prevalence of late-life depression vary widely, from 10% to 15% of older adults in the community (Blazer, 1989) to 17% to 37% of older adult primary care patients (Garrard et al., 1998; Glasser & Gravdal, 1997). It is generally agreed that the highest rates of depression are found in nursing home residents (Masand, 1995), and that a majority of elderly nursing-home residents experience depressive conditions (Jakubiak & Callahan, 1995–1996). Each year, 12% of LTC residents will experience a new episode of major depression; another 18% will develop new depressive symptoms (Reynolds, 1995; Rovner et al., 1991). More than 64% of nursing home residents exhibit at least one depressive symptom (Lair & Lefkowitz, 1990).

Rates of minor depression among LTC residents range from 23% to 40% (Mossey, 1997). Minor depression is a subsyndromal form of depression in which elevated symptoms may be reported by older adults but do not meet diagnostic criteria for major depression or dysthymia. This may signify an early form of major depression, a residual of major depression, a chronic mild form of depression, or a response to an identifiable stressor, that is, loss of independence or illness. Although the *Diagnostic and Statistical Manual of Mental Disorders* (1994 [*DSM-IV*]) does not yet standardize the diagnosis of minor depression (U.S. Surgeon General, 1999), it can be just as disabling as major depression (Unützer et al., 1997). And given the difficulties in defining the milder depressions, they have received even less attention than major depression in terms of case-finding and treatment in LTC (Mossey, 1997). Late-life depression in LTC is of concern in gerontology and health care not only because of its extensiveness, but also due to the lack of efficacious intervention and preventive measures.

There are many barriers to identifying and treating depression in LTC settings. Limitations in diagnosis by professionals is a primary impediment. A lack of geriatric mental health expertise among LTC staff serves as a significant barrier to proper identification and treatment of depression among residents. Many staff members, including social service staff, physicians, rehabilitation therapists, nurses, and nurse aides may perceive depression as a "normal" or expected part of aging or as not being amenable to treatment. In addition, discrepancies in the identification of depression in LTC are common. Studies have documented both low recognition of depression by staff (Bagley et al., 2000) and differential recognition of depression between disciplines (Cohen-Mansfield, Rabinovich, Marx, Braun, & Fleshner, 1991). One study reported only 14% agreement between physicians and psychiatric specialists on both depressive disorders and depressive symptoms of LTC residents (U.S. Surgeon General, 1999). Teresi, Abrams, Holmes, Ramirez, and Eimicke (2001) found that LTC social workers, who do not typically have graduate degrees or licensure, have low recognition of depression. Only one third to fewer than one half of patients diagnosed by psychiatrists were recognized as depressed by other staff. With the low identification of depression by professionals, it is not surprising that older adults themselves and their families often do not recognize depressive symptoms and typically do not ask for professional help.

Concomitantly, late-life depression often coexists with other psychiatric, medical, and neurological conditions. Twenty-five percent of adults diagnosed with Alzheimer's disease meet the diagnostic criteria for major depressive disorder. Forty-six percent of adults with Parkinson's disease and 60% of post-stroke patients are afflicted with depression (Dooneief et al., 1992). Thus, even when symptoms are noted, they may be attributed to coexisting conditions or simply to aging rather than to a treatable depressive disorder. The presence of dementia with depression, in particular, can complicate the diagnosis of depression, further contributing to the lack of treatment.

Inadequate or nontreatment of depression contributes to prolongation of recovery from illnesses and can worsen other chronic conditions, leading to greater physical and cognitive impairment. Non- or undertreatment can lead to serious consequences such as disability, increased psychiatric and medical morbidity, and increased risk of premature death (Ahmed & Takeshita, 1996). Rovner and colleagues (1991) found that nursing home residents with untreated depression are less likely to survive a full year after admission than those without depressive symptoms. Untreated depression also increases the risk of developing irreversible dementia (Abrams, Teresi, & Butin, 1992).

Given the nature of depression among older adults with its multiple, complex contributing factors and the likelihood of concurrent dementia and somatic illnesses, a multidisciplinary team approach to intervention is recommended (NIH Consensus Panel, 1992). Existing models provide some evidence that interdisciplinary, integrated team approaches can improve the delivery of physical and mental health care to geriatric patients in both primary care and inpatient settings (Bultema, Malliard, Getzfrid, Lerner, & Colone, 1996; Eng, Pedulla, Eleazer, McCann, & Fox, 1997; Oxman, 1996). Although the potential for a multidisciplinary response to late-life depression in LTC settings exists, in practice, attending physicians, consulting psychiatrists, and those who provide hands-on care to residents may not actually participate in meetings to plan care with the nursing, social work, and rehabilitation staff, inhibiting a true multidisciplinary approach.

Though federal regulations require that all LTC residents receive appropriate treatment for mental or psychosocial difficulties (Omnibus Budget Reconciliation Act of 1987), the current system of care for older adults is inadequate, fragmented, and passive. An NIH Consensus Panel (1992), convened to review the state of the art in the treatment of geriatric depression, noted a lack of linkages between the health care, mental health, and social service delivery systems. The panel reported that while the picture can be bleak for depressed older adults in the community, "there are even more immediate treatment needs among those in long-term care settings" because "few nursing homes have the staff capability to intervene in appropriate and timely fashions." Although a range of interventions can be used to effectively alleviate late-life depression, according to a recent Administration on Aging (2001) report, generally such interventions are not made available in LTC settings.

Loss of functional independence and control over one's daily routines heightens the risk of depression among LTC residents (Barder, Slimmer, & LeSage, 1994), especially among newly admitted residents (Bagley et al., 2000; Krichbaum et al., 1999). Despite this heightened risk, few facilities seem to offer supportive measures designed to mentor new residents as they transition to a LTC setting. Orientation to a facility may be nonexistent or limited to a tour of the physical facilities and introduction to a few staff members. Few older adults transitioning to living in a LTC facility receive the support necessary for grief and mourning, a common experience of new residents. Unresolved grief, in turn, can lead to depression (Butler & Orrell, 1998).

Despite the recognition that mental and physical health are inextricably linked, the emphasis on medical intervention in LTC settings continues to overshadow attention to older adults' psychosocial needs. Attending primarily to physical needs and even providing a pleasing and pristine living environment are clearly not sufficient to promoting a good quality of life if depression is not recognized or treated.

Effective treatment of depression in LTC residents begins with the recognition of depressive symptoms by helping professionals, the older adults themselves, and the family of the older adult. Depression in older adults is often hidden in psychosomatic complaints, that is, "masked depression." The presentation of depression in older adults may have anxious features and less of the subjective sadness reported by younger adults. The diagnosis of late-life depression may be complicated further by the overlap with symptoms of dementia. An increased opportunity for therapeutic intervention for late-life depression would be possible with greater diagnostic attention to the atypical presentation in older adults.

The diagnosis of depression as defined by the *DSM-IV* requires the presence of at least five of the following symptoms during the same 2-week period: changes in appetite or weight; decrease or increase in sleep; psychomotor agitation or retardation; loss of energy; feelings of worthlessness or guilt; difficulty concentrating; and suicidal thoughts or ideas. Either a depressed mood or loss of interest or pleasure in nearly all activities also must be present. According to the *DSM-IV,* these symptoms must be accompanied by an impairment in function that is not better accounted for by bereavement and not due to a medical condition or substance abuse (American Psychiatric Association, 1994). It is not clear how applicable standard diagnostic criteria are to LTC residents. At least one study (Burrows, Satlin, Salzman, Nobel, & Lipsitz, 1995) raises questions about the application of standard diagnostic categories to late-life depression among LTC residents.

Because many older patients with symptoms of depression do not meet the full criteria for major depression, "minor depression," a subsyndromal form of depression, may be diagnosed. Mossey (1997), noting the prevalence of minor depression among LTC residents, calls for aggressive and comprehensive screening of all residents at regular intervals. Along with a comprehensive psychosocial assessment, a complete medical examination and medical history is important to rule out physical problems, adverse drug interactions, and reactions that may contribute to depressive symptoms. Various assessment tools are available to provide direction for diagnosis and intervention. For the past two decades, the Geriatric Depression Scale (GDS) (Yesavage, 1988) has been widely used to diagnose and assess the severity of depression of older adults. A newer version of this scale was recently developed for use specifically with a residential population (Sutcliffe et al., 2000). Though nursing home residents are regularly evaluated for mood disorders as part of the Minimum Data Set compliance procedures (Burrows, Morris, Simon, Hirdes, & Phillips, 2000), the sensitivity of this tool to depression among LTC residents has been questioned by the National Coalition on Mental Health and Aging (W. Mays, personal communication, June 11, 2000).

PRIOR RESEARCH AND KNOWLEDGE BASE

This section provides a brief review of empirical research on conventional treatments for late-life depression, as well as emerging knowledge about less common approaches (e.g., environmental modifications). Conventional therapies for treating depression can be categorized as biological (pharmacotherapy, electroconvulsive therapy) or psychosocial (individual or group psychotherapies) (Schneider, 1995).

Pharmacotherapy

Intervention for depression in LTC residents commonly involves pharmacologic therapies (Dhooper, Green, Huff, & Austin-Murphy, 1993). Despite a voluminous medical literature on the efficacy of various psychotropic medications for treating geriatric depression (e.g., Mulsant et al., 2001; Reynolds et al., 1999), questions about the use of drugs in nursing homes continue to be raised. The misuse of drug treatment for depression in nursing homes includes both inappropriate underuse (Heston et al., 1992, cited in Lebowitz, 1997) and inappropriate overuse (Beardsley, Larson, Burns, Thompson, & Kamerow 1989; Beers, Avorn, Soumerai, & Everitt, 1988, cited in Lebowitz, 1997). Although older adults have been found to respond to antidepressant medication, only a minority receives adequate dosage and duration of pharmacotherapy (U.S. Surgeon General, 1999). According to a geropsychiatrist who prescribes psychotropic medications to LTC residents (J. Dickens, personal communication, October 18, 2001), special attention is needed when selecting an antidepressant for older adults, due to the physiological changes of aging, increased vulnerability to medication side effects, the impact of polypharmacy, and the interaction with other comorbid disorders. Antidepressants are "fraught with side effects which are often more salient, more intolerable, and more dangerous" in older adults (Payne, 1987, p. 31).

In practice, many LTC facilities do not have physicians or pharmacy consultants who are trained in psychopharmacology, and even fewer have a geropsychiatrist available (Hartz & Splain, 1997). Attending physicians in nursing homes are often not prepared to make psychiatric diagnoses and may or may not follow the recommendations of consulting psychiatrists (Abrams et al., 1992). Consequently, Hartz and Splain (1997) recommend that social service staff learn the basics of psychiatric medication and, further, that medication decisions be monitored by a multidisciplinary psychotropic medication committee. Given that a combined psychosocial-pharmacologic approach is recommended (NIH Consensus Panel, 1992), social workers should be particularly alert to instances where psychotropic medication is the only intervention for depressed LTC residents.

Electroconvulsive Therapy

Electroconvulsive therapy (ECT) is usually reserved for individuals who do not respond well to antidepressants or who are not able to tolerate their adverse effects (Schneider, 1995). ECT is sometimes used as a jump-start when the patient's depression is considered a double or deep major depression (J. Dickens, personal communication, October 18, 2001). The usual course of treatment is a series of 6 to 12 sessions, three times a week, over the course of several weeks. ECT can be given on an outpatient basis and is extremely efficacious due to the short time needed to see improvement in the patient's mood and behavior (Abrams, 1992). It is the preferred treatment for older adults with psychotic depression (Mulsant et al., 2001). Treatments are sometimes followed by a course of antidepressants to prevent relapse. Despite the proven efficacy of ECT, it is interesting that the literature does not address its use with LTC residents.

Psychotherapy

Several types of psychotherapy for treating depression in older adults are mentioned in the literature—psychodynamic, cognitive-behavioral, interpersonal, and reminiscence. According to Hartz and Splain (1997), none of these approaches has been shown to be more effective than the others. Although the largest body of literature on treatment efficacy for depression addresses biological therapies, particularly antidepressants, there is some empirical support for time-limited psychotherapy with older adults (Schneider, 1995).

Psychodynamic approaches focus on internal psychological processes in relation to coping with late-life struggles (Thompson & Gallagher-Thompson, 1997). A variation of psychodynamic therapy is the use of the "life review" to assist residents in finding meaning in the absence of situations and relationships that formerly served this function (Thompson & Gallagher-Thompson, 1997). Key elements of cognitive-behavioral therapy (CBT) include a collaborative therapeutic relationship, a focus on a small number of clearly specified goals, an emphasis on change, and skill training (cognitive, behavioral, and interpersonal). CBT is based on the view that learning is lifelong and people can make important changes in their thoughts, feelings, and actions. Zeiss and Steffen (1996) adapted the basic concepts of CBT to treatment with older adults; their emphasis is on learning to adapt to the challenges of aging rather than on treatment for a mental illness. Core features of the CBT approach to depression are (a) daily self-monitoring, (b) increasing pleasant events, (c) relaxation (to relieve anxiety often accompanying depression), and (d) cognitive restructuring. Efficacy studies have shown favorable results for CBT (e.g., Teri, Curtis, Gallagher-Thompson, & Thompson, 1994) and other psychosocial interventions (e.g., Niederehe, 1994) with elderly outpatients and, more recently, with LTC residents (Thompson & Gallagher-Thompson, 1997). Weiss and Salamon (1987) recommend an eclectic approach to psychotherapeutic intervention with depressed elders in LTC and suggest that practitioners go beyond traditional psychotherapy and use whatever modality best ensures an appropriate outcome for residents.

Thompson and Gallagher-Thompson (1997) describe a number of emerging psychotherapeutic models that target depression of LTC residents, including (a) a pleasant-events model based the work of Lewinsohn, Biglan, and Zeiss (1976); (b) a multifaceted approach developed at Vanderbilt University that focused on improving communication among residents, their families, and staff; (c) simulated presence therapy; and (d) music therapy. Although the efficacy of these approaches has not been thoroughly examined as yet, these authors echo Weiss and Salamon's (1987) recommendation of drawing from a variety of psychotherapeutic interventions, depending on the needs and capabilities of particular residents.

Though many studies have examined treatment response to combined therapeutic intervention for depression using both medication and psychotherapy, such approaches have not been adequately studied with older adults (Schneider, 1995). Gallagher and colleagues have demonstrated success rates of 50% to 70% using CBT or CBT with medication (Gallagher & Thompson, 1982, 1983; Thompson, Gallagher, & Breckenridge, 1987). Schneider (1995) reported similar success rates (61% to 84%) from intervention studies using interpersonal psychotherapy (IPT) or IPT with antidepressants. Although a combined approach of medication and psychotherapy has proven effective with elderly outpatients (Gallagher-Thompson & Steffen, 1994), the relative contributions of each component are not clear (Schneider, 1995). The efficacy of a combined approach with LTC residents has not been studied.

Twenty-five years ago, Ronch and Maizler (1977) called for an end to prejudices that prohibited insight-oriented psychotherapy with institutionalized elders. Despite such pleas and subsequent empirical evidence of the efficacy of psychosocial interventions for depressed LTC residents, the myth persists that older adults are untreatable. The vast majority of LTC residents with depressive symptoms do not receive planned psychosocial intervention.

Group Intervention

The therapeutic factors that operate in group treatment are uniquely suited to the needs of older adults (Meuser, Clower, & Padin-Rivera, 1998), and the LTC setting presents an ideal locale for group intervention. A therapeutic group offers psychosocial support for dealing with the stressors that put LTC residents at increased risk for depression. Therapeutic orientations may include psychodynamic, cognitive, reminiscence, social skills, and eclectic.

The "protective factors" for prevention of depression may include education about depression and its symptoms, social support, acceptance of diminished physical abilities, commitment to seeking help with a change or transition in life, and meeting with a peer group for support. Despite these expected benefits, empirical studies on the efficacy of group treatment for depressed LTC residents are sparse (Abraham, Onega, Reel, & Wofford, 1997). In light of the fact that more than 60% of LTC residents have some cognitive impairment (Parmelee, Katz, & Powell-Lawton, 1989), Lichtenberg (1994) recommends that group intervention with depressed residents emphasize social interaction instead of skill- or knowledge-building. Focusing on social interaction seems appropriate, given that depression in LTC residents is often expressed as a decreased ability to engage, interact, and experience pleasure (Krichbaum et al., 1999). To the extent that depression stems from a lack of connectedness, a group intervention that focuses on relationship-building may prove successful. This premise is supported in part by studies showing a lack of improvement on the depression scores of LTC residents who participated in groups that were focused on skill-building or education (Abraham et al., 1997).

Abraham and colleagues (1997) conducted a series of intervention studies that focused on the efficacy of cognitive group interventions. They compared resident outcomes for three different interventions conducted over a 24-week period: cognitive-behavioral therapy, focused visual-imagery therapy, and educational and discussion groups (the control group). Their study demonstrated improvements in overall cognitive status of nursing home residents, but no significant reduction of depression. Thus, Abraham and colleagues concluded that cognitive group interventions for depressed LTC residents with multiple impairments may help them to *think* better but may not help them to *feel* better. Considering the frailty of many of their group participants, they suggest that the lack of well-being they detected among group participants may not be depression per se, but a realistic acceptance of some of the constraints in their lives. They further surmised that group interventions to alleviate depression may be suited to particular subgroups of LTC residents.

In contrast, a social-skills group intervention with 12 depressed residents yielded improvements in four areas of social interaction (Frazer, 1997). Dhooper and colleagues (1993) successfully demonstrated a reduction in depression of LTC residents using an eclectic group approach. Three fourths of their participants in the treatment group became depression-free and other residents went from moderate to mild depression. Scogin and McElreath (1994) undertook a quantitative review of 17 intervention studies involving depressed older adult outpatients, most of which involved group modalities. Based on their review of existing studies, they concluded that psychotherapy with depressed older adults was as effective as with younger adults. As with individual psychotherapy, group intervention with depressed LTC residents has a growing base of empirical support. However, its implementation in actual practice has not kept pace with the level of need.

Environmental Modification

The source of depression for many older adults is not so much aging itself but their environmental circumstances (Blazer, 1994). To the extent that depressive symptoms of LTC residents are a response to their environment, it follows that alterations in the environment could prevent or alleviate some depression. Environmental modifications encompass alterations to the social environment as well as changes in the physical facility. The Eden Alternative espouses the presence of nature in the form of plants and animals as a means of enhancing LTC residents' well-being (Hamilton & Tesh, 2002; Tavormina, 1999; Weinstein, 1998). Exposure to bright light is another environmental intervention that has proven effective in alleviating depression of LTC residents (Sumaya, Rienzi, Deegan, & Moss, 2001).

Although upgrades to décor and other physical amenities certainly provide benefit to residents, it is the social environment that has a far greater impact on residents' well-being. For example, research has shown that comingling cognitively impaired with noncognitively impaired residents may lead to greater depression among the intact residents (Teresi, Holmes, & Monaco, 1993). Teresi and colleagues (1993) found that cognitively intact residents who roomed with or adjacent to demented residents had higher depression scores than their segregated counterparts. One study showed that residents' perceived social support from family affected depression levels (Commerford & Reznikoff, 1996), yet a more recent study demonstrated that relationships with other residents were a much stronger predictor of depression (Fessman & Lester, 2000). Fessman and Lester (2000) administered the Zung depression scale and the UCLA Loneliness Scale to 170 LTC residents and found that social networks within the facility influenced depression levels more than visits from family and friends. This finding held for both physically disabled residents and those with Alzheimer's disease.

Although relationships with people both outside and inside the nursing home are undoubtedly important, Fessman and Lester (2000) recommend helping residents develop relationships with other residents as a way to improve their emotional and psychological well-being. Gutheil (1991) documented several positive aspects of friendships among residents including social support, companionship, and pleasant interactions. Relationship-building has been identified as one of four phases LTC residents go through in adjusting to institutionalization (Brooke, 1989).

These findings suggest that social workers in LTC settings must be attuned to engendering social relationships of residents, especially within the facility. Based on their study of the factors that contribute to boredom among LTC residents, Ejaz, Schur, and Noelker (1997) recommend that practitioners make an effort to introduce residents with similar interests and backgrounds to each other in order to promote meaningful interactions and positive relationships. They suggest that groups of residents with similar interests could assist in developing innovative programs. In addition, social workers must be sensitive to staff behaviors and facility policies that influence resident well-being. A study conducted in two adult day-care centers demonstrated that social interactions among the elders were negatively affected by infantilizing behaviors of the staff and by procedures that limited elders' autonomy and privacy (Salari & Rich, 2001). One might expect the negative psychosocial effects of a "total institution" such as a nursing home to be even more pervasive.

Innovations in Depression Intervention and Prevention

According to the first Surgeon General's Report on Mental Health (U.S. Surgeon General, 1999), there has been a rapid growth in the number of clinical, research, and training centers dedicated to the mental health–related needs of older adults over the past two decades. Through preventive education and research, more LTC residents could be directed to the intervention that is most effective for their condition. There are several examples of innovative programs aimed at alleviating or preventing depression through valuing and connecting with older adults on a spiritual or relational level: the Eden Alternative (Thomas, 1996); the use of natural helping networks (Cohen, Hyland, & Devlin, 1999); therapeutic-hugging week (Weisberg & Haberman, 1989); reminiscence (Watt & Cappeliez, 2000); everyday activities (Mosher-Ashley & Barrett, 1997); peer counseling (McCurren, Dowe, Rattle, & Looney, 1999); spiritual eldering (Schachter-Shalomi & Miller, 1995); bibliotherapy (Scogin, 1998); and strengths-based approaches such as transpersonal gerontology and narrative therapy (Ronch & Goldfield, 2002). Though not all of the approaches mentioned here have been introduced to the LTC setting as yet, such innovations warrant further study and replication.

Empirically demonstrating the prevention of depression is a formidable research challenge. Consequently, the literature on prevention of late-life depression is fairly limited. One exception is the work of Haight, Michel, and Hendrix (1998, 2000). Based on a 5-year experimental study involving 256 newly relocated nursing home residents, Haight and colleagues (1998) assert that the life review is an effective preventive intervention for clinical depression. Depression scores as measured by the Beck Depression Inventory were significantly lower for residents who were receiving the intervention of life review compared to controls.

Prevention efforts must be grounded in recognition of the centrality of social relationships to LTC residents. Despite being in a group-living situation, LTC residents are susceptible to loneliness, boredom, and helplessness, identified as the three "plagues of nursing home life" by Eden Alternative founder Dr. William Thomas (1996). In an effort to prevent depression, social workers can facilitate relationships not only among residents, but also between residents and staff (Moss & Pfohl, 1988), and with volunteers (Nagel, Cimbolic, & Newlin, 1988), children (Kocarnik & Ponzetti, 1991; Ziemba, Roop, & Wittenberg, 1988), and on-site pets (Thomas, 1996). Having a resident dog at an LTC facility was shown to enhance social interactions among LTC residents and staff (Winkler, Fairnie, Gericevich, & Long, 1989).

With the growing recognition that LTC facilities are a key setting for the study of late-life depression (Rubenstein & Lawton, 1997), there have been attendant gains in our understanding of late-life depression and of efficacious interventions. In contrast to earlier research, for example, a recent study documented a *reduction* of depression within the year after admission to a LTC facility for residents with dementia (Payne et al., 2002). This improvement in residents' depression levels was attributed in part to timely recognition of depressive symptoms followed by appropriate diagnosis and treatment. The incidence of depression for the 201 residents studied declined from 19.9% upon admission to 1.8% at 6 months and 6.4% at 12 months.

CURRENT RESEARCH

It is clear that we need a better understanding of the barriers to implementing recommended interventions for depression in LTC settings. A multimethod study comparing resident, staff, and family views about depression-related treatment, training, and outcomes was conducted by the author (Adamek, 2000). The setting was a 65-bed unit of a large public LTC facility in Indianapolis. Residents were primarily low-income minority elders. The general aim of this project was to better understand current approaches and barriers to identifying and treating depression among LTC residents. Specifically, the study aimed to (a) compare resident, staff, and family views about depression-related treatment, training, and outcomes, and (b) monitor the impact of an MSW mental health clinician's involvement with LTC residents on depression-related care plans, treatments, and outcomes.

The prevalence of depression among residents was attested to, in part, by nearly one third scoring in the depressed range on the GDS (Yesavage, 1988). Responses from residents, family members, and staff members indicate an inconsistent and inadequate approach to identifying and treating depression. Almost all staff members surveyed indicated there was insufficient staff training on geriatric depression and that depressed residents occasionally or frequently went without treatment. Staff respondents estimated that nearly two thirds of the residents were occasionally or frequently overmedicated. There were significant discrepancies in resident, family member, and staff views about such basic issues as whether the resident was depressed or was taking antidepressant medication. This confirms the urgent need for enhanced training about geriatric depression and the involvement of qualified geriatric mental health practitioners in LTC settings.

Direct observation over a 13-month period of care-plan meetings involving 59 residents revealed a casual, routinized approach to addressing depression. Rote verbalization of standard lines about depression (e.g., "potential for signs and symptoms of depression") by social service staff suggested more of a concern for legal compliance than for proactive problem-solving tailored to individual residents. Psychosocial approaches for intervening with depressed residents were rarely suggested. More in-depth problem solving and discussion did occur when a family member or the MSW mental health clinician or both attended care-plan meetings. Anecdotal evidence from interviews with residents suggests that much of the apparent depression stems from a lack of connectedness or social support rather than being primarily a biological condition that is treatable with psychotropic medications.

FURTHER RESEARCH NEEDS

The heavy emphasis on pharmacologic interventions for treating late-life depression has limited the extent of systematic research that is focused on social, behavioral, and psychologically oriented interventions (Rylands & Rickwood, 2001). A study by Rylands and Rickwood (2001) examining the effect of "accepting the past" on depression levels of 73 LTC residents suggests that greater attention is warranted to psychosocial interventions that support personality processes in later life. Clearly, more empirical investigations are needed to identify and describe innovative, nonpharmacological approaches to preventing and alleviating depression. Interestingly, medication remains the primary treatment for depression despite a long-standing recommendation for a combined psychosocial and pharmacologic approach. One study attributed the increased use of antidepressant drugs in residential care to the wider range of such drugs that have become available since 1990 (Arthur, Matthews, Jagger, & Lindesay, 2002).

We know that too few LTC staff persons are trained in geriatric mental health or are skillful in delivering psychosocial interventions, and we need to investigate the extent to which staff attitudes are a barrier to implementing psychosocial interventions. Are professionals pessimistic about the efficacy of nonmedical approaches? Qualitative investigations of staff perceptions may point to ways of overcoming the prevalent view that depression is a normal part of aging. We need to examine innovative approaches to preventing and alleviating late-life depression that can be replicated in the range of settings that make up what Cohen (1997) refers to as the "geriatric landscape." Pruchno and Rose (2000) compared health outcomes of residents in assisted living with those in a nursing home and found that despite the claim of differing philosophies of these two care settings, health outcome patterns of residents, including levels of depression, were similar in both environments.

Research is needed in LTC settings to investigate the barriers to policy and practice innovation in preventing and treating late-life depression. Rowe and Kahn (1987) argue that intervention strategies that address risk factors and have as their goal maintaining health and preventing impairment and disability may reduce the prevalence of depression in older adults. A more in-depth understanding of the risk factors for depression in an LTC population is needed to inform practice innovations.

We need to know more about how residents' social relationships affect their level of depression. Ejaz and colleagues (1997) call for future studies to determine whether depression precedes poorer relationships among LTC residents and less involvement in activities or if the reverse is true. Does participation in a peer support group reduce residents' risk of depression? If so, how? Given the intimate nature of care provided by LTC staff, it may be productive to investigate how the relationships between staff and residents affect residents' emotional well-being. One study documented an association between nurse's aide empathy and depressive symptoms of LTC residents, suggesting that others' views of older adults do affect their level of depression (Hollinger-Samson & Pearson, 2000). Providing staff with training on residents' rights was found to help staff members identify barriers that created conflicts with residents (Brennan et al., 2002). It would be helpful to evaluate whether and how in-service training on topics such as residents' rights, late-life depression, and the psycho-social aspects of aging may lead to enhanced social interaction and improved emotional well-being of residents. Other underresearched issues relevant to depression intervention in LTC are cultural diversity

(Thompson & Gallagher-Thompson, 1997) and spirituality. As the diversity of the older population increases and as spirituality is increasingly recognized as central to the lives of many older adults, the impact of these issues on late-life depression will need to be investigated.

POLICY IMPLICATIONS

Policy decisions at the federal level concerning LTC financing have created a significant barrier to treating mental health conditions in nursing homes (Lebowitz, 1997). As Lebowitz (1997) explains, in order to be eligible for Medicaid reimbursement, nursing homes could not have mental disorder as a primary diagnosis for more than half of their residents. To avoid being reclassified as a mental hospital and risk losing Medicaid dollars, LTC advocates successfully lobbied to relabel Alzheimer's disease as a "neurological and behavioral disorder" rather than as a mental disorder. The unintended consequence of this "victory" was a tacit denial of mental disorders as an issue in LTC institutions (Rubenstein & Lawton, 1997). Describing this quandary as "the nursing home paradox," Cohen (1997) asserts that while mental health diagnoses among LTC residents are the rule rather than the exception, "denial of this reality is still prevalent . . . and, as a consequence, there is insufficient recognition of mental health problems in nursing home settings, or of the associated responsibility to develop effective mental health interventions" (p. 213). Given the nature of the resident population, LTC facilities could be seen as de facto psychiatric hospitals (Abrams et al., 1992) and yet, for the most part, care in nursing homes remains focused on physical illness and disability.

Reimbursement mechanisms often do not support the provision of mental health interventions to older adults—whether they are LTC residents or living in the community. Although group treatment using reminiscence has shown promise in reducing depression (Rattenbury & Stones, 1989), groups whose primary emphasis is social or memory enhancement do not meet the Health Care Financing Administration's criteria for reimbursement (Meuser et al., 1998). Health professionals need to advocate for policy changes that would expand Medicare, Medicaid, and third-party reimbursements for treatment of late-life mental health problems; and for greater emphasis on preventive measures. In addition to equitable reimbursement for mental health services, several policy changes are needed to make mental health services more accessible to older adults.

There seems to be a major disconnect between current reimbursement schemes for mental health treatment, which are tied primarily to pharmacological interventions, and our emerging understanding of the extent to which late-life depression revolves around social connectedness. As members of a profession committed to enhancing human relationships, social workers have an opportunity to broaden policy makers' views of the etiology and, hence, the appropriate response to late-life depression.

Policy makers and insurance providers may perceive geriatric mental-health issues as unimportant, unpopular, or as another drain on the system. They need to be convinced that with proper professional involvement (e.g., aging-competent social workers), mental health outcomes of LTC residents can be enhanced significantly. Empirical studies demonstrating the efficacy of treatments for various mental illnesses, including depression, have gained recognition in the policy arena and, according to Lebowitz (1997), "have provided a scientific rationale for policy discussions of parity in coverage of mental and physical illnesses" (p. 231). Reimbursement mechanisms for designing and implementing training on late-life depression to LTC staff could lead to greater success in properly identifying and treating geriatric depression. Social workers can play a role in informing policy makers that appropriate treatment, in turn, can ultimately prevent further costly disability and morbidity.

The National Coalition on Mental Health and Aging (1999)—a network of 50 organizations committed to improving the mental health of older adults—regularly advocates for "improving the availability and quality of mental health preventive and treatment strategies to older Americans and their families through education, research, and increased public awareness" (p. 1). Rosen and Persky (1997) call for social workers to use their coalition-building skills to replicate such efforts on the state and local levels.

INTEGRATING KNOWLEDGE
INTO THE CURRICULUM

Multiple strategies will be required to avert the projected "impending crisis in geriatric mental health" (Jeste et al., 1999). Central to these strategies is some level of core training in social work, as well as other disciplines, in the provision of mental health care to older adults (Halpain, Harris, McClure, & Jeste, 1999). A critical challenge in educating social workers is overcoming disinterest and lack of accurate information about late-life depression, including its extent, symptoms, causes, consequences, and amenability to treatment. At a minimum, all social workers need to be aware of some key facts about late-life depression; for example, depression is the most common mental health disorder in late life, it is not a normal part of aging, it is especially prevalent in LTC, and left untreated it leads to greater morbidity and mortality. Social workers need to be aware that late-life depression is associated with high rates of elder suicide or, in the case of LTC residents, a higher incidence of indirect self-destructive behavior (McIntosh & Hubbard, 1988; Nelson & Farberow, 1980). Social work students need to learn that late-life depression remains fairly widespread despite being highly amenable to intervention. Through greater awareness of such basic facts, social workers can play a more prominent role in ensuring that late-life depression is more effectively identified, alleviated, and, ideally, prevented. We have the opportunity to build upon our expertise in psychosocial functioning to create and promote intervention models that value and honor older adults.

Mental health issues throughout the life span must be incorporated in MSW course work. Suggestions about content on late-life depression to include throughout the MSW curriculum are given in Table 2.1. We need to distinguish late-life depression from that experienced by children, adolescents, young adults, and middle-aged adults. LTC residents could be used as an example of a vulnerable population in course materials that address underserved and at-risk groups. Given the need for professional social workers in the field of geriatric mental health, MSW students should be encouraged and perhaps given incentives to pursue internships in aging-relevant sites (e.g., LTC and other residential settings, community mental-health centers, home health, geriatric psych units).

CONCLUSION

Perhaps this is the most fundamental question we must ask as professional helpers and aging advocates concerned about geriatric mental health: With late-life depression being so common, why are we not

TABLE 2.1 Curriculum Recommendations for Mastery of Content About Late-Life Depression

	Practice	Policy	HBSE	Research	Field
KNOWLEDGE	Signs & symptoms of depression Efficacious interventions Psychoeducational therapy Reminiscent therapy Preventive measures Discerning depression, dementia, & delirium Suicide warning signs	Medicare/Medicaid & private insurance reimbursement Intersection of mental health/health & LTC systems Treatment barriers	Prevalence of depression Contributing factors Ameliorating factors Social context Losses, grief Long-term care Psychosocial tasks Prevention models	Evidence-based interventions Practice evaluation	Context for the delivery of mental health services to older adults Standards of care for late-life depression

TABLE 2.1 *(continued)*

	Practice	Policy	HBSE	Research	Field
SKILLS	Engaging older adults Assessment & use of screening tools Interviewing skills Lethality assessment	Advocacy Tracking relevant legislation Networking (e.g., state mental health & aging coalition)	Conducting bio-psycho-spiritual-social assessments	Being an informed consumer of emerging research	Interviewing older adults Completing assessments Being a member of a multi-disciplinary team
VALUES	Inherent worth and dignity of each individual, self-determination, confidentiality, honoring of differences, therapeutic optimism, belief in an individual's capacity for change regardless of age, respect for elders' wisdom, autonomy, cultural competence				

Note: HBSE = human behavior and the social environment.

doing more to prevent and alleviate it? If the knowledge base exists to inform us about the nature, causes, and consequences of late-life depression and about the efficacy of various approaches to treatment and prevention, why do we seem to be making so little headway? To a large extent, it seems we are simply not implementing the approaches that have been shown to make a difference. Is the lack of preventive and nonpharmacologic interventions tantamount to a tolerance of depression among older adults? If so, what accounts for that tolerance or allowance, particularly in LTC? Could it be that as a society we are simply more wedded to our outdated notions of later life—notions of boredom, decline, deterioration, loneliness, and depression—than we are to empirical findings of success in ameliorating depression of older adults? The inattention or inadequate response to late-life depression is in many ways a reflection of deep-seated ageism. Despite long-standing evidence that aging is not a disease (Curtin, 1972), as a society we have yet to overcome our negative cultural mind-set about late life. One wonders whether late-life depression would be so pervasive if old age were considered a valued commodity rather than a feared and unwelcome intrusion in life.

Although we would not deny that LTC residents have the same fundamental psychosocial needs as other adults (i.e., the need to feel useful, worthwhile, respected, and acknowledged), we must carefully examine whether our actions and interactions with residents reflect our professed belief that nursing home residents who are frail are worthy human beings. We must consider the ways that LTC residents are devalued and the extent to which this devaluing contributes to an "existential-meaning vacuum" (Lantz, 2002). Perhaps the phenomenon of "failure to thrive," a geriatric syndrome that has been linked to depression (Braun, Wykle, & Cowling, 1988), would be more aptly designated a "failure to be valued" or as "unacknowledged worthiness." Ten years ago, *failure to thrive* was identified as an aging research priority by the Institute of Medicine (National Institutes of Health, 1992). Despite the potential benefit of research focused on this syndrome and its association to late-life depression, Berkman, Foster, and Campion (1989) caution that the use of this term in clinical practice could undermine such benefits if *failure to thrive* becomes a label that reinforces negative stereotypes about aging. In the process of describing and explaining this and other phenomena that contribute to depression of LTC residents, we must guard against the tendency to view depression as inevitable.

Most of the published literature on geriatric depression derives from the medical and nursing fields and hence presents a largely medical perspective. Social workers can offer a critical, holistic, and social-environmental perspective on late-life depression that steps outside the medical model. A strategic broad-based plan for combating depression in LTC is needed (see Figure 2.1). Through designing and implementing innovative psychosocial and preventive intervention models, social workers can play a significant role in carrying out the recommendations of the U.S. Surgeon General (1999). Katon and

---

Improve our understanding of late-life depression including its extent, causes, symptoms, consequences, and amenability to treatment.

Increase acceptance of, and support for, psychosocial interventions among practitioners, policy makers, insurers, family members, and older adults.

Enhance the knowledge and skill level of social workers in implementing efficacious and innovative interventions.

Heighten the extent and impact of prevention strategies aimed at late-life depression.

Promote the use of integrated, multidisciplinary team approaches.

Design and implement creative ways of building and enhancing older adults' social relationships. Recognize the centrality of connectedness to long-term care residents.

Create ways of valuing older adults, particularly those who lack informal supports.

Establish wellness programs that address both mental and physical health.

Partner with older adults in understanding contributing and ameliorating factors.

Advocate for an increased role for professional social workers in long-term care, primary care, and residential settings.

Facilitate older adults' continuing engagement with life and opportunities for creative expression.

Provide leadership in eradicating ageism.

FIGURE 2.1   Combating late-life depression: A social work agenda.

colleagues (1997) suggest that collaborative approaches to addressing geropsychiatric disorders may lead to more efficacious and cost-effective interventions. A multidisciplinary team approach would better facilitate the recommended blend of pharmacological and psychosocial approaches (Reynolds et al., 1999). Social workers can be a catalyst in fostering such multidisciplinary efforts. Given their training and skill in case management and community building, social workers can promote needed linkages among health care, mental health, LTC, and social-service delivery systems. Social workers can make a major impact on LTC environments by educating residents, family members, health professionals, and policy makers about late-life depression and its amenability to a variety of nonpharmacologic interventions that have proven effective in alleviating depression.

Much late-life depression in LTC is avoidable. Greater awareness among professionals as well as among older adults and their families of the extent and nature of late-life depression and of efficacious interventions will go a long way in reducing prevalence rates and improving residents' quality of living. Preventive measures and nonconventional approaches to LTC, such as the Eden Alternative, deserve more widespread attention and study as to their impact on late-life depression. Furthermore, the battle against late-life depression must extend beyond traditional nursing homes to the entire "geriatric landscape" (Cohen, 1997), that is, the growing variety of sites where older adults reside and receive care. Drawing from the premise that no disabled person should be expected to forsake his or her humanity in exchange for care, Kane, Kane, and Ladd (1998) present a range of alternative LTC models for providing both housing and services in a way that preserves the dignity and autonomy of older adults. Finding ways to move beyond the artificial dichotomy between social and medical care will facilitate the provision of high quality LTC without sacrificing quality of living (Kane et al., 1998).

Reflecting the undercurrent of ageism, studies of aging typically focus on the pathological conditions that restrict independence and compromise functioning. Research on geriatric mental health and on LTC has likewise reflected a predominantly problem-based perspective. Although the majority of prior research reflects the psychopathology of depression, emerging work promotes a greater focus on positive living and adaptations to aging, such as "aging well" or "successful aging." Friedrich (2001) predicts that the transition from baby boomers to aging boomers will have a significant impact on views of successful aging and on the availability of preventive interventions for physical, psychological, and social aging. The growth in the older population itself will demand more attention to late-life issues and to both the societal and personal aspects of aging. Though much of the focus of the aging-well movement has been directed at community-dwelling elders (e.g., Ellis & Emmett, 1998; Weiss, 1998), such developments also can be infused in LTC environments. Social workers can help transform our notions about nursing homes as institutions for dying to a view of them as supported-living communities that offer continuing opportunities for residents' growth, creativity, and fulfillment. Noting that the problems of aging can coexist with creative potential, Cohen (1997) asserts that "tapping into this creativity offers important opportunities for innovative clinical practice, new directions in research, and creative social policies" (p. 220).

The future promises a growing demand for LTC. Innovation and creativity are clearly needed (Kane et al., 1998). The need for geriatric mental-health care may reach crisis proportions in the absence of wide-scale change (Koenig, George, & Schneider, 1994). We can no longer afford to overlook how devaluation of elders results in poor quality of care, depression, and other negative outcomes. Our views of aging and of the challenges of late life must be altered. When we progress to the point of accepting that the challenges of aging are actually opportunities for a better understanding and improvement of the whole life process (Jeste, 1999), perhaps then "aging well" will become a universal goal and ageism a thing of the past.

ACKNOWLEDGMENTS

The author would like to acknowledge the valuable input of Gerardine Waggle, MSW, to this chapter and of Celia Sentir, a dear friend and inside source of information on life in a long-term-care facility. Thanks also to Barbara Berkman, DSW, for her tremendous leadership and to Eddie Johnson for his ever-present support.

REFERENCES

Abraham, I. L., Onega, L. L., Reel, S. J., & Wofford, A. B. (1997). Effects of cognitive group interventions on depressed frail nursing home residents. In R. L. Rubenstein & M. P. Lawton (Eds.), *Depression in long-term and residential care: Advances in research and treatment* (pp. 154–168). New York: Springer.

Abrams, R. (1992). Efficacy of electroconvulsive therapy. In R. Abrams (Ed.), *Electroconvulsive therapy* (pp. 10–38). New York: Oxford University Press.

Abrams, R. C., Teresi, J. A., & Butin, D. N. (1992). Depression in nursing home residents. *Clinical Geriatric Medicine, 8,* 309–322.

Adamek, M. (2000, November). *The impact of a social work-managed multidisciplinary team on the treatment of geriatric depression.* Poster presented at the 53rd Annual Scientific Meeting of the Gerontological Society of America, Washington, DC.

Administration on Aging. (2001). *Older adults and mental health: Issues and opportunities.* Washington, DC: Author.

Ahmed, I., & Takeshita, J. (1996). Late life depression. *Generations, 20*(4), 17–22.

American Psychiatric Association. (1994). *Diagnostic and statistical manual of mental disorders* (4th ed.). Washington, DC: Author.

Arthur, A., Matthews, R., Jagger, C., & Lindesay, J. (2002). Factors associated with antidepressant treatment in residential care: Changes between 1990 and 1997. *International Journal of Geriatric Psychiatry, 17,* 54–60.

Bagley, H., Cordingley, L., Burns, A., Mozley, C. G., Sutcliffe, C., Challis, D., et al. (2000). Recognition of depression by staff in nursing and residential homes. *Journal of Clinical Nursing, 9,* 445–450.

Barder, L., Slimmer, L., & LeSage, J. (1994). Depression and issues of control among elderly people in health care settings. *Journal of Advanced Nursing, 20,* 597–604.

Beardsley, R. S., Larson, D. B., Burns, B. J., Thompson, J. W., & Kamerow, D. B. (1989). Prescribing of psychotropics in elderly nursing home patients. *Journal of the American Geriatrics Society, 37,* 327–330.

Beers, M., Avorn, J., Soumerai, S. B., & Everitt, D. E. (1988). Psychoactive medication use in intermediate-care facility residents. *Journal of the American Medical Association, 260,* 3016–3020.

Berkman, B., Foster, L. W. S., & Campion, E. (1989). Failure to thrive: Paradigm for the frail elder. *Gerontologist, 29,* 654–659.

Blazer, D. (1989). Depression in the elderly. *New England Journal of Medicine, 320,* 164–166.

Blazer, D. (1994). Is depression more frequent in late life? An honest look at the evidence. *American Journal of Geriatric Psychiatry, 2,* 193–199.

Braun, J. V., Wykle, M. H., & Cowling, W. R. (1988). Failure to thrive in older adults: A concept derived. *Gerontologist, 28,* 809–812.

Brennan, F., Downes, D., Lubetkin, M., Klein, L., Meyers-DeRosa, E., & Westreich, L. (2002). Whose home is this anyway? Resident rights education. *Journal of Social Work in Long Term Care, 1,* 43–51.

Brooke, V. (1989). How elders adjust: Through what phases do newly admitted residents pass? *Geriatric Nursing, 10,* 66–68.

Buckwalter, K. C., & Piven, M. L. (1999). Depression. In J. T. Stone, J. F. Wyman, & S. A. Salisbury (Eds.), *Clinical gerontological nursing* (pp. 387–412). Philadelphia: W. B. Saunders.

Bultema, J. K., Malliard, L., Getzfrid, M. K., Lerner, R. D., & Colone, M. (1996). Geriatric patients with depression: Improving outcomes using a multidisciplinary clinical path model. *Journal of Nursing Administration, 26,* 31–38.

Burns, B. J., & Taube, C. A. (1990). Mental health services in general medical care and in nursing homes. In B. Fogel, A. Furino, & G. Gottlieb (Eds.), *Mental health policy for older Americans: Protecting minds at risk* (pp. 63–84). Washington, DC: American Psychiatric Press.

Burrows, A. B., Morris, J. N., Simon, S. E., Hirdes, J. P., & Phillips, C. (2000). Development of a Minimum Data Set-based depression rating scale for use in nursing homes. *Age and Ageing, 29,* 165–172.

Burrows, A. B., Satlin, A., Salzman, C., Nobel, K., & Lipsitz, L. A. (1995). Depression in a long-term care facility: Clinical features and discordance between nursing assessment and patient interviews. *Journal of the American Geriatrics Society, 43,* 1118–1122.

Butler, R., & Orrell, M. (1998). Late life depression. *Current Opinion in Psychiatry, 11,* 435–439.

Cohen, C., Hyland, K., & Devlin, M. (1999). An evaluation of the use of the natural helping network model to enhance the well-being of nursing home residents. *Gerontologist, 39,* 426–433.

Cohen, G. D. (1997). Gaps and failures in attending to mental health and aging in long-term care. In R. L. Rubenstein & M. P. Lawton (Eds.), *Depression in long-term and residential care: Advances in research and treatment* (pp. 211–222). New York: Springer.

Cohen-Mansfield, J., Rabinovich, B. A., Marx, M. S., Braun, J., & Fleshner, E. (1991). Nurses' and social workers' perceptions of elderly nursing home residents' well-being. *Journal of Gerontological Social Work, 16,* 135–147.

Comfort, A. (1976). *A good age.* New York: Crown.

Commerford, M. C., & Reznikoff, M. (1996). Relationship of religion and perceived social support to self-esteem and depression in nursing home residents. *Journal of Psychology, 130,* 35–50.

Curtin, S. (1972). *Nobody ever died of old age.* Boston: Little Brown.

Dhooper, S. S., Green, S. M., Huff, M. B., & Austin-Murphy, J. (1993). Efficacy of a group approach to reducing depression in nursing home elderly residents. *Journal of Gerontological Social Work, 20,* 87–100.

Dooneief, G., Mirabello, E., Bell, K., Marder, K., Stern, Y., & Mayeux, R. (1992). An estimate of the incidence of depression in idiopathic Parkinson's disease. *Archives of Neurology, 49,* 305–307.

Ejaz, F. K., Schur, D., & Noelker, L. S. (1997). The effect of activity involvement and social relationships on boredom among nursing home residents. *Activities, Adaptation, and Aging, 21,* 53–66.

Ellis, A., & Emmett, V. (1998). *Optimal aging: Getting over getting older.* Chicago: Open Court.

Eng, C., Pedulla, J., Eleazer, G. P., McCann, R., & Fox, N. (1997). Program of All-inclusive Care for the Elderly (PACE): An innovative model of integrated geriatric care and financing. *Journal of the American Geriatrics Society, 45,* 223–232.

Fessman, N., & Lester, D. (2000). Loneliness and depression among elderly nursing home patients. *International Journal of Aging and Human Development, 51,* 137–141.

Frazer, D. W. (1997). Psychotherapy in residential settings: Preliminary investigations and directions for research. In R. L. Rubenstein & M. P. Lawton (Eds.), *Depression in long-term and residential care: Advances in research and treatment* (pp. 185–207). New York: Springer.

Friedrich, D. D. (2001). *Successful aging: Integrating contemporary ideas, research findings, and intervention strategies.* Springfield, IL: Charles C Thomas.

Gallagher, D. E., & Thompson, L. W. (1982). Treatment of major depressive disorder in older adult outpatients with brief psychotherapies. *Psychotherapy: Theory, Research, and Practice, 19,* 482–490.

Gallagher, D. E., & Thompson, L. W. (1983). Effectiveness of psychotherapy for both endogenous and nonendogenous depression in older adult outpatients. *Journal of Gerontology, 38,* 707–712.

Gallagher-Thompson, D. E., & Steffen, A. M. (1994). Comparative effects of cognitive-behavioral and brief psychodynamic psychotherapies for depressed family caregivers. *Journal of Counseling and Clinical Psychology, 62,* 543–549.

Garrard, J., Rolnick, S. J., Nitz, N. M., Luepke, L., Jackson, J., Fischer, L. R., et al. (1998). Clinical detection of depression among community-based elderly people with self-reported symptoms of depression. *Journal of Gerontology: Medical Sciences, 53A,* M92–M101.

Glasser, M., & Gravdal, J. A. (1997). Assessment and treatment of geriatric depression in primary care settings. *Archives of Family Medicine, 6,* 433–438.

Gutheil, I. A. (1991). Intimacy in nursing home friendships. *Journal of Gerontological Social Work, 17,* 59–73.

Haight, B. K., Michel, Y., & Hendrix, S. (1998). Life review: Preventing despair in newly relocated nursing home residents short and long-term effects. *International Journal of Aging and Human Development, 47,* 119–142.

Haight, B. K., Michel, Y., & Hendrix, S. (2000). The extended effects of the life review in nursing home residents. *International Journal of Aging and Human Development, 50,* 151–168.

Halpain, M. C., Harris, M. J., McClure, F. S., & Jeste, D. V. (1999). Training in geriatric mental health: Needs and strategies. *Psychiatric Services, 50,* 1205–1208.

Hamilton, N., & Tesh, A. S. (2002). The North Carolina Eden Coalition: Facilitating environmental transformation. *Journal of Gerontological Nursing, 28,* 35–40.

Hartz, G. W., & Splain, D. M. (1997). *Psychosocial intervention in long term care: An advanced guide.* New York: Haworth.

Heston, L. L., Garrard, J., Makris, L., Kane, R. L., Cooper, S., Dunham, T., et al. (1992). Inadequate treatment of depressed nursing home elderly. *Journal of the American Geriatrics Society, 40,* 1117–1122.

Hollinger-Samson, N., & Pearson, J. L. (2000). The relationship between staff empathy and depressive symptoms in nursing home residents. *Aging and Mental Health, 4,* 56–65.

Jakubiak, C., & Callahan, J. (1995–1996). Treatment of mental disorders among nursing home residents: Will the market provide? *Generations, 19*(4), 39–42.

Jeste, D. V. (1997). Psychiatry of old age is coming of age. *American Journal of Psychiatry, 154,* 1356–1358.

Jeste, D. V., Alexopoulos, G. S., Bartels, S. J., Cummings, J. L., Gallo, J. J., Gottlieb, G. L., et al. (1999). Consensus statement on the upcoming crisis in geriatric mental health. *Archives of General Psychiatry, 56,* 848–853.

Kane, R. A., Kane, R. L., & Ladd, R. C. (1998). *The heart of long-term care.* New York: Oxford University Press.

Katon, W., Von Korff, M., Lin, E., Simon, G., Walker, E., Bush, T., et al. (1997). Collaborative management to achieve depression treatment guidelines. *Journal of Clinical Psychiatry, 58,* 20–23.

Katz, I. R., & Parmelee, P. A. (1997). Overview. In R. L. Rubenstein & M. P. Lawton (Eds.), *Depression in long-term and residential care: Advances in research and treatment* (pp. 1–25). New York: Springer.

Kocarnik, R. A., & Ponzetti, J. J. (1991). The advantages and challenges of intergenerational programs in long term care facilities. *Journal of Gerontological Social Work, 16,* 97–107.

Koenig, H. G., George, L. K., & Schneider, R. (1994). Mental health care for older adults in the year 2020: A dangerous and avoided topic. *Gerontologist, 34,* 674–679.

Krichbaum, K., Ryden, M., Snyder, M., Pearson, V., Hanscom, J., Lee, H. Y., et al. (1999). The impact of transition to nursing home on elders' cognitive status, well-being, and satisfaction with the nursing home. *Journal of Mental Health and Aging, 5,* 135–150.

Lair, T., & Lefkowitz, D. (1990). *Mental health and functional status of residents of nursing and personal care homes.* National Medical Expenditure Survey Research Findings 7 (DHHS Publication No. 90-3470). Rockville, MD: Agency for Health Care Policy and Research, Public Health Service.

Lantz, J. (2002). Existential therapy with trauma and medical crises. In A. R. Roberts & G. J. Greene (Eds.), *Social workers' desk reference* (pp. 609–612). New York: Oxford University Press.

Lebowitz, B. D. (1997). Depression in the nursing home: Developments and prospects. In R. L. Rubenstein & M. P. Lawton (Eds.), *Depression in long-term and residential care: Advances in research and treatment* (pp. 223–234). New York: Springer.

Lewinsohn, P. M., Biglan, T., & Zeiss, A. (1976). Behavioral treatment of depression. In P. Davidson (Ed.), *Behavioral management of anxiety, depression, and pain* (pp. 91–146). New York: Brunner/Mazel.

Lichtenberg, P. (1994). *A guide to psychological practice in geriatric long-term care.* Binghamton, NY: Haworth.

Masand, P. S. (1995). Depression in long-term care facilities. *Geriatrics, 50*(Suppl. 1), S16–S24.

McCurren, C., Dowe, D., Rattle, D., & Looney, S. (1999). Depression among nursing home elders: Testing an intervention strategy. *Applied Nursing Research, 12,* 185–195.

McIntosh, J. L., & Hubbard, R. W. (1988). Indirect self-destructive behavior among the elderly: A review with case examples. *Journal of Gerontological Social Work, 13,* 37–48.

Meuser, T. M., Clower, M. W., & Padin-Rivera, E. (1998). Group psychotherapy. In P. E. Hartman-Stein (Ed.), *Innovative behavioral healthcare for older adults: A guidebook for changing times* (pp. 103–128). San Francisco: Jossey-Bass.

Mosher-Ashley, P. M., & Barrett, P. W. (1997). *A life worth living: Practical strategies for reducing depression in older adults.* Baltimore: Health Professions Press.

Moss, M. S., & Pfohl, D. C. (1988). New friendships: Staff as visitors of nursing home residents. *Gerontologist, 28,* 263–265.

Mossey, J. M. (1997). Subdysthymic depression and the medically ill elderly. In R. L. Rubenstein & M. P. Lawton (Eds.), *Depression in long-term and residential care: Advances in research and treatment* (pp. 55–74). New York: Springer.

Mulsant, B. H., Sweet, R. A., Rosen, J., Pollock, B. G., Zubenko, G. S., Flynn, T., et al. (2001). A double-blind randomized comparison of nortriptyline plus perphenazine versus nortriptyline plus placebo in the treatment of psychotic depression in late life. *Journal of Clinical Psychiatry, 62,* 597–604.

Nagel, J., Cimbolic, P., & Newlin, M. (1988). Efficacy of elderly and adolescent volunteer counselors in a nursing home setting. *Journal of Counseling Psychology, 35,* 81–86.

National Coalition on Mental Health and Aging. (1999, November). *Actions to improve mental health care for the elderly.* Unpublished conference report.

National Institutes of Health. (1992, November 20). "Failure to thrive" syndrome among older persons. *NIH Guide, 21*(42).

Nelson, F. L., & Farberow, N. L. (1980). Indirect self-destructive behavior in the elderly nursing home resident. *Journal of Gerontology, 35,* 949–957.

Niederehe, G. (1994). Psychosocial therapies with depressed older adults. In L. S. Schneider, C. F. Reynolds, B. D. Lebowitz, & A. J. Friedhoff (Eds.), *Diagnosis and treatment of depression in late life: Results of the NIH Consensus Development Conference* (pp. 293–316). Washington, DC: American Psychiatric Press.

NIH Consensus Development Panel on the Diagnosis and Treatment of Depression in Late Life. (1992). Diagnosis and treatment of depression in late life. *Journal of the American Medical Association, 286,* 1018–1024.

Omnibus Budget Reconciliation Act of 1987, Subtitle C, Pub. L. No. 100-203. The Nursing Home Reform Act, 42 U.S.C. Pt. 2 §4211. 139i(3(a)-(h))(Medicare); 1396r(a)-(h)(Medicaid).

Oxman, T. E. (1996). Geriatric psychiatry at the interface of consultation-liaison psychiatry and primary care. *International Journal of Psychiatry in Medicine, 26*(2), 145–153.

Parmelee, P. A., Katz, I. R., & Powell-Lawton, M. P. (1989). Depression among institutionalized aged: Assessment and prevalence estimation. *Journal of Gerontology: Medical Sciences, 44,* M22–M29.

Payne, D. L. (1987). Antidepressant therapies in the elderly. *Clinical Gerontologist, 7,* 31–41.

Payne, J. L., Sheppard, J. M., Steinberg, M., Warren, A., Baker, A., Steele, C., et al. (2002). Incidence, prevalence, and outcomes of depression in residents of a long-term care facility with dementia. *International Journal of Geriatric Psychiatry, 17,* 247–253.

Pruchno, R. A., & Rose, M. S. (2000). The effect of long-term care environments on health outcomes. *Gerontologist, 40,* 422–428.

Rattenbury, C., & Stones, M. J. (1989). A controlled evaluation of reminiscence and current topics discussion groups in a nursing home context. *Gerontologist, 29,* 768–771.

Reynolds, C. F. (1995). Recognition and differentiation of elderly depression in the clinical setting. *Geriatrics, 50*(Suppl. 1), S6–S15.

Reynolds, C. F., Frank, E., Perel, J. M., Imber, S. D., Cornes, C., Miller, M. D., et al. (1999). Nortriptyline and interpersonal psychotherapy as maintenance therapies for recurrent major depression: A randomized controlled trial in patients older than 59 years. *Journal of the American Medical Association, 281,* 39–45.

Ronch, J. L., & Goldfield, J. (2002). *Mental wellness in aging: Strengths-based approaches.* Baltimore: Health Professions Press.

Ronch, J. L., & Maizler, J. S. (1977). Individual psychotherapy with the institutionalized aged. *American Journal of Orthopsychiatry, 47,* 275–283.

Rosen, A. L., & Persky, T. (1997). Meeting the mental health needs of older people: Policy and practice issues for social work. *Journal of Gerontological Social Work, 27,* 45–54.

Rovner, B. W., German, P. S., Brant, L. J., Clark, R., Burton, L., & Folstein, M. F. (1991). Depression and mortality in nursing homes. *Journal of the American Medical Association, 265,* 993–996.

Rowe, J. W., & Kahn, R. L. (1987). Human aging: Usual and successful. *Science, 237,* 143–149.

Rubenstein, R. L., & Lawton, M. P. (1997). *Depression in long term and residential care: Advances in research and treatment.* New York: Springer.

Rylands, K. J., & Rickwood, D. J. (2001). Ego-integrity versus ego-despair: The effect of "accepting the past" on depression in older women. *International Journal of Aging and Human Development, 53,* 75–89.

Salari, S. M., & Rich, M. (2001). Social and environmental infantilization of aged persons: Observations in two adult day care centers. *International Journal of Aging and Human Development, 52,* 115–134.

Schachter-Shalomi, Z., & Miller, R. S. (1995). *From age-ing to sage-ing: A profound new vision of growing older.* New York: Warner Books.

Schneider, L. S. (1995). Efficacy of clinical treatment for mental disorders among older persons. In M. Gatz (Ed.), *Emerging issues in mental health and aging* (pp. 19–71). Washington, DC: American Psychological Association.

Scogin, F. (1998). Bibliotherapy: A nontraditional intervention for depression. In P. Hartman-Stein (Ed.), *Innovative behavioral healthcare for older adults: A guidebook for changing times* (pp. 129–144). San Francisco: Jossey-Bass.

Scogin, F., & McElreath, L. (1994). Efficacy of psychosocial treatments for geriatric depression: A quantitative review. *Journal of Consulting and Clinical Psychology, 62,* 69–74.

Sumaya, I. C., Rienzi, B. M., Deegan, J. F., & Moss, D. E. (2001). Bright light treatment decreases depression in institutionalized older adults: A placebo-controlled crossover study. *Journal of Gerontology: Medical Sciences, 56A,* M356–M360.

Sutcliffe, C., Cordingley, L., Burns, A., Mozley, C., Bagley, H., Huxley, P., et al. (2000). A new version of the Geriatric Depression Scale for nursing and residential home populations: The Geriatric Depression Scale (residential) (GDS-12R). *International Psychogeriatrics, 12,* 173–181.

Tavormina, C. E. (1999). Embracing the Eden Alternative in long-term care environments. *Geriatric Nursing, 20,* 158–161.

Teresi, J., Abrams, R., Holmes, D., Ramirez, M., & Eimicke, J. (2001). Prevalence of depression and depression recognition in nursing homes. *Social Psychiatry, 36,* 613–620.

Teresi, J., Holmes, D., & Monaco, C. (1993). An evaluation of the effects of commingling cognitively and noncognitively impaired individuals in long-term care facilities. *Gerontologist, 33,* 350–358.

Teri, L., Curtis, J., Gallagher-Thompson, D., & Thompson, L. W. (1994). Cognitive/ behavior therapy with depressed older adults. In L. S. Schneider, C. F. Reynolds, B. D. Lebowitz, & A. J. Friedhoff (Eds.), *Diagnosis and treatment of depression in late life: Results of the NIH Consensus Development Conference* (pp. 279–292). Washington, DC: American Psychiatric Press.

Thomas, W. (1996). *Life worth living: How someone you love can still enjoy life in a nursing home—The Eden Alternative in action.* Acton, MA: VanderWyk & Burnham.

Thompson, L. W., Gallagher, D., & Breckinridge, J. S. (1987). Comparative effectiveness of psychotherapies for depressed elders. *Journal of Consulting and Clinical Psychology, 55,* 385–390.

Thompson, L. W., & Gallagher-Thompson, D. (1997). Psychotherapeutic interventions with older adults in outpatient and extended care settings. In R. L. Rubenstein & M. P. Lawton (Eds.), *Depression in long term and residential care: Advances in research and treatment* (pp. 169–184). New York: Springer.

Unützer, J., Patrick, D. L., Simon, G., Gremeowski, D., Walker, E., Rutter, C., et al. (1997). Depressive symptoms and the cost of health services in HMO patients aged 65 and older: A 4-year prospective study. *Journal of the American Medical Association, 277,* 1618–1623.

U.S. Surgeon General. (1999). *Mental health: A report of the Surgeon General.* Washington, DC: Author.

Watt, L. M., & Cappeliez, P. (2000). Integrative and instrumental reminiscence therapies for depression in older adults: Intervention strategies and treatment effectiveness. *Aging and Mental Health, 4,* 166–177.

Weinstein, L. B. (1998). The Eden Alternative: A new paradigm for nursing homes. *Activities, Adaptation, and Aging, 22,* 1–8.

Weisberg, J., & Haberman, M. (1989). Therapeutic hugging week in a geriatric facility. *Journal of Gerontological Social Work, 13,* 181–185.

Weiss, B. Z., & Salamon, M. J. (1987). Combined intervention: An eclectic approach to the treatment of social phobias and depression in elderly long-term care patients. *Clinical Gerontologist, 7,* 51–62.

Weiss, J. C. (1998). The "Feeling Great" Wellness Program for older adults. *Activities, Adaptation and Aging, 12*(3/4).

Winkler, A., Fairnie, H., Gericevich, F., & Long, M. (1989). The impact of a resident dog on an institution for the elderly: Effects on perceptions and social interactions. *Gerontologist, 29*, 216–223.

Yesavage, J. A. (1988). Geriatric Depression Scale. *Psychopharmacology Bulletin, 24*, 709–711.

Zeiss, A. M., & Steffen, A. (1996). Behavioral and cognitive/behavioral treatments: An overview of social learning. In S. Zarit & B. Knight (Eds.), *A guide to psychotherapy and aging: Effective clinical interventions in a life state context* (pp. 35–60). Washington, DC: American Psychological Association.

Ziemba, J., Roop, K., & Wittenberg, S. (1988). A magic mix: After-school programs in a nursing home. *Children Today, 17*, 9–13.

Chapter 3

OLDER ADULTS WITH DEMENTIA: COMMUNITY-BASED LONG-TERM-CARE ALTERNATIVES

Jeanette Semke

Dementia is society's most costly mental disorder in later life (Zarit & Zarit, 1998), not only in terms of social and health care dollars, but also in emotional costs to those persons who have this condition and their caregivers. The loss of memory and other functional abilities can be devastating. In addition, the emotional and physical burden to those caring for persons with dementia can be considerable and can lead to health problems. Cognitive impairment because of dementia is the leading reason for seeking formal community-based and institutional long-term-care services (Kane, Kane, & Ladd, 1998); a change in symptomatology is a primary reason for older persons who are receiving community-based long-term-care to be transferred to nursing homes.

A major expansion in the population of older adults in need of mental health services and formal long-term care is expected to occur in the United States in the early twenty-first century (Bernstein & Hensley, 1993; Furino & Fogel, 1990; Meeks et al., 1990; Talbott, 1983). A significant proportion of that population will be composed of older adults with dementia. It is estimated that by the year 2050, 14 million

Americans will be diagnosed with some form of dementia (Aronson, 1994). This demographic shift will be accompanied by two emerging trends in service delivery: (a) the growth of community residential care as an alternative to nursing home care, and (b) the adoption of managed systems of mental health and long-term care. The result will be an increasing demand for community residential care by an older and more severely ill population, many of whom experience cognitive impairment accompanied by symptoms of depression and behavioral difficulties (Reichman & Katz, 1996; Tweed, Blazer, & Ciarlo, 1992). Meanwhile, service systems designed to ration social and health service resources proliferate in the public and private sectors. More than ever, social workers with training in gerontology will be important contributors to ensuring an equitable and quality community-based long-term care system.

Many policy observers declare that the United States is in the midst of a health care crisis. At the center of this crisis is the question of how the acute, chronic, and social service systems can be coordinated and designed to effectively and efficiently address the needs of high-cost health care consumers such as those with dementia. Increasingly, community residential care is used as an alternative to nursing home care for this population (Kane et al., 1998). Therefore, the provision of community residential care for older adults with dementia is an area of knowledge that is growing in importance in social gerontology. This topic is important because pressures to save long-term-care costs may overshadow concerns about how the needs of this population can best be met. This chapter discusses issues that must be addressed in order to ensure that community residential-care providers have the capacity to enhance the quality of life of older adults with dementia, a population with complicated and special care needs.

SIGNIFICANCE TO GERONTOLOGY, HEALTH CARE, AND HEALTH PROFESSIONALS

Estimates of the prevalence of dementia in the population as a whole vary considerably. However, it is clear that prevalence increases with age, with rates of 1% for people in their 60s, 7% for people in their 70s, and 20% to 30% for those in their 80s (Jorm, Korten, & Henderson, 1987; Zarit & Zarit, 1998). *Dementia* is "characterized by the development of multiple cognitive deficits that are due to the direct physiological effects of a general medical condition, to the persisting effects of a substance, or to multiple etiologies" (American Psychiatric Association [APA], 1994, p. 133). It is typified by difficulties in intellectual ability, functioning, and behavior that affect an individual's ability to live independently. Symptoms include memory loss, impaired judgment, loss of ability to learn new things, disorientation, loss of language skills, changes in personality, and perceptual difficulties (Aronson, 1994). Individuals with advanced dementia lack the ability to perform the most basic and routine activities of daily living (ADLs). Those with dementia often have behavioral symptoms such as agitation, resistance to care, yelling, and combativeness. Other mental health symptoms that may be experienced are depression and paranoia; insomnia and wandering are also common.

The dementia syndrome can develop from many different disorders. Several types of dementia, referred to as *primary dementias,* are not reversible and worsen and persist over time. Approximately 50% of cases of primary dementia are associated with Alzheimer's disease; 10% are dementias of the frontal lobe type; 8% to 18% have characteristics of both Alzheimer's disease (AD) and vascular dementia; and 8% to 12% of the cases are caused by vascular disease. Other less prevalent causes of primary dementia that are not reversible include Parkinson's disease, AIDS, Creutzfeldt-Jacob disease, Huntington's chorea, Pick's disease, and substance-induced persisting dementia (APA, 1994; Bachman et al., 1993; Cummings & Jeste, 1999). Finally, a number of dementia symptoms, that may or may not be reversible, are associated with other medical disorders. These *secondary dementias* can be caused by a variety of illnesses including depression, acute medical or psychosocial stressors, nutritional deficits, medications, environmental poisons, and chronic alcoholism.

The most prevalent form of dementia is Alzheimer's disease. A positive diagnosis of Alzheimer's disease is achievable only through microscopic examination of the brain postmortem. Such examination usually shows senile plaques, neurofibrillary tangles, granulovascular degeneration, neuronal loss, astrocytic gliosis, and amyloid angiopathy (APA, 1994). Life span from the time Alzheimer's disease is diagnosed until death averages about 9 years.

Alzheimer's disease is insidious and begins with almost imperceptible changes in a person's ability to function and to manage. Subtle changes include the gradual reduction in the ability to remember recent events; to learn or remember new information; to recall names of familiar persons or objects; to maintain personal appearance and hygiene; and to concentrate on such activities as watching television or reading. There also may be changes in mood not typical of past behaviors. As the disease progresses, tasks that require judgment (such as driving a vehicle) or abstract thinking (such as balancing a checkbook) become more difficult. As deficits in cognitive functioning become more pronounced, frustration, anger, and depression may be experienced. In late stages, the ability to recognize loved ones and perform basic ADLs is lost, including walking, eating, and dressing (Dixon, 1991).

Community Residential Care and Dementia

When informal and formal care providers are unable to meet the care needs of older adults in a person's home, community residential care is increasingly used as a substitute for nursing home care. Most clients prefer homelike settings to the medicalized, institutional environments typical of nursing homes. Potentially, health care services in community-based care can be individualized in a social environment that offers more choices in day-to-day living than in institutional settings.

Community residential care refers to a form of long-term care that includes shelter, food, and a number of supportive social and health services. Across the states, there is no consistent nomenclature that distinguishes one type of community residential care from another; however, terms such as *assisted living, congregate care, boarding homes, adult foster care, adult family homes, and personal care homes* are commonly used for community residential care. The settings range from large institutional-type buildings to small homelike abodes. Although skilled nursing and nurse monitoring are sometimes provided as part of a package of community residential-care services, personal care workers provide the greatest amount of care. Services include, for example, assistance with bathing, transferring, supervision of medications, shopping, meal preparation, and laundry. Other social health-care services that are important for long-term care of clients with dementia, but not necessarily administered under the auspices of the residential care provider, include outpatient mental-health services and inpatient services provided in community hospitals and state mental hospitals. Housing and service requirements for community residential settings can be categorized as follows: (a) a homelike environment that encompasses homelike public space and homelike private space; (b) a capacity for service that meets routine or regular needs of the consumer, as well as specialized needs that might arise; and (c) a philosophy that promotes maximum client choice and control (Wilson, 1996).

In the past, it was commonly accepted that community residential care was intended for persons who could no longer stay with their natural families, but were not so disabled as to require nursing home care. More recently, however, it has been seen as an alternative for nursing home care for a more disabled population who in the past would have been placed in a nursing home. Older persons with dementia seem to thrive in normal living environments that are prosthetic in the sense that they are designed to compensate for cognitive deficits and provide opportunities to socialize and to experience appropriate stimulation (Kane et al., 1998). The preference for community alternatives to nursing home care is in keeping with a philosophy referred to as *aging in place* (Klein, 1994; Rowles, 1994), a concept that refers to residential stability in one's home or a homelike milieu with minimal disruptions.

Aging in place is made possible with the aid of a range of social, health, and personal care services that maximize residential stability without compromising quality of life and health outcomes. The concept has great appeal for care recipients, families, providers, and funders because of its potential to provide cost-effective services in a homelike setting while enhancing an individual's independence. Typically, health and social services can be provided more flexibly in the community than in nursing homes and other institutional settings. Different types and amounts of services can be bundled or unbundled, depending upon the differing and changing health circumstances of long-term-care clients. Thus, there is the potential to match services more closely to the needs of the client than is possible in institutional settings where a one-size-fits-all approach tends to dominate. As Kane and colleagues (1998) state, "Assuming that some long-term care clients will need to move away from their current home, an ideal long-term care system would present a range of options for new living quarters where services could be received and daily life would still go on in a normal manner" (p. 160).

SIGNIFICANCE FOR HEALTH CARE

Community residential care has the potential to affect health outcomes for both older adults with dementia and their family members. In many instances, such care is sought for a loved one when the stress and burden to the family caregiver has reached the point that the caregiver's health is compromised. Many families struggle against great odds to maintain family members with dementia at home as long as possible (Dixon, 1991). A potential for improved care exists once placement in community residential care has been made and the formal care provider takes over the care responsibilities that, up to that time, belonged to the family caregiver. A family caregiver, who heretofore only had the time and physical or emotional resources to attend to basic care needs, is now free to engage in a more normalized relationship with the loved one. Time and energy can be spent on such things as visits together into the community and involvement in leisure activities within the community residence. Community residential care also fulfills care needs for older adults who have no family or friends to provide care.

One challenge for health care service providers is that of differentially diagnosing the specific type of dementia. Because there are no definitive markers for diagnosis of dementing illnesses such as Alzheimer's disease, diagnosticians use behavioral, neuropsychological, and medical data (Aronson, 1994; Dixon, 1991; Zarit & Zarit, 1998). As Cummings and Jeste (1999) state, "The current approach to diagnosing Alzheimer's disease is time-intensive, labor-intensive, and costly. Its sensitivity and specificity are largely dependent on the expertise of the examiner. Improvements in detection, diagnosis, and treatment are needed" (p. 1175). Detection of mild cases of dementia is especially unreliable (Callahan, Hendrie, & Tierney, 1995). Therefore, one can infer that among the population of older adults with symptoms of dementia, there will be a number of individuals for whom a specific dementia diagnosis may not be well established.

Nonetheless, differential diagnosis is important because symptoms for some types of dementia may be treatable. For example, memory impairment occurs in both delirium and dementia. They can be differentiated by observing evidence about the clinical course. According to the *Diagnostic and Statistical Manual of Mental Disorders (DSM-IV*, 1994),

> Typically, symptoms in delirium fluctuate and symptoms in dementia are relatively stable. Multiple cognitive impairments that persist in an unchanged form for more than a few months suggest dementia rather than delirium. Delirium may be superimposed on a dementia, in which case both disorders are diagnosed. In situations in which it is unclear whether the cognitive deficits are due to a delirium or a dementia, it may be useful to

make a provisional diagnosis of delirium and observe the person carefully while continuing efforts to identify the nature of the disturbance. (p. 138)

Delirium caused by a general medical condition that is induced by toxicity from intake of alcohol, drugs, or medication side effects can be reversed when treated appropriately. The same may be true for schizophrenia and major depression.

Another reason that differential diagnosis is important is because the course of specific dementia diagnoses may differ. Knowledge of whether the course is progressive, static, or remitting is critical for the individual, family, and caregivers as they develop care-planning strategies into the future. For example, the clinical course of vascular dementia is variable and typically progresses in stepwise fashion, whereas the severity of impairment in cognitive functioning after stroke often remains static. Until diagnostic technology improves, dementia of the Alzheimer's type is treated as a diagnosis of exclusion where other causes for the cognitive deficits must first be ruled out.

The high prevalence of co-occurring medical and mental health problems among older adults adds to the complexity of service provision for those with dementia. The individual client may lack the awareness and vigilance necessary to manage medical conditions without help and supervision. Most individuals with Alzheimer's disease experience symptoms of behavioral dysfunction, including withdrawal, apathy, depression, hostility, anger, and aggression. Symptoms of depression are common in Alzheimer's disease patients (17% to 30%) and are associated with broad behavioral dysfunction and increased functional disability (Teri, Logsdon, Uomoto, & McCurry, 1997). Behavioral dysfunction is a major influence on the morbidity and disability of patients and is central to decisions on patient institutionalization.

There is considerable variation in comorbidity among this population, suggesting that a one-size-fits-all approach to community care is inadequate. For some persons, cognitive impairment may be the main factor that limits independent functioning. For others, the need for assistance with ADLs is due to a combination of physical disability and cognitive impairment. An example would be an individual with middle-stage Alzheimer's dementia, a heart condition, diabetes, and skin problems. Someone with multiple needs would require combinations of several types of services and, in fact, may be at exponentially increased risk of being admitted to a nursing home.

For most people with dementia, the condition changes over time with a decline in functioning. However, abrupt deterioration can be due to causes that are treatable. For example, delirium in reaction to other disease conditions or to medication and depression are common among older persons. Thus, it is very important that persons with dementia have thorough medical evaluations and periodic reevaluations (Aronson, 1994; Berg, 1994). Also, programs must be designed so that they are adaptable to changing and fluctuating needs. People with dementia have good days and bad days. Ideally, a program will have the capacity to be responsive to a person whose needs for personal attention by caregivers increases dramatically on a given day.

SIGNIFICANCE TO HEALTH PROFESSIONALS

Dementia is devastating to the ones who have it and to families and friends who experience the loss of their loved ones as they had known them. However, an individual's quality of life remains something to be cherished and concerned about no matter how ill that person is. Grandma is still grandma. Auntie is still auntie. Although the person with dementia will experience memory loss and personality changes, love can be felt and received, and the human spirit of the loved one can be accessed. Thus, relocation to community residential care need not be synonymous with giving in or giving up.

Long-term care is connected with many aspects of life including physical functioning, mental health, family relationships, social life, and basic needs for food and shelter. Likewise, it spans historically distinct areas of professional expertise. Therefore, several professions are key to an effective community-based long-term-care system for older adults with dementia. In the field of long-term care, physicians who practice geriatric medicine, a subspecialty of internal medicine and family practice, act as consultants. They can provide brief clinical assessments that include diagnosis and medical intervention. However, because of the limited number of these geriatricians, they typically provide consultation and training to others who work with older adults.

Nonspecialty primary-care physicians, nurse practitioners, and registered nurses also play a critical role in effective care for this population. The need for their ongoing involvement with individuals with dementia is conspicuous, because people receiving long-term care are more likely to need medical treatment than the average older person. Physical therapists, speech therapists, and occupational therapists contribute substantially to improving and maintaining optimal levels of functioning for persons with dementia. Also, when new levels of disability are encountered, these professionals can help the individual and caregivers understand facts of the condition and how to deal with them. Mental health professionals, including psychiatrists, psychologists, and social workers, offer expertise about how caregivers can manage behavioral symptoms that often accompany dementing diseases.

Working with older persons who have dementia requires advanced interpersonal skills and special training. Staff and family can help the individual to maintain a sense of mastery with environmental cues and adaptations that help compensate for loss of orientation and other cognitive deficits that accompany dementia. In many cases, careful monitoring of an individual's health condition, good nutrition, exercise, and stimulation can help slow the decline in functioning. Staff in prosthetic environments does not demand functioning beyond a person's capacity and, when appropriate, provide cues for daily activities. Individuals with dementia do better when activities occur in smaller areas where there is noise control. Signage and wandering areas are helpful. These measures engender a sense of mastery while protecting clients' safety (Kane et al., 1998). Recognition of the cultural norms of persons with dementia and their families will help in arriving at appropriate plans of care. Living situations with shared language and culturally based food preferences have the potential to greatly increase a sense of home.

Standards of care across disciplines and carefully conceived mechanisms for coordinating care of the multiple professions are essential to maintaining health and functioning of this population. Agreement upon a common system of record keeping is crucial to the successful functioning of interdisciplinary teams that serve this population. Teamwork among the many professionals involved with the client who has dementia potentially will ensure that the various actors work together toward the same goal (Kane et al., 1998). Although roles are differentiated, based on the specific expertise of the different professions, a successful team approach requires the willingness of those from the different professions to have intimate knowledge of the work of the other professionals and to share roles when needed and appropriate. The quality of the work environment for staff also is an important concern and can indirectly influence quality of life for the resident. Because this work is emotionally demanding, administrators must attend to the emotional and physical needs of staff to prevent staff burnout.

Of necessity, disability and frailty bring persons with dementia into long-term-care systems and community residential care. Typically, eligibility for services is determined on the basis of health problems, an inevitably deficit approach. The medical field is oriented toward identifying a health problem and fixing it or at least preventing avoidable decline among those with chronic disease. Often, the whole person is forgotten when the focus of assessment and intervention is on unmet need. This circumstance offers an opportunity for social workers to intervene, because expectations for their involvement stress the social and psychological aspects of a problem more than the medical. Although assessment and intervention are focused upon medical problems and care needs, outcomes for clients can be enhanced when practice is embedded in a philosophy that recognizes and builds upon strengths of the individual and his or her social system. The value base of the social work profession supports such a strength-based approach to practice. A holistic approach to individual community residential clients with dementia, their families, and other loved ones can be promoted by skilled, culturally competent social workers. A strength-based approach by social workers emphasizes the positive aspect of life in the residence and the fact that quality of life is an important concern for those with dementia, just as it is for all long-term-care clients. In addition, because many social workers are trained to intervene at multiple systems levels and to take a holistic approach to individual clients, families, and organizational systems, they can be expected to contribute significantly to team building and coordination and integration of care.

PRIOR RESEARCH AND KNOWLEDGE BASE

There is considerable uncertainty about the place of community-based services in the long-term-care system for dementia patients and in ongoing health care reforms (Bartels, Levine, & Shea, 1999; Kane, Kane, Illston, Nyman, & Finch, 1991; Mehrotra & Kosloski, 1991; Thompson, 1999; Weissert & Hedrick, 1994). This uncertainty is especially salient when the clients' needs are complicated by multiple and co-occurring cognitive, behavioral, and somatic conditions that require interventions by more than one service system. There is some indication that, to date, necessary community systems may not be in place to support frail elders with serious cognitive impairment or behavioral problems (Bernstein & Hensley, 1993; Hastings, 1993; Semke & Jensen, 1996). One concern is that community residential care may not be conducive to the coordination of the distinct service sectors required for individuals with multiple, chronic, and varied health and mental health problems (Boyer, McAlpine, Pottick, & Olfson, 2000; Florio et al., 1996; Patterson, Higgins, & Dyck, 1995; Proctor, Morrow-Howell, Rubin, & Ringenburg, 1999). This concern may be warranted by the fact that there has been little involvement of psychiatrists and other mental health specialists in nursing facility care (Borson, Liptzin, Nininger, & Rabins, 1987; Tourigny-Rivard & Drury, 1987) or in home and community-based care (Lebowitz, Light, & Bailey, 1987; Light, Lebowitz, & Bailey, 1986).

Variations in service provision do not arise only from differences in patient care needs; they also attest to the uncertainties about the place of community residential care in the long-term-care system. Other causes of those variations include (a) prevailing views in a community about what it takes to care for people with varying characteristics (Capitman & Sciegaj, 1995; Hennessy, 1989); (b) health care resources within a community such as availability of health care professionals and nursing home beds (Cohen et al., 1986,1988, 1988; Greene & Ondrich, 1990); and (c) uncertainty among direct-care decision makers and program administrators about what types and amounts of services to authorize (Eddy, 1994; Wallace, 1990; Wennberg & Gittelsohn, 1973; Wolff, 1989). For example, providers of community residential care may be unprepared to care for individuals with behavioral problems. This may be especially true among the Mom-and-Pop type of personal care homes. Responsibility for identifying need and arranging for additional behavioral health-care services may not be clear and, therefore, may be overlooked. Those persons with the greatest needs are typically the least able to articulate their needs and the most difficult to assess and engage (Raschko, 1985). This is compounded by the lack of training of some providers in identification and management of emotional and behavioral problems (Badger et al., 1994; Carney, Dietrich, Eliassen, Owen, & Badger, 1999; Olfson, Sing, & Schlesinger, 1999). For example, several studies indicate that depression is related to increased disability caused by chronic medical illness (Evans, 1993; Katon, 1998; Sullivan, Katon, Rosso, Dobie, & Sakai, 1992). It can be inferred that untreated depression may contribute to an increased likelihood of institutionalization in these circumstances.

Most studies in this area have been experimental or quasi-experimental evaluations of demonstrations that measured the average or programmatic effect of supportive community services to a treatment group. All but one of a group of rigorous studies reviewed by Greene, Lovely, and Ondrich (1993) found that the community services did not sufficiently offset nursing home use to cover costs of operations. Most studies of the effectiveness of home and community-based services have focused on the ability of home care services to delay and prevent nursing home admission. Some studies have found a positive relationship between personal care services and delay or prevention of nursing home admission (Hughes et al., 1992; Hughes, Manheim, Edelman, & Conrad, 1987; Nielsen, Blenkner, Bloom, Downs, & Beggs, 1972; Nocks, Learner, Blackman, & Brown, 1986) and others have not (Wooldridge & Schore, 1986; Zimmer, Groth-Junker, & McCusker, 1985). After a review of previous studies of risk of nursing home placement for dementia patients, Tsuji, Whalen, and Finucane (1995) and Weissert and Hedrick (1994) concluded that differences in findings could be attributable to differences in research designs, nature of services received, long-term-care eligibility criteria, and client characteristics. Although a review of the research literature by Weissert and Hedrick (1994) agrees with these studies, they aptly point out that the popularity of home and community-based programs, despite the absence of empirical evidence of effectiveness, suggests that prior and future research be used to identify ways of making it cost-effective.

CURRENT RESEARCH

The fact that contemporary community residential care clients are likely to suffer from co-occurring health conditions and require intervention from multiple service organizations raises the question of whether they receive care in accordance with their multiple needs. This question is of particular concern for older adults with dementia, because mental health services may be a key component in successful community living.

Recognizing these concerns, I conducted a study of social and health service use by older adult residents of adult family homes who had symptoms of mental disorders including dementia (Semke, 2002). The study occurred in the State of Washington in cooperation with the Washington Department of Social and Health Services. I used automated clinical and service records for calendar year 1998 for the analyses. (Adult family homes in Washington are similar to care settings that are called personal care homes and adult foster care in other states.) Although some adult family homes are run by registered nurses, most are run by individuals who have no professional background, but have enough training in the fundamentals of caregiving to qualify as providers. Several additional days of training are required to be designated as a mental health or dementia-care specialty home. In addition, 10 hours a year of continuing education are required on topics relevant to giving adult family home care.

The study population was composed of 2,051 adults aged 60 years or older who had symptoms of a mental disorder and resided in an adult family for 6 or more months in calendar year 1998; 77% of the study population were women. Most or all of the care was paid for by the State of Washington and Medicaid funds. Forty-four percent of this group had symptoms of dementia, 42% had behavioral symptoms, and 53% had symptoms of depression. Aside from dementia, depression, schizophrenia, and other forms of mental illness, the most prevalent diagnoses for the study population were cardiovascular disease, arthritis, musculoskeletal disability, respiratory disease, and stroke.

Results of the study showed that a majority (62%) of the study population received outpatient medical services during the period of the study, and a minority received mental health services (21%). Three different types of providers provided mental health services: (a) 11% received services from specialty mental health staff funded by the Washington State Mental Health Division, (b) 11% received services from outpatient nonspecialty medical practitioners, and (c) 4% received services from psychiatrists. Some clients received mental health services from more than one type of provider. These results, although inconclusive, raise questions about access to mental health services by this population and suggest that further research examine details about the mental health needs of older adult family-home residents and the barriers to receiving needed mental health care.

FURTHER RESEARCH NEEDS

In order to be cost-effective, appropriate types of services are provided to those who need them, unnecessary services are not provided, and services are delivered in the least costly setting. Greene and colleagues (1993) and other researchers recommend more study of cost-effectiveness at the individual level of analysis. For example, they found that additional home-health-aide hours per week significantly reduced the likelihood of institutionalization and reduced the predicted overall cost of long-term care for older adults with cognitive impairment. Increases in personal care hours, however, had no significant effect. Future studies need to examine whether services from mental health professionals and mental health services that are provided by primary care physicians reduce the likelihood of institutionalization and improve quality of life for individuals with cognitive impairment.

In addition, because the types of settings and services required for individuals with different sets of problems vary, they need to be more clearly articulated in future research (Kruzich & Kruzich, 1985). Further research must begin by identifying characteristics of individual community-residential-care clients that predict positive outcomes when receiving specific service packages. Service packages must be broadly defined to consider the role of community health services outside of the community-residential-care program in prolonging community tenure and client well-being.

At this early stage in the development of a community-residential-care-system, one appropriate and cost-effective research approach is to use secondary clinical and service data to identify which community-residential-care service attributes are associated with better outcomes. The fact that older adults with similar illness profiles vary significantly in types, volume, and mix of services they receive *within* and *across* regions and states creates, in effect, a natural experiment. The natural experiment allows for the testing of hypotheses about relationships between social and health service provision and client outcomes.

Qualitative studies about the process of care and the experiences of older adults with dementia living in community-based residential care settings would provide in-depth knowledge that would complement the studies that use administrative data. In addition, studies of the effect of staff training programs on the quality of community residential care will be important to address the challenges faced by paraprofessional caregivers who are trying to meet the complex care needs of individuals with dementia.

POLICY IMPLICATIONS

National, state, and local governments increasingly are adopting managed care approaches to long-term care in an attempt to control the costs of social and health services. It will be important for policy makers to keep abreast of accumulating evidence about what types of community-based care and social and health services at varying levels of intensity produce the best outcomes for a variety of citizens with diverse needs. This information will be critical to planning and administering systems of social services, health care services, and long-term-care services that are coordinated, that recognize the diversity of the population in need, and that use client outcomes as the measure of success. Older adults who are frail and who suffer from dementia compose one important group whose well-being may be significantly affected by the design and implementation of these systems.

The need for specific social and health services varies among older adults with dementia. The current system of care can be improved by increasing its responsiveness to patients' diverse needs. There are a variety of specialized services that when tailored to the individual symptoms of the patient have the potential to improve quality of life and slow functional decline (e.g., treatment of depression).

A better understanding of community residential care in the context of the larger social and health service systems and the cultural context of communities in which they are embedded is required if the care needs of this population are to be appropriately addressed. To improve the provision of services to diverse populations of older persons with dementia, several policy goals must be met: (a) increased coordination of existing social and health service systems, (b) increased emphasis on the cultural context of different communities in which long-term-care services are provided, (c) dramatic development of the community-based long-term-care workforce, and (d) increased institutional support to case managers that will enable them to accurately assess need for care.

An important barrier to meeting these goals is the fragmented long-term-care system, characterized by multiple payers and organizations. Fragments include different payers such as Medicare, Medicaid, and private insurance. Fragments also include different systems for mental health, primary care, long-term care, specialty medical care, inpatient services, and home health care. As the care needs of older people in long-term care change, immediate access to an array of services with varied and flexible levels of intensity will enhance the likelihood of achieving optimum outcomes, preventing health care crises, and avoiding premature decline in health and well-being (Lebowitz et al., 1987). Often the fragmentation that is typical of most health care systems creates barriers to timely and appropriate responses to clients' complex and changing needs (Estes & Swan, 1993). Although providers of day-to-day personal care may be in the best position to detect the need for early interventions with community-residential-care patients, the knowledge and skills of residential care providers may not be sufficient to the ongoing assessment task. Also, a lack of coordination of services among multiple providers within the fragmented social and health service systems in most communities may result in significant deficiencies. These include (a) insufficient follow-up and monitoring of chronic conditions, (b) poor communication about co-occurring illnesses and the potential interactions of medications, and (c) redundancy in care and subsequent cost inefficiencies, all of which are a burden to the patient, the system, and the caregivers.

Serious health conditions might be prevented by early detection and referral to the appropriate health care professional service. Therefore, it is critical to a long-term care-system that policy measures increase the incentives and capacity for coordinating disparate service delivery organizations, of which community residential care is one important component. Several policy areas stand out as fundamental to improving community residential care for persons with dementia: (a) raising public awareness, (b) improving standards of care, (c) developing the personal care workforce, and (d) testing models of social service integration.

Public Awareness

Although they support research that may lead to a cure for Alzheimer's disease (the leading cause of cognitive dysfunction in older adults), policy initiatives at the national and local levels must address the stigma attached to dementia. The prevalent all-is-lost attitude can be countered with public information campaigns that stress the importance of maintaining dignity regardless of cognitive status and with media stories about successful and positive aspects of dementia care. Also, it is important to provide more public education about the array of choices available in dementia care. Persons with dementia may successfully live in their own homes with a combination of formal and informal care; in family-like homes where room, board, and personal care are provided by a nonrelative; in assisted living facilities or boarding homes; and in nursing homes. The individual preferences, personal strengths, needs, and cultural context of persons with dementia will lead to a variety of housing arrangements. An important consideration for all those who are anticipating formal long-term care for themselves or their loved ones is the chosen facility's capacity to adapt care to the changing needs of the client. Too many older persons have moved into a particular community-based facility, dazzled by its offerings, only to find out that they must move when their care needs increase.

Standards of Care

Unlike nursing homes, community residential care has not been highly regulated. Therefore, accountability and standards for appropriate care are of great concern to consumers, their families, professionals, and policy makers. Several commonly used vehicles for assuring quality care are (a) education of consumers about their rights, (b) programs that would be responsible for taking complaints and mediating problems on behalf of residents of personal care homes, boarding homes, and nursing homes, (c) criminal checks of employees and licensing requirements for professionals and agencies, (d) systems of continuous quality improvement initiated by providers that are designed to identify problems in the delivery of services and then to take corrective action, (e) case management by personnel outside the provider agencies, and (f) systems of monetary rewards and penalties to providers. In the evolving long-term-care industry, new mechanisms for regulation will be needed to allow for flexibility and to support innovation in care. Currently, regulations that specify the qualifications of direct care providers who are allowed to provide different types of services often constrain and limit flexibility in caregiving. To encourage the development of innovative, cost-effective approaches to care in community residential settings, mechanisms for assuring quality of care and safety for older persons with dementia must be designed in a such a way to allow for creativity and flexibility.

Development of the Workforce

The long-term personal-care labor market is characterized by part-time jobs, low wages, and low benefit packages (Estes & Swan, 1993). Attrition is high. To increase the quality of personal care workers, policies must be made that increase wages and benefits, training, and supervision for this important work force.

Models of Service System Integration

Integration and coordination of services have the potential to improve long-term-care systems by increasing availability, accessibility, and acceptability (Wallace, 1990). Planning and structuring an array of services at the macro level is important to ensure the availability of different types of services. If services that meet the special needs of persons with dementia are not provided in the first place, then the system of care is incomplete. Accessibility of services to those who need them, when they need them, can be improved through integration and coordination efforts. Putting a professional in charge of care management for patients with multiple needs who require multiple providers is one way to accomplish accessibility (Yordi, 1990). Consumers are more likely to use and gain maximum benefit from services that they perceive as acceptable. Certainly, different types of living situations appeal to different people. An ability to honor the preferences of individual consumers for particular types of residential care will increase acceptability of long-term-care services.

Long-term-care service systems in the United States can be improved through vertical integration of different levels of long-term care and horizontal integration among acute- and long-term-care providers. The goal of integrating levels of care is to provide continuity in persons who interact with consumers over time, regardless of the level of care they are receiving. Policies designed to promote integration have the potential to avoid situations where, for example, a man with dementia is abruptly moved from a community residential setting that has become his home to a completely unfamiliar environment elsewhere because his care needs have increased. Also, coordination of primary medical care and long-term care potentially can prevent avoidable functional decline that can result from unmet needs (Weiner & Illston, 1994). A number of exemplary systems of care management include the Program for All Inclusive Care for the Elderly, Social Health Maintenance Organizations (Kane et al., 1998), and the New York State "Commonwealth" Managed Long Term Care Demonstration.

INTEGRATING KNOWLEDGE INTO THE CURRICULUM

Community residential care for older adults with dementia can be addressed in bachelor's and master's social-work practice and policy courses. Social work practice in the area of dementia care is challenging and can be rewarding. The work may be difficult, but with it comes the opportunity to increase the quality of life significantly for individuals with dementia, caregivers, and family members. Specialized skills are required for direct practice and can be integrated into a variety of direct practice courses. Students will learn that much can be done to maintain the dignity of a person with dementia and to prevent excessive disability from occurring. Key components of this knowledge and skill area include (a) guidelines for providing a safe environment, (b) guidelines for setting realistic goals that maximize independence and health for each person, (c) understanding the course of different types of dementias (e.g., Alzheimer's disease progresses through phases and cognitive changes are accompanied by behavior changes and losses in functional ability), (d) provision of meaningful and doable activities, (e) ways to successfully communicate with an individual with dementia, (f) how to manage problematic behavioral symptoms, and (g) establishing competency in communicating with family members.

Important topics to be included in health-care-policy courses are health insurance policy, including Medicare, Medicaid, and private insurance; and long-term-care insurance. Every citizen faces the possibility of needing care for a chronic illness and for long-term care. The prospect of dementia brings to the forefront the importance of including a behavioral-health benefit that is in parity with a physical-health care benefit in both medical health insurance policies and in long-term-care insurance policies.

Courses on mental health policy should include dementia as one important form of cognitive impairment. They should also address the issue of how individuals with dementia often are underserved in a bifurcated, fragmented social- and health care system. Too often medical practitioners view dementia as the responsibility of the mental health system, whereas mental health professionals view it as the responsibility of the medical field or of long-term-care providers. Meanwhile, the person who has dementia may not receive needed services.

CONCLUSION

This chapter has introduced the issue of dementia among older adults, a condition that is creating an increasing demand for dedicated, highly skilled practitioners at the micro, meso, and macro levels of social work practice. Community residential care has the potential to enhance the quality of life for individuals with dementia by enhancing independence and dignity in a homelike milieu that is safe. The fact that this type of care is increasingly used as an alternative to nursing home care for individuals with dementia heightens its importance as a focus in social work training.

The most important concern that this trend raises is that, in some communities, the move away from institutional-type care towards community residential care may be premature. Care providers who use models of care that were designed for a more able and healthy population may not be prepared to address medical needs of the changing community long-term care population. It is important that policy planners assure that models of community care accommodate the needs of a population that is increasingly more physically and mentally ill. This chapter has introduced some important clinical assessment and treatment issues and stressed the importance of an integrated approach to care for persons with chronic and complex health and mental health needs.

Intervention in community long-term care involves working with the person with dementia, with family systems, organizations, social and health service systems, and state and national policy makers. To optimize the likelihood of older persons with dementia living in dignity with maximum health and well-being, work must occur at all of these levels. Social workers are change agents and are in a good position to bring to the table issues of quality of life and social and emotional issues for persons with dementia, their families, and their caregivers. They are trained to consider the whole person within his or her cultural context and community. They bring a social justice perspective to their work, which is an important contribution in this area of practice, because individuals with dementia may be especially vulnerable to social injustices. This group is highly vulnerable to abuse and neglect from those caring for them. Also, families need support to counter the stigma surrounding dementia and to cope with the sometimes overwhelming burden of caregiving. Therefore, there is critical need for social workers as advocates for clients with dementia and their families.

REFERENCES

American Psychiatric Association. (1994). *Diagnostic and statistical manual of mental disorders* (4th ed.). Washington, DC: Author.

Aronson, M. K. (1994). Overview of dementia and the nursing home. In M. K. Aronson (Ed.), *Reshaping dementia care: Practice and policy in long-term care* (pp. 1–14). Thousand Oaks, CA: Sage.

Bachman, D. L., Wolf, P. A., Linn, R. T., Knoefel, J. E., Cobb, J. L., Belanger, A. J., et al. (1993). Incidence of dementia and probable Alzheimer's disease in a general population: The Framingham Study. *Neurology, 44,* 1892–1900.

Badger, L. W., deGruy, F. V., Hartman, J., Plant, M. A., Leeper, J., Ficket, R., et al. (1994). Psychosocial interest, medical interviews, and the recognition of depression. *Archives of Family Medicine, 3,* 899–907.

Bartels, S. J., Levine, K. J., & Shea, D. (1999). Community-based long-term care for older persons with severe and persistent mental illness in an era of managed care. *Psychiatric Services, 50,* 1189–1197.

Berg, L. (1994). Current challenges in dementia care. In M. K. Aronson (Ed.), *Reshaping dementia care: Practice and policy in long-term care* (pp. 15–30). Thousand Oaks, CA: Sage.

Bernstein, M. A., & Hensley, R. (1993). Developing community-based program alternatives for the seriously and persistently mentally ill elderly. *Journal of Mental Health Administration, 20,* 201–207.

Borson, S., Liptzin, B., Nininger, J., & Rabins, P. (1987). Psychiatry and the nursing home. *American Journal of Psychiatry, 144,* 1412–1418.

Boyer, C. A., McAlpine, D. D., Pottick, K. J., & Olfson, M. (2000). Identifying risk factors and key strategies in linkage to outpatient psychiatric care. *American Journal of Psychiatry, 157,* 1592–1598.

Callahan, C. M., Hendrie, H. D., & Tierney, W. M. (1995). Documentation and evaluation of cognitive impairment in elderly primary care patients. *Annals of Internal Medicine, 122,* 422–429.

Capitman, J., & Sciegaj, M. (1995). A contextual approach for understanding individual autonomy in managed community long-term care. *Gerontologist, 35,* 533–540.

Carney, P. A., Dietrich, A. J., Eliassen, M. S., Owen, M., & Badger, L. W. (1999). Recognizing and managing depression in primary care: A standardized patient study. *Journal of Family Practice, 48,* 965–972.

Cohen, M. A., Tell, E. J., & Wallack, S. S. (1986). Client-related risk factors of nursing home entry among elderly adults. *Journal of Gerontology, 41,* 785–792.

Cohen, M. A., Tell, E. J., & Wallack, S. S. (1988). The risk factors of nursing home entry among residents of six continuing care retirement communities. *Journal of Gerontology: Social Sciences, 43,* S15–S21.

Cummings, J. L., & Jeste, D. V. (1999). Alzheimer's disease and its management in the year 2010. *Psychiatric Services, 50,* 1173–1177.

Dixon, M. A. (1991). In M. S. Harper (Ed.), *Management and care of the elderly* (pp. 247–255). Newbury Park, CA: Sage.

Eddy, D. M. (1994). Clinical decision-making: From theory to practice. Principles for making difficult decisions in difficult times. *Journal of the American Medical Association, 271*, 1792–1798.

Estes, C., & Swan, J. H. (1993). *The long term care crisis: Elders trapped in the no-care zone*. Newbury Park, CA: Sage.

Evans, M. (1993). Depression in elderly physically ill in-patients: A 12-month prospective study. *International Clinical Psychopharmacology, 8*, 333–336.

Florio, E. R., Rockwood, T. H., Hendryx, M. S., Jensen, J. E., Raschko, R., & Dyck, D. G. (1996). A model gatekeeper program to find the at-risk elderly. *Journal of Case Management, 5*, 106–114.

Furino, A., & Fogel, B. S. (1990). The economic perspective. In B. S. Fogel, A. Furino, & G. L. Gottlieb (Eds.), *Mental health policy for older Americans: Protecting minds at risk* (pp. 257–277). Washington, DC: American Psychiatric Press.

Greene, V. L., Lovely, M. E., & Ondrich, J. I. (1993). The cost-effectiveness of community services in a frail elderly population. *Gerontologist, 33*, 177–189.

Greene, V. L., & Ondrich, J. I. (1990). Risk factors for nursing home admission and exits: A discrete-time hazard function approach. *Journal of Gerontology: Social Sciences, 45*, S250–S258.

Hastings, M. M. (1993). Aging and mental health services: An introduction. *Journal of Mental Health Administration, 20*, 186–189.

Hennessy, C. (1989). Autonomy and risk: The role of client wishes in community-based long-term care. *Gerontologist, 19*, 633–639.

Hughes, S. L., Cummings, J., Weaver, F., Manheim, L., Braun, B., & Conrad, K. (1992). A randomized trial of the cost effectiveness of VA hospital-based home care for the terminally ill. *Health Services Research, 26*, 801–817.

Hughes, S. L., Manheim, L. M., Edelman, P. L., & Conrad, K. J. (1987). Impact of long-term home care on hospital and nursing home use and cost. *Health Services Research, 22*, 19–47.

Jorm, A. F., Korten, A. E., & Henderson, A. S. (1987). The prevalence of dementia: A quantitative integration of the literature. *Activa Psychiatrica Scandinavica, 76*, 465–479.

Kane, R. A., Kane, R. L., Illston, L. H., Nyman, J. A., & Finch, M. D. (1991). Adult foster care for the elderly in Oregon: A mainstream alternative to nursing homes? *American Journal of Public Health, 81*, 1113–1120.

Kane, R. A., Kane, R. L., & Ladd, R. C. (1998). *The heart of long-term care*. New York: Oxford University Press.

Katon, W. (1998). The effect of major depression on chronic medical illness. *Seminars in Clinical Neuropsychiatry, 3*, 82–86.

Klein, H. A. (1994). Aging in place: Adjusting to late life changes. *Journal of Social Behavior and Personality, 9* [Special issue], 153–168.

Kruzich, J. M., & Kruzich, S. J. (1985). Milieu factors influencing patients' integration into community residential facilities. *Hospital and Community Psychiatry, 36*, 378–382.

Lebowitz, B. D., Light, E., & Bailey, F. (1987). Mental health center services for the elderly: The impact of coordination with area agencies on aging. *Gerontologist, 27*, 699–702.

Light, E., Lebowitz, B. D., & Bailey, F. (1986). CMHC's and elderly services: An analysis of direct and indirect services and service delivery sites. *Community Mental Health Journal, 22,* 294–302.

Meeks, S., Carstensen, L. L., Stafford, P. B., Brenner, L. L., Weathers, F., Welch, R., et al. (1990). Mental health needs of the chronically mentally ill elderly. *Psychology and Aging, 5,* 163–171.

Mehrotra, C. M., & Kosloski, K. (1991). Foster care for older adults: Issues and evaluations. *Home Health Care Service Quarterly, 12,* 115–136.

Nielsen, M., Blenkner, M., Bloom, M., Downs, T., & Beggs, H. (1972). Older persons after hospitalization: A controlled study of home aide service. *American Journal of Public Health, 62,* 1094–1101.

Nocks, B. C., Learner, R. M., Blackman, D., & Brown, T. E. (1986). The effects of community-based long term care project on nursing home utilization. *Gerontologist, 26,* 150–157.

Olfson, M., Sing, M., & Schlesinger, H. S. (1999). Mental health/medical care cost offsets: Opportunities for managed care. *Health Affairs (Millwood), 18,* 79–90.

Patterson, T., Higgins, M., & Dyck, D. G. (1995). A collaborative approach to reduce hospitalization of developmentally disabled clients with mental illness. *Psychiatric Services, 46,* 243–247.

Proctor, E. K., Morrow-Howell, N., Rubin, E., & Ringenburg, M. (1999). Service use by elderly patients after psychiatric hospitalization. *Psychiatric Services, 50,* 553–555.

Raschko, R. (1985). Systems integration at the program level: Aging and mental health. *Gerontologist, 25,* 460–463.

Reichman, W. E., & Katz, P. R. (Eds.). (1996). [Preface.] In W. E. Reichmond & P. R. Katz (Eds.), *Psychiatric care in the nursing home* (pp. vii–ix). New York: Oxford University Press.

Rowles, G. D. (1994). Evolving images of place in aging and 'aging in place.' In D. Sheck & W. Achenbaum (Eds.), *Changing perceptions of aging and the aged* (pp. 115–125). New York: Springer.

Semke, J. (2002). *Examining adult family home care for frail older adults with mental health problems.* Unsubmitted manuscript. University of Washington at Seattle.

Semke, J., & Jensen, J. (1996). High utilization of inpatient psychiatric services by older adults: Analyses of available data. *Psychiatric Services, 48,* 172–174.

Sullivan, M., Katon, W. J., Rosso, J., Dobie, R., & Sakai, C. (1992). Somatization, co-morbidity, and the quality of life. Measuring the effect of depression upon chronic medical illness. *Psychiatry in Medicine, 10,* 61–76.

Talbott, J. A. (1983). A special population: The elderly deinstitutionalized chronically mentally ill patient. *Psychiatric Quarterly, 55,* 90–105.

Teri, L., Logsdon, R. G., Uomoto, J., & McCurry, S. M. (1997). Behavioral treatment of depression in dementia patients: A controlled clinical trial. *Journal of Gerontology: Psychological Sciences, 52B,* P159–P166.

Thompson, J. M. (1999). Understanding variation in resident needs and services in homes for adults. *Social Work in Health Care, 30,* 49–63.

Tourigny-Rivard, M. F., & Drury, M. (1987). The effects of monthly psychiatric consultation in a nursing home. *Gerontologist, 27,* 363–366.

Tsuji, I., Whalen, S., & Finucane, T. E. (1995). Predictors of nursing home placement in community-based long-term care. *Journal of the American Geriatrics Society, 43*, 761–766.

Tweed, D. L., Blazer, D. G., & Ciarlo J. A. (1992). Psychiatric epidemiology in elderly populations. In R. B. Wallace & R. F. Woolson (Eds.), *The epidemiologic study of the elderly* (pp. 213–233). New York: Oxford University Press.

Wallace, S. P. (1990). The no-care zone: Availability, accessibility, and acceptability in community-based long-term care. *Gerontologist, 30*, 254–261.

Weissert, W. G., & Hedrick, S. C. (1994). Lessons learned from research on effects of community-based long-term care. *Journal of the American Geriatrics Society, 42*, 348–353.

Wennberg, J., & Gittelsohn, A. (1973). Small area variations in health care delivery. *Science, 182*, 1102–1108.

Wiener, J. M., & Illston, L. H. (1994). Health care reform in the 1990's: Where does long-term care fit in? *Gerontologist, 34*, 402–408.

Wilson, K. B. (1996). *Assisted living: Reconceptualized regulation to meet consumers' needs and preferences.* Washington, DC: American Association of Retired Persons.

Wolff, N. (1989). Professional uncertainty and physician medical decision-making in a multiple treatment framework. *Social Science and Medicine, 28*, 99–107.

Wooldridge, J., & Schore, J. (1986). *Evaluation of the national long term care demonstration: Channeling effects on hospital, nursing home, and other medical services.* Washington, DC: U.S. Department of Health and Human Services.

Yordi, C. (1990). *Case management practice in S/HMO demonstrations.* Oakland, CA: Berkeley Planning Associates.

Zarit, S. H., & Zarit, J. M. (1998). *Mental disorders in older adults: Fundamentals of assessment and treatment.* New York: Guilford Press.

Zimmer, J. G., Groth-Junker, A., & McCusker, J. (1985). A randomized controlled study of a home health care team. *American Journal of Public Health, 75*, 134–141.

Chapter 4

THE OLDER PATIENT AT HOME: SOCIAL WORK SERVICES AND HOME HEALTH CARE

Ji Seon Lee and Irene A. Gutheil

As the population ages, many older persons face living with a disability that limits their activity. In 1997, more than 4.5 million elders reported having difficulty with carrying out their activities of daily living (ADLs) (Administration on Aging [AOA], 2001). Many of these elders, who are frail and coping with chronic illness, live in their homes and are in need of supportive services. Home health care (HHC) has been an important source of services available to older patients since the inception of the Medicare program.

HHC is a benefit widely used by Medicare beneficiaries. In 1999, about 8 million individuals in the United States received services from more than 20,000 home care providers, with an estimated $36 billion in annual HHC expenditures (National Association of Home Care [NAHC], 2001). Medicare home-health use grew rapidly in the 1990s. The proportion of Medicare beneficiaries using home health increased from 5.8% in 1990 to 10.8% in 1997. Between 1987 and 1997, the annual average number of home health visits per patient rose from 23 visits to 73 visits per user. In addition, there was a significant increase of patients who received more than 200 visits, rising from less than 1% in 1987 to 10% in 1997 (Health Care Financing Administration [HCFA], 1999). These heavy-use patients represent more than 46% of the total Medicare expenditures for HHC (HCFA, 1999).

The types of home-health-visits have also changed since 1987, when about 51% were for skilled nursing care and 33% were for home-health-aide services. Types of visits shifted by 1997, where skilled nursing services fell to 41% and home-health-aide services rose to 48%. This shift may reflect older patients using HHC for long-term care services rather than using it for a short-term service focused on patient with skilled nursing care needs (HCFA, 1999). Medicare spending on HHC has also grown rapidly, reflecting the growth in utilization. Total Medicare home-health expenditures increased at an annual rate of 21% between 1987 and 1997, from 2% of total Medicare spending in 1987 to 9% in 1997 (HCFA, 1999).

To curb the rise in HHC expenditures, the Centers for Medicare and Medicaid Services implemented a new payment system in October 2000. A prospective-payment system (PPS) was implemented to replace the traditional cost-based reimbursement system and focus on improving patient outcomes while motivating HHC providers to control costs. Under PPS, the ways in which social work can help with the recovery process provide opportunities to better integrate social work into the HHC service delivery system and effectively respond to the emerging needs of patients. To capture these unique opportunities, social work must demonstrate effectiveness in impacting patient outcomes.

SIGNIFICANCE TO GERONTOLOGY, HEALTH CARE, AND HEALTH PROFESSIONALS

Older consumers of HHC are most commonly diagnosed with a chronic illness, which often requires help with disease management and psychosocial support. In 1998, more than half (50.6%) of persons aged 75 and older reported a limitation caused by a chronic illness compared with 28.8% aged 65–74 (AOA, 2001). For these older adults, HHC provides important services to those who wish to receive care at home. Medicare home-health users tend to be older than the overall Medicare population. Proportionately, the largest users of Medicare home health are beneficiaries aged 85 and older (HCFA, 1999). Although those who are aged 85 years and older only represent 11% of all Medicare beneficiaries, they represent 26% of all home health users (HCFA, 1999). Between 1987 and 1997 home health users have increased rapidly across all age groups, yet HHC use has increased the most among the oldest (85 and older) and youngest (disabled) beneficiaries.

Medicare home-health users are also likely to be female. Sixty-seven percent of all Medicare home-health users are women, compared with 55% of Medicare home-health nonusers (HCFA, 1999). Home health users are also poorer than nonusers and are more likely to be dually eligible for Medicare and Medicaid. Home health users are more likely to live alone (40%) compared with nonusers (30%) (HCFA, 1999). Medicare beneficiaries who use HHC also have more limitations in their ADLs than nonusers of HHC. As shown in Figure 4.1, compared

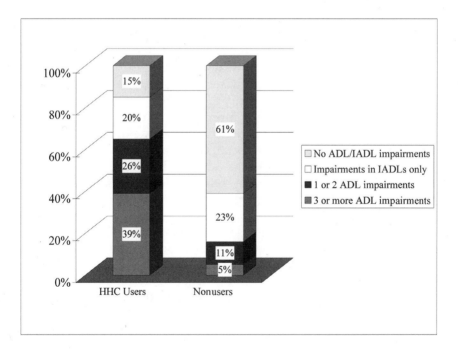

FIGURE 4.1 Activities of daily living (ADLs) impairments of medicare home health care users and nonusers.

Note: From Health Care Financing Administration (1999).

with 5% of Medicare nonusers of HHC, 39% of HHC users have three or more limitations in their ADLs (HCFA, 1999). Although Medicare beneficiaries utilize home health services for a variety of diagnoses, the 10 most common diagnoses in 1997 in order of prevalence were diabetes, hypertension, heart failure, osteoarthrosis and allied disorders, cerebrovascular disease, chronic skin ulcers, chronic airway obstruction, other forms of chronic ischemic heart disease, cardiac disrhythmias, and general symptoms (HCFA, 1999). Thus, these users of HHC, who are mostly elderly, often enter HHC due to an acute episode of a chronic illness, such as diabetes, hypertension, or heart failure, and have psychosocial issues that compound their illness, requiring care from multiple care professionals including social workers.

The various care professionals in HHC may consist of a skilled nurse who is the primary care coordinator, a physical therapist, a speech therapist, and a social worker. The chronic nature of the elderly HHC patient's illness raises the need to address psychosocial factors, which are closely related to improving patient outcomes. This is where social work can add significant value to the HHC team. With the implementation of PPS in Medicare HHC, it has become critical for home health providers to find ways to improve patient outcomes under an episodic case payment system. To care effectively for patients under PPS, it is essential to identify factors that contribute to negative outcomes and to intervene with appropriate help in a timely manner. In addition to the medically oriented services, elderly patients can benefit from complementary social work services, which can help reduce negative outcomes such as rehospitalization (Berkman & Abrams, 1986). To address the psychosocial factors effectively, social workers require efficient screening methods to determine patient needs. Early screening and true integration of social work services are the keys to helping older patients and their families, which adds value to the health care and well-being of older adults and to the broader health community (Berkman, Millar, Holmes, & Bonander, 1990).

Social work in HHC can be a valuable part of the HHC team, improving patient outcomes and benefitting not only the patient but also other health professionals. Social workers, who are trained to view their patients from a systems perspective, assess their patients as "person-in-environment." They understand that the patient and family are within a system that influences how they function. Thus social workers can provide a wide range of services that are helpful to both patients and the system that serves them.

Although social workers perform various functions in HHC (Table 4.1), there are four primary ways in which a social worker can help other members of the HHC team reach their patient outcome goals. First, social workers can help reduce social and emotional problems that may hinder the patients' ability to follow treatment recommendations (Abel-Vacula, Nathans, Phillips, & Robbins, 2000). Social workers can assist patients in developing better coping skills to help them focus on the treatment of their illness. Second, it has been shown that early intervention of social work services can reduce the length of time a patient spends in HHC (Blanchard, Gill, & Williams, 1991). Under PPS, positive outcomes combined with shorter length of stay may be the ultimate goal for the patient and for all members of the HHC team. Third, addressing the social and emotional needs can support a patient's ability to remain at home (Abel-Vacula et al., 2000). Acute relapses that can result in rehospitalizations or institutional admissions may be prevented if the patient is able to cope and focus on his or her treatment. Fourth, social workers can help mediate between the patient and family and other health care professionals. Often a patient receives multiple services but is unable to cope with

TABLE 4.1 Current Roles of Social Workers in Home Health Care

Direct Patient Activities	Indirect Patient Activities	Organizational/ Professional Activities
Counseling patients and family members: • Short-term therapy • Placement of patients after discharge Crisis intervention Education of patients about services Counseling about legal rights	Coordination of services: • Referrals to other community services • Placement of patients after discharge Completing applications for government benefits Collaboration with other health care professionals Advocating for patients Dealing with managed care organizations	Education of other professionals in home health about the roles of social work

managing the conflicts in personality and care that frequently occur with multiple caregivers.

With proper and timely assessment of the older patient, social work services can help the elderly person cope with and manage the limitations associated with their chronic illness. For example, a major issue for older patients receiving home health services following a hospital discharge is in the understanding of, and compliance with, medication needs (Gray, Mahoney, & Blough, 2001). Furthermore, home health users are primarily older women who live alone and face psychosocial problems related to isolation or lack of social support. Not only can social work services help patients, but they can also help caregivers of chronically ill elders, who may be especially vulnerable to caregiver fatigue, anger, and depression, which leads to a complex problem of caregiver burden (Pilisuk & Parks, 1988). Caregiver burden is a main predictor of posthospital functioning of elderly adults. Elderly patients with caregivers who have high levels of burden are more likely to be rehospitalized than patients who have caregivers with less burden (Marely, 1993). Both caregivers and older patients can therefore benefit from social work services that provide psychosocial support, thereby reducing caregiver burden and improving the caregivers' ability to care for their loved ones. Thus, social work services in HHC are vital in helping reduce the vulnerability of elderly patients and family caregivers, which can improve their health and well-being (Kerson & Michelsen, 1995). By helping the patient or family communicate more effectively, the care can be better coordinated, which may result in better patient cooperation with the treatment plan.

PRIOR RESEARCH AND KNOWLEDGE BASE

The home care literature has been widely reviewed (Hedrick & Inui, 1986; Hughes, 1985; R. A. Kane & Kane, 1987; Salisbury et al., 1999; Williams, Lyons, & Rowland, 1997), however, the body of research in this area is broad and diffused. Typically, home health agencies, home-care-aide organizations, and hospices are grouped together in databases and are known as "home care organizations" (NAHC, 2001). Benjamin, Fox, and Swan (1993) point out that much of the home care literature does not distinguish between skilled and nonskilled services in their analyses, which does not reflect the multifaceted and diverse service needs of frail elders at home. Given the various types and financing of home care services, it is important to examine the specifics in more detail in order to understand the effect of individual programs on patient care.

Although HHC expenditures are the largest within home care, studies specifically examining "home health care" have been sparse (Benjamin et al., 1993; R. L. Kane, 1989; McAuley & Arling, 1984) and the topics covered are broad (e.g., caregiver issues, home health aides, case management, compliance with medication). Starting from the mid-1990s, the policy changes in HHC increased the literature in this area and studies began to focus more on service use and patient outcomes (Chen, Kane, & Finch, 2000; R. L. Kane et al., 1998; Shaughnessy, Crisler, & Schlenker, 1998; Shaughnessy, Schlenker, & Hittle, 1995).

Compared with the growth of the literature on HHC, studies focusing on social services in HHC have been stagnant, mostly limited to roles of social work, barriers to social work services, nurse and social worker conflict, or ethical concerns of social work in home health care (Berger, 1988; Egan & Kadushin, 1999; Fessler & Adams, 1985; Lee, 2002; Levande, Bowden, & Mollema, 1987; Vincent & Davis, 1987). A small subset of studies has included social work services when examining the effectiveness of interdisciplinary teams in HHC (Fessler & Adams, 1985). However, new empirical research is limited on psychosocial interventions and social work–related outcomes, even with recent changes in the reimbursement policies in HHC. This may reflect the heavy emphasis on medically oriented outcomes in HHC and the relatively low status of social work and psychosocial outcomes. Furthermore, the difficulty in developing meaningful social work–related outcomes measurements in HHC also contributes to problems in conducting empirically based social-work outcomes research.

CURRENT RESEARCH AND RESEARCH AGENDA

A study on social work and patient outcomes was conducted during the year 2001, which was supported by the J. A. Hartford Foundation. There were three major phases to this study: documenting social work roles in HHC; study of social work and patient outcomes in HHC; and a policy roundtable. In the following section, findings from these three components will be briefly reported as an exemplar of a study that shows the importance of the intersection between home health, aging, and social work practice that is influenced by a changing policy environment—the implementation of PPS in HHC.

Phase 1: Documenting Social Work Roles in HHC

Focus groups with home health nurses and social workers were conducted to document the current roles of social work in HHC and to identify barriers related to social work practice in HHC (Lee, 2001). Using Egan and Kadushin's (1999) model, current social work roles were categorized into three areas—direct, indirect, and organizational/professional activities. These activities are summarized in Table 4.1, with the identified roles consistent with the prior literature (Egan & Kadushin, 1999). However, the findings of this study also identified three types of barriers—informational, systems, and organizational and interprofessional (Lee, 2002)—posing challenges to providing care for both social workers and nurses.

Informational Barriers

The focus group revealed HHC nurses' lack of understanding of social work roles. Home health nurses and social workers have different perceptions of the actual functions of social workers, leading to differences in identifying patients who need social work services. Both groups agreed that social workers were needed to help patients with dementia, those who had caregiver issues, and those who were victims of abuse or neglect. The nurses, who are the case managers in HHC, also identified patients with administrative issues (e.g., repeat patients) as needing social work services, whereas social workers wanted referrals of patients with depression, those who had financial needs, and those who lived alone.

Systems Barriers

Two systems barriers were identified. First, Medicare takes a medical model orientation to home health benefits, which makes the psychosocial aspects of care a secondary service. This further creates "turf" battles between the nurses and social workers, especially under PPS, where it does not matter who provides the services as long as positive patient outcomes are achieved under a set rate. Second, organizationally, the high percentage of per diem social workers creates communication barriers in managing patient needs between the case manager—the nurse—and the social worker.

Interprofessional Barriers

Due to the differences in their education and orientation, the approaches to patient treatment differ between social workers, who use a psychosocial and patient empowerment model, and nurses, who use a medical treatment model. This can create interprofessional conflicts when developing a coherent treatment plan for patients.

Phase 2: Social Work Outcomes Study

Based on the findings from phase 1, this exploratory study examined the relationship between social work and patient outcomes using diabetes as an exemplar. Because diabetes can strain elders' biopsychosocial functioning, social workers can make a difference in helping them cope with their illness (DeCoster, 2001). In addition, social workers can help diabetic patients by identifying and helping with psychosocial factors that affect outcomes (Auslander, Bubb, Rogge, & Santiago, 1993). Two questions were explored. First, does the sociodemographic profile of diabetic elderly patients who are receiving social work services in HHC differ from diabetic elderly patients who did not receive social work services? Second, is there a relationship between social work services and patient outcomes in HHC?

The study used elders with diabetes (50 and older) who received no social work services as the control group ($n = 100$) and elders with diabetes who received social work services while in HHC as the comparison group ($n = 32$). These patients were interviewed 30 days postdischarge from HHC. Although differences existed in the profiles of elders who received social work services and those who did not, there were no statistically significant differences between the two groups in age or in perceptions of unmet needs. However, interesting differences were found in the number of patients who were rehospitalized or used the emergency room. Although not statistically significant, about 14% of patients who did not receive social work services had rehospitalizations or emergency room visits, compared to less than 7% of patients who received social work services. These data indicate that there may be some relationship between social work services and these patient outcomes. The small number of patients in the sample who received social work services may contribute to this lack of significant difference found between the two groups. Further study needs to be conducted to see whether social work visitation is indeed a significant factor that contributes to better patient outcomes.

Phase 3: Policy Roundtable

A policy advocacy roundtable discussion on the "Impact of Prospective Payment System (PPS) on Social Work Services in Home Health Care" was held in April 2001 at Fordham University to learn about PPS and its impact on social work services as well as to set an agenda that can influence policy changes. Three major challenges for social work were identified. First, under PPS, it is critical that social workers demonstrate that their efficiency and effectiveness in improving patient outcomes contributes to the revenue of an agency. Second, it is critical to improve communications with other health care professionals in HHC (Lee, 2002). Because social work relies on referrals from other health care professionals within HHC, social work needs to view not only the patients as their consumers and stakeholders, but also the nurses, physical therapists, and speech therapists. Third, social work must advocate to become an equal member of the interdisciplinary HHC team. In both hospital and primary care settings, social workers have been incorporated into interdisciplinary teams and have been shown to improve patient outcomes (Sommers, Marton, Barbaccia, & Randolph, 2000). However, in HHC, social work still struggles to be accepted by other health care professionals despite the contribution of social workers to patient care (Baer, Blackmore, Foster, Rose, & Trafon, 1984).

Nine action steps were developed from this roundtable to advocate policy changes and address the various issues related to social work and the implementation of PPS (Lee & Rock, 2001). The steps are as follows:

1.   An integrated health care system with seamless transition between acute care and long-term care should be created.

2.   Caregiver/natural-helping-network education and support should be integrated into the HHC PPS case-mix methodology.

3.   Independent case findings should be established for social work services, in place of the current system that depends on nurses and physicians for referrals.

4. An HCFA (Medicare, Medicaid, and State Children's Health Insurance Program Agency) waiver program should be established, allowing for demonstrations of alternative case-mix models. Social care models and models incorporating caregivers should be demonstrated and researched.

5. In order to deal with the opportunities endemic to PPS and capitation for stinting on or rationing care, it is proposed that a systematic mechanism be created to safeguard against such practices, including comprehensive quality-assurance programs. Mechanisms such as "trip wires," which immediately detect a potential problem and notify administrators for change, should be established for additional case reimbursement when the cost of care of complex cases exceeds the PPS case mix. Mechanisms must also be established to counter the potential for abuse of such trip wires.

6. Social work roles should be clearly defined in HHC and understood by other health care professionals.

7. Development of true interdisciplinary HHC teams (which include social work) will be the key to successful patient care under PPS.

8. Evidence-based research on the effectiveness of social work services must be conducted for the survival of social work in HHC.

9. Screening instruments for social work services should be developed for use in HHC to ensure that all patients will receive timely social work services.

FURTHER RESEARCH NEEDS

Research on social work services in HHC is still in its infancy. However, there are four major areas in which social work can focus its research to support its services under the new PPS environment.

1. *Conduct evidence-based research on patient outcomes related to social work services in HHC:* Given the current reimbursement environment in health care, advocacy for changes to include social work services can only begin with the social work profession's ability to demonstrate its capacity to improve patient outcomes in HHC.

2. *Validate the importance of including caregiver supports in the HHC PPS case-mix methodology:* Similar to what had happened with diagnostic related groups (DRGs), there is concern that PPS is based on a biomedical view of health care and ignores or limits social and psychosocial factors. Systematic attention to these factors has been demon-

strated to be value-added to both cost containment and quality. Large-scale waivers may be the way to test out different models for PPS that include caregiver supports.

3. *Develop social work screening to help other professionals in HHC identify high-risk patients:* To address the psychosocial needs of home health patients appropriately, effective screening is the key to determining which patients need social work intervention. As nurses continue as the case managers under PPS, it is critical to provide easy-to-use tools to help nurses identify patients in need of social work services. Early identification and intervention will be critical to address the patients' psychosocial needs while they receive medical care, as well as to plan for their discharge.

4. *Conduct cost-effectiveness studies related to social work services in HHC:* It is critical to demonstrate social work's effectiveness on the traditional cost-based outcomes, such as length of stay, hospitalization, and readmission, as agencies are looking toward all professionals in home health to show their cost-effectiveness and efficiency related to positive patient outcomes.

POLICY IMPLICATIONS

On October 1, 2000, a change in the reimbursement system for HHC was implemented to curb the rising cost of Medicare HHC and to improve patient outcomes (St. Pierre & Dombi, 2000). Similar to what had happened to Medicare's hospital reimbursement system, home health agencies (HHA) now have to provide adequate and appropriate care under a set rate for each patient. This major change can pose both an opportunity and a threat to social work and to the older patients receiving HHC.

The new reimbursement system links patient outcomes to reimbursement. The reimbursement system has changed from a cost-based system to PPS. PPS sets a rate for each type of patient before services are provided. The payment calculation for HHC patients is based on a 60-day episode and then case-mix adjusted. The purpose of using a case-mix adjustor is to recognize the differences in costs of caring for various types of patients and to control for the difference in types of caseload for each HHA. Case mix was created using *OASIS* (Outcomes Assessment Information Set) data collected by the HHAs and is based on clinical, functional, and service utilization dimensions (Goldberg &

Delargy, 2000). Using these dimensions, a patient can be assigned to 1 of 80 possible groups. The payment is also adjusted for geographic differences by applying a wage index. Although payment for each patient is adjusted for various patient characteristics, a special outlier provision exists to ensure appropriate payment for those beneficiaries who have the most expensive care needs. It is hoped that by adjusting for payment to reflect the HHA's cost in caring for each beneficiary, including the sickest, all beneficiaries will be ensured access to the HHC services for which they are eligible. This case-mix system works for the patient, HHA, and Medicare. PPS provides higher payments for high-need patients, which may make accepting these patients more attractive to HHAs. Also, with various payment groups, PPS reduces the average difference between set payment and actual cost, which is good for Medicare and HHAs (Goldberg & Delargy, 2000). There are six main features to HHC PPS:

- Payment is for a 60-day episode.
- It is case-mix adjusted.
- It provides outlier payments.
- Adjustment is made for beneficiaries who only require a few visits during a 60-day episode.
- Adjustments are made for beneficiaries who experience a significant change in their condition.
- Adjustments are made for beneficiaries who change HHAs.

PPS and Social Work

PPS poses both opportunities and threats to social work services. Medicare requires that every HHA make social work services available to patients (HCFA, 1992). However, under the previous cost-based system, there was no requirement that social workers see patients or participate in the planning of their care (Dhooper, 1997). Furthermore, the home health nurse, usually the case manager, determines the need for and referral to social work services. Because reimbursement is no longer based on the type of professional visit and it rewards care that promotes positive patient outcomes, social work can be more aggressive in its offerings to address the psychosocial needs of the patient. To capture this opportunity, social work must demonstrate a relationship between positive outcomes and social work services. Social work needs to document efficiency and effectiveness and correlate them to agency revenues. In addition, PPS provides an opportunity for social work services to be truly integrated in the HHC system rather than just being a secondary service. As agencies try to find an optimal mix of services for each patient that yields positive outcomes, agencies may be more open to social work's becoming a part of the core services HHC offers. However, if social work cannot capture this opportunity, PPS may be a threat. Given the current outcomes-focused health-care policy environment, any service that cannot document its effectiveness to patient care will be pushed aside.

As PPS is being implemented, policies that deal with rationing of care must be in place. Similar to what happened with inpatient care when the DRGs were introduced in the early 1980s, there is a clear danger of rationing of care for the most vulnerable (often the most expensive) patient population. Although it is clear that cost containment is necessary, it must take place in the context of building on comprehensive policy provision and a seamless, continuous delivery system, with the protection to ensure the highest quality of care. Therefore, quality assurance programs must accompany all HHC programs under PPS.

Furthermore, social workers must advocate for a biopsychosocial approach to HHC under Medicare. In order to fully incorporate this aspect of care, policy makers need to understand clearly and integrate into Medicare policy that HHC for patients should not be limited to medical considerations, but that Medicare fully recognizes the importance of addressing the psychosocial needs of the patient. Without this understanding, patients may not receive needed services.

INTEGRATING KNOWLEDGE INTO THE CURRICULUM

The current situation in HHC provides a lens for considering ways to enhance the gerontological base in social work education. Social work experience in HHC provides an avenue for increasing gerontological content in the social work curriculum through a focus on health care. There are many avenues for addressing evidence-based knowledge priorities through courses in both the foundation and in the advanced curricula. The following suggestions are the most apparent, but certainly not the only, choices:

- Policy courses provide a good context to introduce material about the role of social work services in controlling or reducing costs of care, as well as an understanding of ways to effectively convey this information to the larger health care community. Changes in HHC are a significant example to use in a primary course.

- Practice courses are the choice for material on HHC assessment and treatment of psychological factors and social factors that affect, or are affected by, physical health or illness. In addition, practice courses should integrate material on assessing caregivers' capacities and needs and enhancement of their ability to sustain caregiving.
- Research courses are a good forum for examining HHC interventions that have been shown effective in enhancing psychological and social functioning or ameliorating the negative effects of impairment.
- Practice, research, and human behavior and the social environment courses all provide good forums for understanding the contributions of social workers to HHC interdisciplinary teams and factors that support effective teamwork.

One of the most effective ways to introduce and examine this material is by using case studies. Cases can be introduced through material that is developed prior to class by the faculty, or they can emerge from students' own field experiences. The most effective cases may be those with an intergenerational focus because the material will feel relevant to students and faculty who do not have expertise or even an interest in aging. Intergenerational cases demonstrate the integration of aging issues into the larger contexts of families and communities, which helps counteract a tendency to marginalize aging issues.

Cases can be used in individual classes or on a school-wide basis. For example, Fordham University's Graduate School of Social Service holds an annual case-study event that brings together all foundation students around the use of a single case (Cohen, Koch, & DiDonna, 2002). During the class day, the case is used in both a large gathering of all students and in individual courses. The overall purpose of the case study event is to demonstrate the integration of all courses in the foundation curriculum. The case-study-event model can provide an effective avenue for introducing additional gerontological content into the social work curriculum.

CONCLUSION

Social work service is an essential component in HHC. This is especially true for older patients who are facing chronic illnesses and may have many psychological and social needs. However, social workers need to be acutely aware of the changes they will encounter in the new health-policy environment, where producing positive outcomes is the ultimate goal. For home health social workers, this change may present opportunities to be better integrated into the service delivery system. Conversely, this opportunity can only be capitalized on by demonstrating social work's value in contributing to positive patient outcomes. Research on the effectiveness of social work in HHC is currently limited. Much more research is needed to demonstrate social work's effectiveness with older patients in HHC by capturing accurately, and meaningfully tapping into, the relevant dimensions of social work outcomes. As with any area in health care, social work services in HHC will be in jeopardy without active outcomes research.

These difficult realities also come at a time when social work students are not being prepared adequately to serve older clients. This is especially true in health care settings where social workers may not directly work in a setting that serves only elderly patients but frequently encounters older patients as their clients. As the baby boomers enter older adulthood, the future of social work's ability to provide much-needed services rests on how well social workers will be educated, By first acknowledging the enormous population shift that is currently taking place and infusing gerontological knowledge into all aspects of the social work curriculum is an essential step in helping older adults and their families maneuver through the current health-care maze in the United States.

To bring about these vital changes, social workers need to tap into their heritage and be more involved in social action. With the implementation of PPS, partnerships with various organizations—such as community and health care organizations, the National Association of Social Workers, the Council on Social Work Education, and the American Network of Home Health Social Workers—are essential to creating the strong alliances needed to advocate for social work services in HHC.

REFERENCES

Abel-Vacula, C., Nathans, D., Phillips, K., & Robbins, J. (2000). *Home health care social work: Guidelines for practitioners and agencies*. Chicago: American Network of Home Health Care Social Workers.

Administration on Aging. (2001). *A profile of older Americans: 2001*. [On-line]. Available: http://www.aoa.gov/aoa/STATS/profile/2001/12.html. Accessed April 27, 2002.

Auslander, W. F., Bubb, J., Rogge, M., & Santiago, J. V. (1993). Mothers' satisfaction with medical care: Perceptions of racism, family stress, and medical outcomes in children with diabetes. *Health and Social Work, 22,* 190–199.

Baer, N., Blackmore, R., Foster, J., Rose, J., & Trafon, J. (1984). Home health services social work treatment protocol. *Home Healthcare Nurse, 2*(4), 43–49.

Benjamin, A. E., Fox, P. J., & Swan, J. H. (1993). The posthospital experience of elderly Medicare home health users. *Home Health Care Service Quarterly, 14*(2/3), 19–35.

Berger, R. M. (1988). Making home health social work more effective. *Home Health Care Services Quarterly, 9*(1), 63–75.

Berkman, B., & Abrams, R. (1986). Factors related to hospital readmission of elderly cardiac patients. *Social Work, 31,* 99–103.

Berkman, B., Millar, S., Holmes, W., & Bonader, E. (1990). Screening elder cardiac patients to identify need for social work services. *Health & Social Work, 15*(1), 64–72.

Blanchard, L., Gill, G., & Williams, E. (1991). *Guidelines for documentation requirements for social workers in home health care.* Washington, DC: National Association of Social Workers.

Chen, Q., Kane, R. L., & Finch, M. D. (2000). The cost effectiveness of post-acute care for elderly Medicare beneficiaries. *Inquiry, 37,* 359–375.

Cohen, C. S., Koch, D., & DiDonna, G. (2002, February). *Integrating curriculum and community: Educational innovation using a case study model case study week.* Paper presented at Council on Social Work Education Annual Program Meeting, Nashville, TN.

DeCoster, V. A. (2001). Challenges of type 2 diabetes and role of health care social work: A neglected area of practice. *Health and Social Work, 26,* 26–37.

Egan, M., & Kadushin, G. (1999). The social worker in the emerging field of home care: Professional activities and ethical concerns. *Health and Social Work, 24,* 43–55.

Fessler, S. R., & Adams, C. G. (1985). Nurse/social work role conflict in home health care. *Journal of Gerontological Social Work, 9*(1), 113–123.

Goldberg, H. B., & Delargy, D. (2000). Developing a case-mix model for PPS: Everything you ever wanted to know about case mix but were afraid to ask. *Caring, 19*(1), 16–19.

Gray, S. L., Mahoney, J. E., & Blough, D. K. (2001). Medication adherence in elderly patients receiving home health services following hospital discharge. *Annals of Pharmacotherapy, 35,* 539–545.

Health Care Financing Administration. (1992). *Medicare home health agency manual* (HCFA Publication No. 11). Washington, DC: U.S. Government Printing Office.

Health Care Financing Administration. (1999). *A profile of Medicare home health: Chart book* (Publication No. HCFA-10138). Washington, DC: U.S. Government Printing Office.

Hedrick, S. C., & Inui, T. S. (1986). The effectiveness and cost of home care: An information synthesis. *Health Services Research, 20,* 851–880.

Hughes, S. L. (1985). Apples and oranges? A review of evaluations of community-based long-term care. *Health Services Research, 20,* 461–488.

Kane, R. A., & Kane, R. L. (1987). *Long-term care: principles, programs, and policies.* New York: Springer.

Kane, R. L. (1989). *PAC: A national study of post-acute care.* Minneapolis: University of Minnesota.

Kane, R. L., Chen, Q., Finch, M., Blewett, L., Burns, R., & Moskowitz, M. (1998). Functional outcomes of posthospital care for stroke and hip fracture patients under Medicare. *Journal of American Geriatrics Society, 46,* 1525–1533.

Kerson, T. S., & Michelsen, R. W. (1995). Counseling homebound clients and their families. *Journal of Gerontological Social Work, 24*(3/4), 159–190.

Lee, J. S. (2002). Social work services in home health care: Challenges for the new prospective payment system era. *Social Work in Health Care, 35*(3), 23–36.

Lee, J. S., & Rock, B. D. (2001). Social work in home health care: Challenges in the new prospective payment system: A policy action paper. *Occasional Paper of the Ravazzin Center for Social Work Research in Aging* (Serial No. 2). Tarrytown, NY: Ravazzin Center for Social Work Research in Aging.

Levande, R., Bowden, S. W., & Mollema, J. (1987). Home health services for dependent elders: The social work dimension. *Journal of Gerontological Social Work, 11*(3/4), 5–17.

Marely, M. A. (1993). *Caregiver strain as a predictor of posthospital functioning of the elderly.* Unpublished doctoral dissertation, Tulane University, New Orleans, LA.

McAuley, J. W., & Arling, G. (1984). Use of in-home care by very old people. *Journal of Health and Social Behavior, 25,* 54–64.

National Association of Home Care. (2001). *Basic statistics about home care.* [On-line]. Available: http://www.nahc.org/consumer/hcstats.html. Accessed December 19, 2001.

Pilisuk, M., & Parks, S. H. (1988). Caregiving: Where families need help. *Social Work, 35,* 436–440.

Salisbury, C., Bosanquet, N., Wilkinson, E. K., Franks, P. J., Kite, S., Lorentzon, M., et al. (1999). The impact of different models of specialist palliative care on patient's quality of life: A systematic literature review. *Palliative Medicine, 13,* 3–17.

Shaughnessy, P. W., Crisler, K. S., & Schlenker, R. E. (1998). Outcomes-based quality improvement in home health care: The OASIS indicators. *Quality Management in Health Care, 7*(1), 58–67.

Shaughnessy, P. W., Schlenker, R. E., & Hittle, D. F. (1995). Case mix of home health patients under capitated and fee-for-service payment. *Health Services Research, 30,* 79–113.

Sommers, L. S., Marton, K. I., Barbaccia, J. C., & Randolph, J. (2000). Physican, nurse and social worker collaboration in primary care for chronically ill seniors. *Archives of Internal Medicine, 160,* 1825–1833.

St. Pierre, M., & Dombi, W. A. (2000). Home health PPS: New payment system, new hope. *Caring, 19*(1), 6–11.

Vincent, P. A., & Davis, J. M. (1987). Functions of social workers in a home health agency. *Health and Social Work, 12,* 213–219.

Williams, J., Lyons, B., & Rowland, D. (1997). Unmet long term care needs of the elderly in the community: A review of the literature. *Home Health Care Services Quarterly, 16*(1/2), 93–119.

APPENDIX A. MAJOR BIBLIOGRAPHIC REFERENCES

Policy and PPS

Berke, D., & St. Pierre, M. (1998). Toward more reasoned home health payment reform. Industry, legislative, and regulatory proposals to modify IPS. *Caring, 17*(2), 54–55.

Bishop, C. E., Kerwin, J., & Wallack, S. S. (1999). The Medicare home health benefit implications of recent payment changes. *Journal of Care Management, 1*(3), 189–196.

Bishop, C. E., & Stassen, M. (1986). Prospective reimbursement for home health care: Context for an evolving policy. *Pride Institute Journal of Long Term Home Health Care, 5*(1), 17–26.

Cohen, M. A., & Tumlinson, A. (1997). Understanding the state variation in Medicare home health care. The impact of Medicaid program characteristics, state policy, and provider attitude. *Medical Care, 35*, 618–633.

Conely, V. M., & Walker, M. K. (1998). National health policy influence on Medicare home health. *Home Health Care Services Quarterly, 17*(3), 1–15.

Dombi, W. A. (2001). Quality of care compliance plans under PPS. *Caring, 20*(3), 32–36.

Fazzi, A. (2000). Balancing books and balancing values: The hidden threat of PPS. *Caring, 19*(8), 30–32.

Forster, T. M. (1998). Home care, the Balanced Budget Act of 1997, and IPS. *Caring, 17*(2), 8–13.

Gage, B. (1999). Impact of the BBA on post-acute utilization. *Health Care Financing Review, 20*(4), 103–126.

Goldberg, H. B. (1997). Prospective payment in action. The National Home Health Agency Demonstration. *Caring, 16*(2), 14–19, 21–22, 24–27.

Goldberg, H. B., & Delargy, D. (2000). Developing a case-mix model for PPS: Everything you ever wanted to know about case mix but were afraid to ask. *Caring, 19*(1), 16–19.

Grazier, K. L. (1986). The impact of reimbursement policy on home health care. *Pride Institute Journal of Long Term Home Health Care, 5*(1), 12–16.

Grimaldi, P. L. (2000). Medicare's new home health prospective payment system explained. *Healthcare Financial Management, 54*(11), 46–56.

Lui, K., Wissoker, D., & Rimes, C. (1998). Determinants and costs of Medicare post-acute care provided by SNFs and HHAs. *Inquiry, 35*, 49–61.

Mauser, E. (1997). Medicare home health initiative: Current activities and future directions. *Health Care Financing Review, 18*, 275–291.

McSpedon, C. (1999). The transition to prospective payment changes the face of home care. *Managed Care Interface, 12,* 77–80, 82–83.

Seifer, S. (1987). The impact of PPS on home health care: A survey of thirty-five home health agencies. *Caring, 6*(4), 10–12.

St. Pierre, M. (1999). A look to the future. Home health PPS. *Caring, 18*(3), 16–19.

St. Pierre, M., & Dombi, W. A. (2000). Home Health PPS: New payment system, new hope. *Caring, 19*(1), 6–11.

Sullivan, C. (1998). The impact of the interim payment system: Agency expectations. *Caring, 17*(2), 56–60.

Torrez, D. J., Estes, C., & Linkens, K. (1998). The impact of a decade of policy on home health care utilization. *Home Health Care Services Quarterly, 16*(4), 35–56.

HHC: Service Use and Outcomes

Anderson, M. A., Pena, R. A., & Helms, L. B. (1998). Home care utilization by congestive heart failure patients: A pilot study. *Public Health Nursing, 15,* 146–162.

Barker, J. C., Mitteness, L. S., & Muller, H. B. (1998). Older home health care patients and their physicians: Assessment of functional ability. *Home Health Care Services Quarterly, 17*(2), 21–39.

Brown, M. G. (1995). Cost-effectiveness: The case of home health care physician services in New Brunswick, Canada. *Journal of Ambulatory Care Management, 19*(1), 13–28.

Brown, N. J., Griffin, M. R., Ray, W. A., Meredith, S., Beers, M. H., Marren, J., et al. (1998). A model for improving medication use in home health care patients. *Journal of the American Pharmaceutical Association, 38,* 696–702.

Chen, Q., Kane, R. L., & Finch, M. D. (2000). The cost effectiveness of post-acute care for elderly Medicare beneficiaries. *Inquiry, 37,* 359–375.

Crisler, K. S., Baillie, L. L., & Richard, A. A. (2000). Integrating OASIS data collection into a comprehensive assessment. *Home Healthcare Nurse, 18,* 249–254.

Dansky, K. H., Dellaasega, C., Shellenbarger, T., & Russo, P. C. (1996). After hospitalization: Home health care for elderly persons. *Clinical Nursing Research, 5,* 185–198.

Donelson, S. M., & Feldman, P. H. (2000). How to determine if PPS will provide adequate resources for your population: One agency's experience. *Home Healthcare Nurse, 18,* 363–369.

Dyeson, T. B., Murphy, J., & Stryker, K. (1999). Demographic and psychosocial characteristics of cognitively-intact chronically ill elders receiving home health services. *Home Health Care Services Quarterly, 18*(2), 1–25.

Fortinsky, R. H., & Madigan, E. A. (1997). Home care resource consumption and patient outcomes: What are the relationships? *Home Health Care Services Quarterly, 16*(3), 55–73.

Gray, S. L., Mahoney, J. E., & Blough, D. K. (2001). Medication adherence in elderly patients receiving home health services following hospital discharge. *Annals of Pharmacotherapy, 35,* 539–545.

Hadley, J., Rabin, D., Epstein, A., Stein, S., & Rimes, C. (2000). Posthospitalization home health care use and changes in functional status in a Medicare population. *Medical Care, 38,* 494–507.

Health Care Financing Administration. (1992). *Medicare home health agency manual* (HCFA Publication No. 11). Washington, DC: U.S. Government Printing Office.

Health Care Financing Administration. (1999). *A profile of Medicare home health: Chart book* (Publication No. HCFA-10138). Washington, DC: U.S. Government Printing Office.

Hedrick, S. C., & Inui, T. S. (1986). The effectiveness and cost of home care: An information synthesis. *Health Services Research, 20,* 851–880.

Hughes, S. L. (1985). Apples and oranges? A review of evaluations of community-based long-term care. *Health Services Research, 20,* 461–488.

Intrator, O., & Berg, K. (1998). Benefits of home health care after inpatient rehabilitation for hip fracture: Health service use by Medicare beneficiaries, 1987–1992. *Archives of Physical Medicine and Rehabilitation, 79,* 1195–1199.

Jette, A. M., Smith, K. W., & McDermott, S. M. (1996). Quality of Medicare-reimbursed home health care. *Gerontologist, 36,* 492–501.

Kane, R. A., Kane, R. L., Illston, L. H., & Eustis, N. N. (1994). Perspectives on home care quality. *Health Care Financing Review, 16*(1), 69–89.

Kane, R. L., Chen, Q., Finch, M., Blewett, L., Burns, R., & Moskowitz, M. (1998). Functional outcomes of posthospital care for stroke and hip fracture patients under Medicare. *Journal of the American Geriatrics Society, 46,* 1525–1533.

Kane, R. L., Chen, Q., Finch, M., Blewett, L., Burns, R., & Moskowitz, M. (2000). The optimal outcomes of posthospital care under Medicare. *Health Services Research, 35*(3), 615–661.

Krulish, L. H. (2001). 101 uses for OASIS? *Home Healthcare Nurse, 19,* 113–114.

Langa, K. M., Chernew, M. E., Kabeto, M. U., & Katz, S. J. (2001). The explosion in paid home health care in the 1990s: Who received the additional services? *Medical Care, 39,* 147–157.

Manley, J. (1996). Home health care in the continuum: A review. *Continuum, 16*(5), 1, 3–9.

Mullner, R. M., Jewell, M. A., & Mease, M. A. (1999). Monitoring changes in home health care: A comparison of two national surveys. *Journal of Medical Systems, 23,* 21–26.

Munson, M. L. (1999). Characteristics of elderly home health care users: Data from the 1996 National Home and Hospice Care Survey. *Advance Data, 309,* 1–11.

Murtaugh, C. M., & Litke, A. (2002). Transitions through postacute and long-term care settings: Patterns of use and outcomes for a national cohort of elders. *Medical Care, 40*(3), 227–236.

Navaie-Waliser, M., Feldman, P. H., Gould, D. A., Levine, C., Kuerbis, A. N., & Donelan, K. (2001). The experiences and challenges of informal caregivers: Common themes and differences among Whites, Blacks, and Hispanics. *Gerontologist, 41,* 733–741.

Navaie-Waliser, M., Feldman, P. H., Gould, D. A., Levine, C., Kuerbis, A. N., & Donelan, K. (2002). When the caregiver needs care: The plight of vulnerable caregivers. *American Journal of Public Health, 92,* 409–413.

Peters, D. A., & Eigsti, D. (1991). Utilizing outcomes in home care. *Caring, 10*(10), 44–46, 48, 50–51.

Redeker, N. S., & Brassard, A. B. (1996). Health patterns of cardiac surgery clients using home health care nursing services. *Public Health Nursing, 13,* 394–403.

Richard, A. A., Crisler, K. S., & Stearns, P. M. (2000). Using OASIS for outcome-based quality improvement. *Home Healthcare Nurse, 18,* 232–237.

Schlenker, R. E., Shaughnessy, P. W., & Hittle, D. F. (1995). Patient-level cost of home health care under capitated and fee-for-service payment. *Inquiry, 32,* 252–270.

Shaughnessy, P. W., Crisler, K. S., & Bennett, R. E. (2000). We've collected the OASIS data, now what? *Home Healthcare Nurse, 18,* 258–265.

Shaughnessy, P. W., Crisler, K. S., & Schlenker, R. E. (1998). Outcomes-based quality improvement in home health care: The OASIS indicators. *Quality Management in Health Care, 7*(1), 58–67.

Shaughnessy, P. W., Crisler, K. S., Schlenker, R. E., Arnold, A. G., Kramer, A. M., Powell, M. C., et al. (1994). Measuring and assuring the quality of home health care. *Health Care Financing Review, 16*(1), 35–67.

Shaughnessy, P. W., Schlenker, R. E., & Hittle, D. F. (1995). Case mix of home health patients under capitated and fee-for-service payment. *Health Services Research, 30,* 79–113.

Stewart, C. J., Blaha, A. J., Weissfeld, L., & Yaun, W. (1995). Discharge planning from home health care and patient status post-discharge. *Public Health Nursing,* 12(2), 90–98.

Weiler, R. M. (1998). Home health care workers' attitudes toward the elderly. *Home Health Care Services Quarterly, 16*(4), 1–13.

Williams, J., Lyons, B., & Rowland, D. (1997). Unmet long term care needs of the elderly in the community: A review of the literature. *Home Health Care Services Quarterly, 16*(1/2), 93–119.

Wilson, J. R., Smith, J. S., Dahle, K. L., & Ingersoll, G. L. (1999). Impact of home heath care on health care costs and hospitalization frequency in patients with health failure. *American Journal of Cardiology, 83,* 615–617. A10.

Social Work and HHC

Auerbach, D., Bann, R., Davis, D., Sassi, S., Straus, R., & Felsen, S. (1984). The social worker in home health care. *Caring, 3*(10), 71–76.

Baer, N., Blakemore, R., Foster, J., Rose, J., & Trafon, J. (1984). Home health services social work treatment protocol. *Home Healthcare Nurse, 2*(4), 43–49.

Berger, R. M. (1988). Making home health social work more effective. *Home Health Care Service Quarterly, 9*(1), 63–75.

Bonner, J. P., Sacia, J. M., Rowlands, E., & Snouffer, K. (1978). Medical social services in home health agency: Luxury or necessity. *Home Health Review,* 1(2), 28–34.

Claiborne, N., & Vandenburgh, H. (2001). Social workers' role in disease management. *Health and Social Work, 26,* 217–225.

Egan, M., & Kadushin, G. (1999). The social worker in the emerging field of home care: Professional activities and ethical concerns. *Health and Social Work, 24,* 43–55.

Fessler, S. R., & Adams, C. G. (1985). Nurse/social work role conflict in home health care. *Journal of Gerontological Social Work, 9*(1), 113–123.

Harris, M. D., & Diodato, J. (1997). The medical social worker: Member of the home healthcare team. *Home Healthcare Nurse, 15,* 327–328.

Healy, T. C. (1998). The complexity of everyday ethics in home health care: An analysis of social workers' decisions regarding frail elders' autonomy. *Social Work in Health Care, 27*(4), 19–37.

Healy, T. C. (1999). Community-dwelling cognitively impaired frail elders: An analysis of social workers' decisions concerning support for autonomy. *Social Work in Health Care, 30*(2), 27–47.

Jackson, J. A. (1997). Medical social work's contribution to home care. *Caring, 16*(9), 28–31.

Lee, J. S. (in press). Social work services in home health care: Challenges for the new prospective payment system era. *Social Work in Health Care.*

Lee, J. S., & Rock, B. D. (2001). Social work in home health care: Challenges in the new prospective payment system: A policy action paper. *Occasional Paper of the Ravazzin Center for Social Work Research in Aging* (Serial No. 2). Tarrytown, NY: Ravazzin Center for Social Work Research in Aging.

Levande, R., Bowden, S. W., & Mollema, J. (1987). Home health services for dependent elders: The social work dimension. *Journal of Gerontological Social Work, 11*(3/4), 5–17.

Sommers, L. S., Marton, K. I., Barbaccia, J. C., & Randolph, J. (2000). Physician, nurse and social worker collaboration in primary care for chronically ill seniors. *Archives of Internal Medicine, 160,* 1825–1833.

Vincient, P. A., & Davis, J. M. (1987). Functions of social workers in a home health agency. *Health and Social Work, 12,* 213–219.

Chapter 5

GERONTOLOGICAL SOCIAL WORK AND CASE MANAGEMENT

Matthias J. Naleppa

As the elderly population increases within the overall population, there will be an increasing number of persons who have chronic health conditions related to age. This will be compounded as the baby boom generation enters this life stage. Currently, more than 40% of those who suffer from chronic conditions have more than one such condition (Institute of Medicine, 2001), and some form of assistance with everyday activities is required by about one third of persons older than age 75 and half of those older than 85 (U.S. Bureau of the Census, 2000). This poses a considerable challenge to the health care and service delivery system, as elderly persons and their caregivers frequently require help in negotiating complex and fragmented service delivery systems (Applebaum & Austin, 1990; Austin, 1993; Quinn, 1995). Case management is an approach that was developed in response to the need to assist people in accessing and coordinating services.

SIGNIFICANCE TO GERONTOLOGY, HEALTH CARE, AND PROFESSIONALS

Many services for older adults are part of a continuum of care, a concept that has been developed as a result of provisions in the Older

Americans Act of 1965 (Wacker, Roberto, & Piper, 1997). The contin-uum of care consists of a graded continuum of services, including social, financial, medical, mental health, and personal care. It grew out of efforts to control growing health care costs in the 1980s as part of a shift from fee-for-service to prospective payment systems (Pu, 2001). Typically, the term *continuum of care* is used to describe the range of types of services as well as the mechanisms to integrate them. The goal of the continuum of care is to match a person's individual needs with the appropriate level of care and services. Community-based in-home services, which typically focus on assisting with activities of daily living, are at one end of the spectrum. At the other end are acute care hospitals and long-term-care facilities. Some of the more common services in the continuum of care are senior centers, legal services, nutritional services, nonmedical home care, skilled home-health care, respite care, adult day care, assisted living, hospitals, nursing homes, and hospice care. This wide range of service in the continuum of care can result in difficulties for elderly clients and caregivers in finding and accessing appropriate resources. Case management is embedded in this system of services.

A trademark of case management is interdisciplinary or multidisci-plinary practice. Case management teams can include social workers, nurses, physicians, and other therapeutic staff collaborating on a case (Austin, 2001). There are many models of interdisciplinary and multi-disciplinary case management. Although findings on the effectiveness of case management teams are inconclusive (Schofield & Amodeo, 1999), teams are typically valued by their members (McClaran, Lam, Snell, & Franco, 1998). After social workers, nurses are the most common professional group in case management.

Social work plays an important role in the continuum of care. In addition to being one of the primary professional reference groups for case management, social workers assume numerous roles, ranging from clinical therapist in the community to hospital social worker and discharge planner to nursing home administrator. Clinical case management has been identified as a hallmark of gerontological social work practice (Morrow-Howell, 1992). Many clinical social workers who practice with elderly clients assume some case management func-tions, including conducting assessments, helping clients access and link to services, monitoring service delivery, and providing important counseling functions. A growing number of social workers now spe-cialize as private geriatric case managers.

Background

Although many of its concepts date back to the beginnings of social work, case management became popular in gerontological social work in the early 1970s. Previously, institutionally based health care services were the primary services for which costs were reimbursed. Consequently, many community programs such as home health care and outpatient mental-health services did not receive adequate funding and attention (Quinn, 1993). Escalating medical costs and sophisticated technologies that could be delivered on an outpatient basis led to a reexamination of the focus of service delivery and a consideration of new ways of financing, coordination, and providing care. In 1975, the Social Security Act and the Older Americans Act led to increased funding for home and community-based services, a trend that continued throughout the 1980s (Quinn, 1993). The Omnibus Reconciliation Act of 1981 included a mechanism for waiver programs that enabled states to incorporate health care, personal care, and case management expenditures in one funding source (Quinn, 1993). The ensuing waiver demonstration projects evaluated various innovative approaches to integrating and coordinating services, systems of case management and care coordination, financing schemes, and service eligibility criteria. The more prominent demonstration projects included On Lok (California), Nursing Homes Without Walls (New York), ACCESS (New York), Triage (Connecticut), and the Multiservice Senior Project (California). Some of these programs are still in existence, including some of the channeling demonstrations (see below) and On Lok, which continues as PACE replication projects in several states (Branch, Coulam, & Zimmerman, 1995; Rich, 1999).

In 1980, the federal government, concurrently with the state Medicaid waivers, initiated the National Long-Term Channeling Demonstrations at 10 sites across the country. At the center of these projects were two approaches for channeling services to elderly persons who are at risk for entering a nursing home. In the financial channeling model, case managers worked with pooled funding, which included money from Medicaid, Medicare, Title III of the Older Americans Act, and Title XX of the Social Service Block Grant (Applebaum & Austin, 1990). Case managers could purchase an extensive range of services for their clients with these funds. They were allowed to expend up to 85% of the comparable nursing home costs per client, as long as they stayed within 60% of those costs for the total caseload served by the program

(Applebaum & Austin, 1990). Except for services funded through waiver funds, case managers had the authority to authorize services. The second approach, basic channeling, used a broker model, in which case managers primarily accessed and coordinated services already existing in the community. In addition, they had access to some Social Service Block Grant and Title III funding (Quinn, 1993), as well as funds to establish services to fill existing gaps (Applebaum & Austin, 1990).

In 1984, the Deficit Reduction Act made possible the Social/Health Maintenance Organizations (S/HMOs) (Applebaum & Austin, 1990). Similar to an HMO, the S/HMO unites services and providers under the same auspices, but adds chronic care and case management to the service mix (Quinn, 1993). In the 1990s, the Health Care Financing Administration implemented the Medicare Alzheimer's Disease Demonstrations to apply some of the findings from other demonstration projects to case management with cognitively impaired clients (Arnsberger, Fox, & Xiulan, 1999).

Since its inception in 1978 as one of the early demonstration projects, On Lok and its successor PACE have moved through several stages of development. Interdisciplinary team members function as case managers, administering intake, assessing, monitoring, and directly providing some of the services (Rich, 1999). The program provides all medical, health-related, and social services in one consolidated provider system. Sources of funding are Medicare, Medicaid, private insurers, and individual copayments (Branch et al., 1995).

S/HMOs function on a prepaid, capitated payment system, financed through Medicaid, Medicare, and enrollee fees. Contrary to many demonstration projects, S/HMOs include acute care and long-term care in their program. They also differ in terms of participants, because members of SHM/Os include elderly clients with all different levels of functioning. Services offered include all regular HMO services, as well as expanded community care and nursing care services.

Consumer-directed case management programs have recently received significant attention. Although most programs still focus on younger Medicaid-eligible persons with disabilities, efforts have been undertaken to extend consumer-directed care to older adults. Consumer-directed programs focus primarily on social and supportive services such as homemaker and personal assistance, rather than highly skilled services (Benjamin & Matthias, 2001). Using this approach, the client recruits, selects, hires, supervises, and fires providers of services. Research from the Cash and Counseling Demonstration and Evaluation, a consumer-directed program initiative, indicates that at least one third of older adults would be interested in such models of accessing and coordinating services (Mahoney et al., 1998).

A case management model based on the strengths perspective has been presented by Tice and Perkins (1998). This model follows the regular case management structure (intake, assessment, case planning, etc.), but rather than focusing on client problems, it emphasizes client strengths and the uniqueness of their situations. The partnership between client and case manager is collaborative in nature and includes client needs and wants as the treatment focus.

Several implementation projects made an effort to integrate case management into physicians' practices (Netting & Williams, 1999a). These projects employed teams that consisted of nurse and social worker case managers who partnered with physicians in conducting in-home assessments, linkage, and coordination of services. The "physician ownership" was found to be a critical factor for success (Anker-Unnever, 1999). In another noteworthy project, family members were trained as case managers. This study found that training increased the amount of caregiving tasks that family members undertook, compared with those families that received only the regular caregiving supports (Seltzer, Litchfield, Kapust, & Mayer, 1992; Seltzer, Litchfield, Lowy, & Levin, 1989).

GERIATRIC TASK-CENTERED CASE MANAGEMENT

In this section, a detailed discussion of the processes involved in geriatric task-centered case management is given. The geriatric task-centered case management model is a synthesis of three practice concepts: (a) empirically based case-management core functions (Rothman, 1991); (b) task-centered practice (Reid, 1978, 1992); and (c) modular treatment (Dupree, 1994). Ample research supports the effectiveness of task-centered practice (Reid, 1997). Before inclusion in the newly developed model, it was successfully applied to geriatric social work practice (Dierking, Brown, & Fortune, 1980; Fortune & Rathbone-McCuan, 1981; Scharlach, 1985). Geriatric task-centered case management consists of a core intervention model (initial, middle, and termination phases), parallel functions, and practice guidelines (see Figure 5.1).

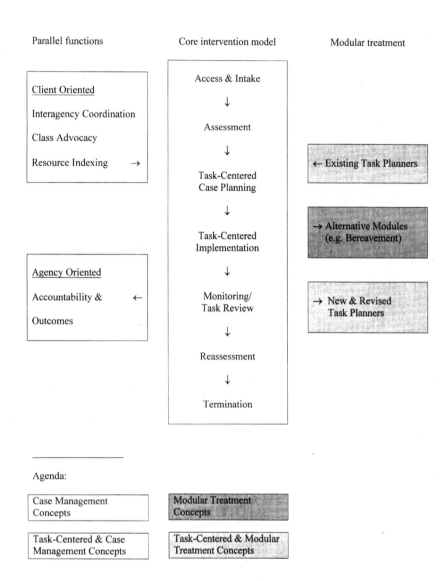

FIGURE 5.1   The task-centered case management model.
Source: Naleppa and Reid, 2000, p. 6.

Initial Phase: Access, Intake, and Assessment

Outreach to potential clients occurs through various channels, including networking with other providers, marketing, and active collaboration with physicians and primary care providers. When clients come to the attention of the case management program—through a provider or a self-referral—an intake interview to assess the appropriateness for the case management program is conducted. A determination is made as to whether the client may be participating in another case management program already or whether he or she may be better suited for a different service provider. If a client is deemed appropriate, an assessment interview is scheduled. The assessment visit begins with an explanation of the general procedures and a time frame for the intervention. In order for clients to participate actively, they need to know what the treatment process will involve. Thus, the purpose of intervention is explained and an overview of the steps that the practitioner and client will undertake is provided. The respective roles of all involved are clarified, and the active client role in making and implementing care decisions is emphasized. Task-centered case management uses time limits in a slightly different way than task-centered practice. Rather than contracting for a specific number of sessions, as is common in the clinical practice utilization of the model, the time-delimited nature of client problems in geriatric case management often does not call for efforts to control the length of service. Thus, an estimate of the overall length of the case management process, as well as time frames for addressing needs, are provided at the onset of treatment. These time frames may range from a few days to a few months, depending on the type of problem or need that is being addressed.

The initial assessment includes the client-centered problem assessment process of the task-centered practice model and standardized multidimensional assessment instruments. Case management programs often utilize comprehensive multidimensional assessments, and some programs and jurisdictions mandate specific multidimensional tools like Uniform Assessment Instruments (UAI) and the Minimum Data Set (MDS). As in regular task-centered practice, geriatric task-centered case management places much weight on client-defined problems and goals. Autonomy and active involvement in client decision-making and implementation of care-related actions are always at the forefront of the case manager's planning. The focus of task-centered case management is on client-acknowledged problems (Naleppa & Reid, 2000). Thus, in addition to completing a standardized assessment, the practitioner requests that the client describe the presenting problems in general terms and in his or her own words.

Middle Phase: Task-Centered Case Planning

Case planning begins with a detailed exploration of the identified target problems. Although some information about the client's problems and needs has been collected at this time, more comprehensive knowledge is needed for treatment planning, for example, factual description and frequency of typical occurrences, duration of the problem, the seriousness or severity of the problem, previous client problem-solving attempts, and context of the problem. At the end of this process, the client is asked for explicit acknowledgement of his or her problems and an agreement that he or she will become the focus of their collaborative work. Next, all client problems are prioritized, that is, the client is asked to list the sequence in which they should be addressed. The case manager guides this process and contributes information that may help in developing the priorities. If required, the case manager should also express concerns about the way priorities are set. In general, however, client choices for setting priorities should be respected. Finally, all identified problems and needs are included in the initial case plan. The case plan should include information on the time frame in which they will be addressed and the short-term and long-term goals.

Developing Tasks

The client and case manager begin to develop tasks to address the problems. Task alternatives are generated through brainstorming by the client and case manager. This process focuses on identifying actions that could change the problem or need. Once task alternatives are developed, potential obstacles to their implementation are reviewed. Obstacles can be defined as whatever prevents clients from solving their problems (Reid, 1992). Together, the case manager and client think through any eventuality that could hinder task implementation. After devising plans to deal with such contingencies, an agreement is made on one or more tasks. Clients should be willing to implement tasks or agree that another person will carry them out on their behalf. At the end of this process of generating, selecting, and agreeing on them, tasks are operationalized—a statement is developed that includes a description of who will do what, how, and by when. Common case-management tasks focus on care planning, home and personal safety, caregiving, respite, living and care arrangements, health, and mental health. It should be noted that occasionally situations exist in which the task-centered structure is not followed, for example when working on issues of loss and grief.

Task-Centered Implementation

Case management tasks are implemented during or between sessions. Clients should take on at least some tasks, but caregivers or case managers may assume tasks on their behalf, if clients are not able to do so or clearly express that they want help. Client or collaborative task-performance is preferable to tasks completed by the case manager. The more frail a client, the more tasks will have to be assumed by caregivers and case managers. Practice experience and data from a field test indicate that case manager tasks led to only slightly higher levels of completion than shared or client tasks, whereas caregiver tasks received the lowest completion ratings (Naleppa, 1996).

Monitoring

Monitoring occurs through an ongoing review of task achievements and problem changes at the beginning of each client contact. The client and case manager review the tasks that were implemented and rate their completion. This review may call for further action. In such cases, any encountered obstacles are reviewed and another task is planned that takes this new information into account. Concurrently, changes in the client's problems are evaluated.

Reassessment

In addition to ongoing monitoring, a formal reassessment is regularly conducted. This reassessment includes an evaluation of all problems and needs, as well as whether any changes in their status and severity occurred.

Termination Phase

Task-centered case management is the bridge between the short-term requirements for direct interventions and the long-term case management relationship. Consequently, termination differs slightly from regular task-centered practice. Time limits (or time frames) concentrate on the current service episodes. Once that episode is completed, an assessment is made as to whether any other needs exist that require immediate attention. If not, the case management affiliation either becomes dormant or is terminated. In the first scenario, the case manager indicates the continued availability and that services can be started whenever new needs arise. A complete termination occurs when the client moves to a service provider that does not require case management (e.g., skilled nursing facility) or if the client dies.

Parallel Functions

Parallel functions cover those activities that a case manager carries out on behalf of a client but, differing from the core intervention model, may not ask for the client's explicit agreement. Such activities may be client-oriented or agency-oriented. Parallel intervention functions in this practice model include resource indexing, interagency coordination, class advocacy, and outcome evaluation. The last of these parallel functions, outcome evaluation, is increasingly important. Measuring changes in problem status and task completion is a routine accountability activity and is integrated into regular practice. Changes in problem status do not always take place at the same time that tasks are completed. Tracking provides a measure of the process of case management as well as the outcomes. For example, while a significant amount of task work may have been completed toward moving into an assisted living facility, the actual placement (change in problem status) may not occur until a few weeks later due to a lack of open apartments.

Practice Guidelines

The purpose of practice guidelines has recently received attention in the gerontological and social work research community (e.g., Dupree, 1994; Howard & Jenson, 1999; Reid, 2000). Practice guidelines are typically a described set of practice procedures that practitioners undertake to address a client problem or need. They are "based on research findings and the consensus of experienced clinicians" (Howard & Jenson, 1999, p. 285). Practice guidelines assist social workers in day-to-day practice by reducing clinical uncertainty and supporting scientifically based decision making (Howard & Jenson, 1999). One type of practice guideline that is developed for specific problem situations is the *task planner*. The development of these task planners is based on a systematic review of the research and practice literature, as well as practice evidence (Reid, 2000). Thus, they follow the call by Howard and Jenson (1999) that practice guidelines should be based on empirical evidence, practice experience, and social work values. The task-planning practice guidelines are descriptive in nature, describing task alternatives that have been shown to work for addressing specific problems or needs.

Each task planner comprises a description of the problem or need, references to relevant literature and research, and a menu of possible actions that can be completed to resolve the problem (Reid, 2000). They also describe how a practitioner can facilitate these problem-solving actions. Because each case and situation differs, they need to be modified to reflect the client's reality. To date, more than 50 task planners have been developed for geriatric case management, focusing on resources and care planning, home and personal safety, living and care arrangements, caregiving, respite, health and mental health, and end-of-life decision making (Naleppa & Reid, in press). Case management lends itself to practice guidelines, as it addresses a wide range of problems and needs through a multitude of differential interventions. The case manager uses a variety of skills and techniques to address the need for linkage and brokering, education, clinical intervention, and so on. Task planners can help in developing tasks that fit the individual case, thus assisting the planning and decision-making process.

PRIOR RESEARCH AND KNOWLEDGE BASE

Research on the previously discussed demonstration projects focused primarily on evaluating and improving systems-level aspects of accessing, financing, and coordinating care. Recent studies and publications have increasingly emphasized research on direct practice issues (e.g., Geron & Chassler, 1994; Hennessy, 1993; Netting & Williams, 1999b; Raiff & Shore, 1993; Soares & Rose, 1994; Vourlekis & Greene, 1992). Several studies have looked at new ways of collaborating on the delivery of case management interventions. Examples are the training of family members as case managers (Seltzer et al., 1989) and the interdisciplinary collaboration between physicians, social workers, and nurses (Netting & Williams, 1999a, 1999b). However, despite the knowledge gained through these projects, a need continues to exist for empirically tested clinical-practice strategies for case management with older adults and their caregivers. Available research has focused on case management core functions, time limits, and consumer-directed care.

Core Functions

Although a range of structural models for case management exists, there is agreement on the core functions that any model should address. At a minimum, case management core functions include screening, assessment, planning, linking, monitoring, advocacy, and evaluation (Austin & McClelland, 1996; Moxley, 1989; Rubin, 1987; Weil, 1985). Rothman (1991) presents an empirically developed set of case-management core functions that integrates a client and systems perspective through a primary intervention model and several parallel practice functions. The geriatric task-centered case management model, presented earlier in this chapter, includes this dual focus on client and systems-level practice considerations (Naleppa & Reid, 2000).

Time Limits

Ample research has demonstrated that outcomes for short-term time-limited case management interventions are usually as effective as long-term interventions (Bloom, 2000; Koss & Shiang, 1994; Reid & Shyne, 1969). Time limits help to mobilize and motivate clients and practitioners alike. Thus, they lead to a more effective use of time. Moreover, client motivation has a positive impact on reaching treatment goals.

The pace and brevity of interventions with elderly clients deserve special attention. Although case management usually takes place over long periods of time, a case manager is likely to intervene during an acute crisis when there is limited time to intervene and a need for quick action. Although short-term treatment models and the long-term goals of case management might seem to be conflicting, time-limited interventions can be successfully integrated within case management (Naleppa & Reid, 1998, 2000). New problems and needs can be conceptualized as recurring service episodes (Naleppa & Reid, in press). Problems that are identified for help in case management are often specific and their course delimited, thus they may be dealt with in short-term treatment.

Consumer-Directed Care

Systems-level considerations have long been at the forefront of the development and evaluation of new ways of delivering case management services. Demonstration projects have looked at issues such as cost containment, gatekeeping, and increasing efficiency. At times, these efforts overlooked the quality of life and the wishes of the elderly clients on whose behalf case management occurs. Active client involvement has recently received increased attention. Consumer-directed personal assistance programs are a way to enhance the involvement of clients (National Institute of Consumer Directed Long-Term Care Services, 1996).

> Consumer direction is a philosophy and orientation to the delivery of home and community-based service whereby informed consumers make choices about the services they receive. . . . Consumer direction ranges from the individual independently making all decisions and managing services directly, to an individual using a representative to manage needed services. (p. 4)

Consumer direction may seem most challenging in those service delivery arrangements that focus primarily on cost containment, such as managed care organizations (MCOs). Evaluating a national sample of MCOs, Meiners and associates determined that significant variations exist in the amount of client participation and consumer direction in making decisions (Meiners, Mahoney, Shoop, & Squillace, 2002). Their study also found that consumer direction and managed care are compatible and can be integrated. Another study evaluated whether the age of clients had an impact on service outcomes (Benjamin & Matthias, 2001). It found that younger clients were more favorable toward consumer direction. However, service outcomes were found to be similar among both younger and older clients. Although research on the effectiveness of consumer-directed care is still limited, several state and federal agencies are planning the implementation of demonstration projects (Benjamin & Matthias, 2001).

CURRENT RESEARCH

The geriatric task-centered case management model has been developed following the intervention research paradigm set forth by Thomas and Rothman (Rothman & Thomas, 1994; Thomas, 1984). The goal of model development and intervention research is to generate concrete strategies for practice utilization. Intervention research is presented as typically going through a sequence of six stages: problem analysis and project planning; information gathering and synthesis; design; early development and pilot testing; evaluation and advanced development; and dissemination (Rothman & Thomas, 1994). To date, the model has been taken through the first four stages. A systematic review has been completed of research and practice literature as well as existing programs that address community-based practice with older adults. An initial practice model has been designed and tested in an exploratory field trial (Naleppa, 1996; Naleppa & Reid, 1998). Revisions have been made to the practice model to address the findings from the field trial. Two projects have looked at the adaptability of the model to German and Korean social work practice (Huh, 1998; Naleppa, 1999). An ongoing project is implementing another field test of the model with an older adult client population (Naleppa, 2002).

Continued development and revisions of the practice guidelines are integrated into the current practice model. Tasks carried out by clients and case managers are recorded as part of the regular practice activities. These records of task completion are reviewed on a regular basis. If a task planner already exists, it is updated with any additional new information from these task records. Updates also include a review of the literature for recent developments relating to the treatment module. Tasks that were not successfully completed are not added, but the existing task planners are reviewed to assess whether they need to be changed in light of the new information. Successful tasks that are not yet covered by a task planner are the basis for new practice guidelines, which are developed in the same way as was described previously.

During the most recent geriatric task-centered case management project, the task planners were also redesigned to fit a Web-based format, in which they were cross-linked to related treatment modules as well as to a Website with contact information for continuum of care programs. When logging off a Web-based task planner, users are asked to provide feedback on several aspects and, after implementing tasks with their clients in the field, are requested to provide any additional useful information for the task planner. This information is used in the ongoing improvement of the structure and content of the task planners.

FURTHER RESEARCH NEEDS

Case management has become a widely utilized approach for negotiating and coordinating services for elderly clients and their families. A review of the literature and research indicates that most attention has been given to systems-level aspects, such as funding, targeting, gatekeeping, and system coordination. Less consideration has been placed on the practice of case management and the skills that case managers utilize. Although general agreement exists as to the core functions of case management models, the structure of the delivery systems into which these core functions are embedded varies significantly across specific client populations, regions, and types of problems.

Because of changing policies and service delivery systems a continued focus on the improvement of case management delivery systems is required. Many managed care providers include case management as part of service delivery and care coordination. As new ways of financing and managing care continue to be implemented, it is critical to ensure that case management practice is provided by qualified professionals and that access to services is not based solely on cost considerations. The professional literature indicates the need for multiple qualified professionals to carry out case management. At the same time, a conflict is emerging in the field concerning which professional reference group is best suited to provide case management. In this context, it is important to test the benefits of interdisciplinary teams in providing case management.

The primary focus of research on case management has been on improving the effectiveness of systems of care delivery and coordination and evaluating mezzo- and macro-level factors, to some extent neglecting clinical micro-level aspects of case management. Although demonstration projects evaluated case management in long-term care for the elderly, the focus was almost exclusively on macro-level issues. This points to a continued need for intervention research, the development of innovative models of case management practice, and the evaluation of their effectiveness. Improving the practice knowledge and the skills that case managers utilize should be considered as important as improving the systems in which these practitioners and clients interact.

Little attention has been given to the intervention skills that practitioners employ within the core functions and frameworks of case management. Because the frameworks, and the policies that dictate them, change over time and across settings for case management, preference should be given to case management practice approaches that are flexible enough to be implemented in diverse situations and settings. Special attention should be given to the growing influence of managed care approaches on social work and case management practice. This will require an increased emphasis on the development and evaluation of case management models that foster accountability and easy access to outcomes-related information. Short-term interventions that can be applied within long-term case management are promising because they combine time limits with established effectiveness, but should be studied further.

Geriatric task-centered case management is a model that includes the client in making and implementing care decisions. Although it uses a professional case manager to guide the treatment process, active client participation is one of the basic tenets. Future research should focus on a controlled evaluation of the model's effectiveness, the optimum levels of client direction, and which clients are best suited for this practice approach. Research has begun to look at consumer-directed care models. Clients vary greatly in their abilities to actively participate in consumer-directed care, so research should look at client involvement as a continuum and evaluate which mix would best fit which client and problem situation.

Generating and evaluating practice guidelines such as the geriatric task planners merits more attention in geriatric social work research. One stringent approach to generating such practice guidelines would be to take only practice approaches that have been validated through empirical research and systematically develop them using panels of expert scholars. Evidenced-based intervention should be the priority and serve as the foundation of practice guidelines. If no empirical evidence is available, no practice guideline is developed. Case management must be able to address a wide range of problems, which requires the availability of sufficient research in each area. Currently, many gaps in the research exist.

A second approach to developing practice guidelines is through experts, including representatives from the research and scholarship community as well as experienced practitioners. If no empirical evidence exists, the information is supplemented by knowledge and evidence that is transferred from other research as well as from practice experience. If the source of practice knowledge is clarified, that is, an indication is made whether the module is based on empirical evidence, knowledge transfer, or practice experience, the user can make an informed decision about whether and how to apply it.

A third approach to developing practice guidelines is to integrate research and knowledge building into geriatric practice. The practice guidelines of the task-centered case management model are an example of how this could be accomplished. As practice guidelines are used by practitioners, they are continuously updated and improved. However, this integration into practice enhances the development, but cannot replace the inclusion, of research-based knowledge.

POLICY IMPLICATIONS

Case management practice is strongly shaped through social and economic policy. In few areas of social work practice is this connection more obvious than in geriatric case management. Whether policies increase or restrict services through adjusting eligibility criteria, provide open-ended funding or cap costs, or make service available only in certain catchment areas, these factors influence the way case management practice occurs.

Primary Mission

When looking at the primary mission of a case management program, it is important to establish the program's orientation: Is the intention of policy to contain cost or to facilitate client access to needed services? The former is a systems-level goal, whereas the latter is a client-oriented goal. When client access is the primary goal, the focus is on optimizing the care package a client receives. The amount of gatekeeping, expressed in the extent to which a case manager has control over resources, continues to vary greatly. In some programs, the main goal is to manage costs. Gatekeeping mechanisms serve to control the amount of services that are accessible, usually by using narrow eligibility criteria (Applebaum & Austin, 1990).

Targeting Criteria

Programs are mandated by policies to specify the target group eligible for their services. Some programs cover only certain catchment areas. Some programs have broad disability criteria, serving clients with a wide range of needs, whereas other programs employ narrow disability-based eligibility requirements, such as being at risk of nursing home placement as in the National Channeling Demonstration (Applebaum & Austin, 1990). Other programs use needs-based eligibility criteria, focusing on clients with specific functional impairments. Recent discussion in several programs has focused on increasing efficiency by further narrowing the functional-needs requirements for eligibility.

Systems of Service Delivery

Case management is employed in various parts of the service delivery system, from long-term care to MCOs and health care providers to private practitioners. Each of these areas demands different policy and program decisions. The priority areas for improving health care identified by the Institute of Medicine (2001) are relevant for developing programs and policies for case management and care coordination. Service delivery systems should be safe and avoid additional harm to the client. Decisions on whether to provide specific services should be based on empirical evidence about their effectiveness for the particular client and problem (Institute of Medicine, 2001). Developing and evaluating programs that provide services in a client-centered manner should continue. A client's personal preferences, needs, and values should be taken into consideration when making care and service decisions. The consumer-directed care models and the Cash and Counseling Demonstration and Evaluation projects mentioned earlier are a first step in this direction. Future policies should continue to balance the consumer's involvement with the system's requirements.

Policies should foster the delivery of services in a timely and efficient way. Services and programs should be equitable, reducing fluctuations in quality and coverage of services due to geographic, racial, gender, and socioeconomic factors. Information and knowledge should flow freely, allowing client access to all relevant information. To facilitate this process, Kane (2001) proposes developing sources of consumer information as a policy priority. In a similar vein, the various professionals who coordinate care should be supported in better communicating, collaborating, and accessing the information they need (Institute of Medicine, 2001).

Policy priorities for systems of service delivery:

1. Increase availability of noninstitutional programs and services.
2. Streamline and improve access to services.
3. Improve quality of home and community-based services.
4. Develop and evaluate programs that foster client-centered decision making.
5. Include a focus on micro-level practice of case management when developing and evaluating programs.
6. Include quality of care as a major evaluative component when designing case management services and long-term-care programs.

Funding of Case Management

Funding has a significant impact on the practice of case management. Despite the creation of the continuum of care, the system of services for older adults continues to be fragmented and difficult to navigate: "Form follows funding . . . splintered funding produces disconnected and discontinuous service delivery" (Austin & McClelland, 1996, p. 267). Reducing fragmentation should become an overarching goal of policy and funding decisions. Case management can assist in bringing pieces of this system together on behalf of clients. However, as Austin and McClelland (1996) caution, the individual case-manager's role in changing systems should not be overstated. They assert that meaningful changes can only come about through a substantial policy and organizational reform of the service delivery systems and the current funding structures. The way a funding system is set up influences the case management provider's capability to control costs. Experimentation with different systems of funding was the main objective of many demonstration projects.

There are significant variations in how case management programs and the services they coordinate are financed. The funding for services is as fragmented as the service system. One way this fragmentation can be decreased is by pooling funds, an approach that integrates various funding sources into one pool, out of which services are financed (Austin, 1990). In a second approach, prospective financing, a fixed amount of funds is established and made available to the provider a priori. The provider has to offer services within these preset limits. In contrast to this is a third variation, retrospective reimbursement, based on the actual services provided. When funding is capped, a per-client limit of expenditures exists. A final alternative is open-ended funding, which takes into account each individual client's eligibility for services (Applebaum & Austin, 1990). Although cost containment is of prime interest to the funding system, it can have disadvantages for clients, for example, when certain services are not provided because they are out of the financial range of a prospective capitated pool of funds. Furthermore, pooling finances establishes a new fund that is easy to truncate (Kane, 1988).

Each of these funding approaches has direct consequences for case managers and their clients. From a systems and policy perspective, "cost containment and quality services are usually twin goals in case management systems" (Austin & McClelland, 1996, p. 12). Until now, the focus has typically been on the development and evaluation of one funding approach at a time. An alternative approach to current funding mechanisms would be the utilization of blended methods of payment (Institute of Medicine, 2001). Rather than providing only retrospective reimbursement, pooling all funds, or capping all expenses, alternative approaches could differentiate between certain conditions for which bundled payments would be provided and others that would be reimbursed in a retrospective manner.

Policy priorities for funding of case management:

1. Increase coordination between various sources of program and service funding.
2. Develop and evaluate blended funding approaches.

3. Evaluate costs and effectiveness of consumer-directed care.
4. Evaluate which services and delivery approaches work best for whom and improve targeting them to those clients.
5. Improve screening and targeting of services to those at high risk of institutionalization.
6. Develop and evaluate mechanisms to better match clients with appropriate services, especially for high-cost services.
7. Balance cost-containment requirements and improvements of the quality of care.

Payment policies should be realigned with improved quality of care; they should eliminate obstacles to quality improvement and create incentives for the enhancement of quality (Institute of Medicine, 2001). Kane (2001) concurs that client quality-of-life issues deserve a more prominent place in any initiatives to reform the system. Programs and policies for case management continue to face a difficult balancing act between good access to high-quality services and low costs of service delivery to older adults. In this environment we have to make sure that

> policy efforts to contain expenses, to limit care to the most-in-need, and to create ambitious schema for forging community-wide relationships do not lose sight of the importance of the individual, the much larger scope of unfunded need, and the obligation to integrate case management with actual support for direct service delivery. (Raiff & Shore, 1993, p. 154)

INTEGRATING KNOWLEDGE INTO THE CURRICULUM

Geriatric task-centered case management is still in the early to middle stages of development. Although this model incorporates empirically based case management core functions (Rothman, 1991) and task-centered practice, one of the most researched and empirically validated social work models (Reid, 1992)—the integrated geriatric task-centered case-management model—still has to undergo empirical testing through controlled research studies. Initial evidence points to the applicability and positive outcomes of the geriatric task-centered case-management model (Naleppa & Reid, 1998, 2000). Furthermore, it is one of the few case-management practice models that is being evaluated from a micro practice perspective, rather than from a systems-level perspective.

The best-practice treatment modules are in an early stage of development in social work and case management practice. The medical field has applied such practice modules with great success. Efforts to replicate such models in social work are underway (Howard & Jenson, 1999). As more best-practice treatment modules become available, they will make a significant contribution to social work practice and field-based education.

Case management lends itself well to serving as a foundation practice model for gerontological social-work elective courses as well as for inclusion into the regular foundation practice curriculum. The geriatric task-centered case-management practice model provides clearly structured and easy-to-implement intervention guidelines. Case management also can serve as the basis from which to integrate knowledge and skills specific to geriatric assessment: communication with elderly clients, practice with caregivers, the continuum of care and service delivery systems, and so on. The inclusion of task-centered practice—a mainstream social-work practice model—into case management practice should facilitate student learning. Empirical evidence on the effectiveness of task-centered practice, as well as the inclusion of outcome measures in the case management model, can serve as an example of evidence-based social work practice in the foundation practice curriculum and in gerontological social-work elective courses.

The task planners or practice guidelines also are well suited for integration in foundation practice. More important, however, they can aid students in their field-based education. Through their design—basic knowledge on problems, needs, and resources—they can assist students and beginning practitioners in identifying and implementing change strategies. In addition, they provide a guideline for developing interventions with elderly clients.

Finally, the impact of policy decisions on the realities of practice is very evident in geriatric case management. How a program is funded, who can access which programs and services, and who coordinates care in which way are all affected by policy and systems-level decisions. The demonstration projects can serve as an example of how policy can influence research, practice, and future policy decisions.

CONCLUSION

As the older adult population continues to increase, a growing number of elderly clients will experience problems with accessing required assistance in a service delivery system that is fragmented and difficult to navigate. This chapter has presented several ways of characterizing case management. Research and demonstration projects have evaluated numerous ways of providing case management; however, the findings are often mixed and do not provide clear endorsement for any one approach. Moreover, evaluations of demonstration projects have generally focused attention on systems-level aspects of service delivery such as targeting, funding, and coordinating care. A need for more knowledge about the practice of case management continues to exist.

In should be reiterated that elderly clients in case management vary greatly in their level of cognitive, physical, psychological, and emotional functioning. Moreover, many elderly clients who are frail have caregivers who participate in the intervention, either as providers of informal services or as corecipients of treatment. Thus, case-management practice models should be flexible to adapt to various levels of client participation. Because a case manager, just as any other gerontological practitioner, will encounter clients with and without caregiver involvement, treatment models should accommodate both practice situations.

The discussion in this chapter has also highlighted how policies influence case management, for example, by mandating case management activities, funding only certain services, or requiring practitioners to serve as gatekeepers. Case management has been applied in a range of service environments, from health, mental health, and managed care to long-term care and private practice. Although the general approach to case management is similar in these service environments, the specifics of implementation vary greatly. Future research on case management will continue to face the dilemma of significant differences in these various service delivery systems. As one of the primary intervention modalities in practice with older adults, knowledge and skills in geriatric case management should be a major focus in training future social workers.

REFERENCES

Anker-Unnever, L. (1999). An effective managed care strategy: Case managers in partnership with primary care physicians. In F. E. Netting & F. G. Williams (Eds.), *Enhancing primary care of elderly people* (pp. 151–169). New York: Garland.

Applebaum, R. A., & Austin, C. D. (1990). *Long-term care case management: Design and evaluation.* New York: Springer.

Arnsberger, P., Fox, P., & Xiulan, Z. (1999). Case manager-defined roles in the Medicare Alzheimer's Disease Demonstration: Relationship to client and caregiver outcomes. *Care Management Journals, 1,* 29–37.

Austin, C. D. (1990). Case management: Myths and reality. *Families in Society, 71,* 398–407.

Austin, C. D. (1993). Case management: A systems perspective. *Families in Society, 74,* 451–459.

Austin, C. D. (2001). Case management. In M. E. Mezey (Ed.), *The encyclopedia of elder care: The comprehensive resource on geriatric and social care* (pp. 121–124). New York: Springer.

Austin, C. D., & McClelland, R. W. (Eds.). (1996). *Case management practice.* Milwaukee, WI: Families International.

Benjamin, A. E., & Matthias, R. E. (2001). Age, consumer direction, and outcomes of supportive services at home. *Gerontologist, 41,* 632–642.

Bloom, B. (2000). Planned short-term psychotherapies. In C. R. Snyder & R. E. Ingram (Eds.), *Handbook of psychological change* (pp. 429–454). New York: Wiley.

Branch, L. G., Coulam, R. F., & Zimmerman, Y. A. (1995). The PACE evaluation: Initial findings. *Gerontologist, 35,* 349–359.

Dierking, B., Brown, M., & Fortune, A. E. (1980). Task-centered treatment in a residential facility for the elderly: A clinical trial. *Journal of Gerontological Social Work, 2,* 225–240.

Dupree, L. W. (1994). Geropsychological modular treatment: Back to the future. *Journal of Gerontological Social Work, 22,* 211–220.

Fortune, A. E., & Rathbone-McCuan, E. (1981). Education in gerontological social work: Application of the task-centered model. *Journal of Education for Social Work, 17,* 98–105.

Geron, S. M., & Chassler, D. (1994). *Guidelines for case management practice across the long-term care continuum.* Bristol, CT: Connecticut Community Care.

Hennessy, C. H. (1993). Modeling case management decision making in a consolidated long-term care program. *Gerontologist, 33,* 333–341.

Howard, M. O., & Jenson, J. M. (1999). Clinical practice guidelines: Who should develop them? *Research on Social Work Practice, 9,* 283–301.

Huh, N. S. (1998). A task-centered approach for the elderly in the community: Case management. *Korean Journal of Social Welfare, 35,* 399–427.

Institute of Medicine. (2001). *Crossing the quality chasm: A new health system for the 21st century.* Washington, DC: National Academy Press.

Kane, R. A. (1988). Case management: Ethical pitfalls on the road to high-quality managed care. *Quality Review Bulletin, 14,* 161–165.

Kane, R. A. (2001). Long-term care and good quality of life: Bringing them closer together. *Gerontologist, 41,* 293–304.

Koss, M. P., & Shiang, J. (1994). Research on brief psychotherapy. In A. Bergin & S. Garfield (Eds.), *Handbook of psychotherapy and behavior change* (4th ed., pp. 664–700). New York: Wiley.

Mahoney, K. J., Simon-Rusinowitz, L., Desmond, S. M., Shoop, D. M., Squillace, M. A., & Fay, R. A. (1998). Determining consumers' preferences for a cash option: New York telephone survey findings. *American Rehabilitation, 24,* 24–36.

McClaran, J., Lam, Z., Snell, L., & Franco, E. (1998). The importance of the case management approach: Perceptions of multidisciplinary team members. *Journal of Case Management, 7*, 117–126.

Meiners, M. R., Mahoney, K. J., Shoop, D. M., & Squillace, M. R. (2002). Consumer direction in managed long-term care: An exploratory survey of practices and perceptions. *Gerontologist, 42*, 32–38.

Morrow-Howell, N. (1992). Clinical case management: The hallmark of gerontological social work. *Journal of Gerontological Social Work, 18*, 119–131.

Moxley, D. P. (1989). *The practice of case management.* Newbury Park, CA: Sage.

Naleppa, M. J. (1996). *Task-centered case management for the elderly in the community: Developing a practice model.* Unpublished doctoral dissertation, University at Albany, New York.

Naleppa, M. J. (1999). *Das Münchener Task-Centered Projekt [The Munich Task-Centered Project].* Unpublished manuscript, Deutscher Berufverband der Sozialarbeiter, Sozialpädagogen und Heilpädagogen, Munich, Germany.

Naleppa, M. J. (2002). *An evaluation of geriatric task-centered case management.* Unpublished manuscript.

Naleppa, M. J., & Reid, W. J. (1998). Task-centered case management for the elderly: Developing a practice model. *Research on Social Work Practice, 8*, 63–85.

Naleppa, M. J., & Reid, W. J. (2000). Integrating case management and brief-treatment strategies: A hospital-based geriatric program. *Social Work in Health Care, 31*, 1–23.

Naleppa, M. J., & Reid, W. J. (in press). *Gerontological practice: A task-centered approach.* New York: Columbia University Press.

National Institute of Consumer Directed Long-Term Care Services. (1996). *Principles of consumer-directed home and community-based services.* Washington, DC: National Council on Aging.

Netting, F. E., & Williams, F. G. (Eds.). (1999a). *Enhancing primary care of elderly people.* New York: Garland.

Netting, F. E., & Williams, F. G. (1999b). Implementing a case management program designed to enhance primary care physician practice with older persons. *Journal of Applied Gerontology, 18*, 24–45.

Pu, C. T. (2001). Continuum of care. In M. E. Mezey (Ed.), *The encyclopedia of elder care: The comprehensive resource on geriatric and social care* (pp. 158–161). New York: Springer.

Quinn, J. (1993). *Successful case management in long-term care.* New York: Springer.

Quinn, J. (1995). Case management in home and community care. *Journal of Gerontological Social Work, 24*, 233–248.

Raiff, N. R., & Shore, B. K. (1993). *Advanced case management: New strategies for the nineties.* Newbury Park, CA: Sage.

Reid, W. J. (1978). *The task-centered system.* New York: Columbia University Press.

Reid, W. J. (1992). *Task strategies: An empirical approach to clinical social work.* New York: Columbia University Press.

Reid, W. J. (1997). Research on task-centered practice. *Social Work Research, 21*, 132–137.

Reid, W. J. (2000). *The task planner.* New York: Columbia University Press.

Reid, W. J., & Shyne, A. (1969). *Brief and extended casework.* New York: Columbia University Press.

Rich, M. L. (1999). The PACE model: Description and impressions of a capitated model of long-term care for the elderly. *Care Management Journals, 1,* 62–70.

Rothman, J. (1991). A model of case management: Toward empirically based practice. *Social Work, 36,* 520–528.

Rothman, J., & Thomas, E. J. (Eds.). (1994). *Intervention research: Design and development for human service.* Binghamton, NY: Haworth Press.

Rubin, A. (1987). Case management. *Social Work, 28,* 49–54.

Scharlach, A. E. (1985). Social group work with institutionalized elders: A task-centered approach. *Social Work With Groups, 8,* 33–47.

Schofield, R. F., & Amodeo, M. (1999). Interdisciplinary teams in health care and human service settings: Are they effective? *Health and Social Work, 24,* 210–219.

Seltzer, M. M., Litchfield, L. C., Kapust, L. R., & Mayer, J. B. (1992). Professional and family collaboration in case management: A hospital-based replication of a community-based study. *Social Work in Health Care, 17,* 1–22.

Seltzer, M. M., Litchfield, L. C., Lowy, L., & Levin, R. J. (1989). Families as case managers: A longitudinal study. *Family Relations, 38,* 332–336.

Soares, H. H., & Rose, M. K. (1994). Clinical aspects of case management with the elderly. *Journal of Gerontological Social Work, 22,* 143–156.

Thomas, E. J. (1984). *Designing interventions for the helping professions.* Beverly Hills, CA: Sage.

Tice, C., & Perkins, K. (1998). Case management for the baby boom generation: A strengths perspective. *Journal of Case Management, 7,* 3–9.

U.S. Bureau of the Census. (2000). *The Census 2000 brief series: Population change and distribution: 1990–2000.* [On-line]. Available: http://www.census.gov/prod/2001 pubs/c2kbr01-2.pdf. Retrieved October 15, 2000.

Vourlekis, B. S., & Greene, R. R. (Eds.). (1992). *Social work case management.* New York: Aldine De Gruyter.

Wacker, R. R., Roberto, K. A., & Piper, L. E. (1997). *Community resources for older adults: Programs and services in an era of change.* Thousand Oaks, CA: Pine Forge.

Weil, M. (1985). Key components in providing efficient and effective services. In M. Weil & J. M. Karls (Eds.), *Case management in human service practice: A systematic approach to mobilizing resources for clients* (pp. 29–72). San Francisco: Jossey-Bass.

Chapter 6

SELF-HEALTH CARE
BY URBAN, AFRICAN
AMERICAN ELDERS

Denise Burnette and Suk-Young Kang

The National Center for Chronic Disease Prevention and Health Promotion of the Centers for Disease Control defines *chronic diseases* as illnesses that are prolonged, do not resolve spontaneously, and are rarely completely cured. An estimated 100 million Americans have at least one chronic health condition, and these conditions limit the routine activities of one in six, or 41 million, persons. Barring unforeseen biomedical advances that might eradicate or appreciably ameliorate these diseases, their prevalence will continue to increase as a function of population aging, and individual and societal objectives will remain focused on managing their progression and impact.

The first and foremost strategy for managing these conditions is the complex, still poorly understood process of self-care. Although often posited as the antithesis of formal medical care and associated with less informed treatment (lay, folk, traditional), studies routinely show that (a) self-evaluations of symptoms and self-treatment are both the basic and predominant form of primary health care across age groups and cultures (medical consultation, when sought, tends to be contingent on lay symptom evaluation and decision making and to be preceded and followed by self-treatment); and (b) most self-care strategies are appropriate and effective (Dean, 1986a, 1986b; Eisenberg et al., 1993; Hickey, Akiyama, & Rakowski, 1991).

According to Haug, Wykle, and Namazi (1989, p. 171), Levin, Katz, and Holst (1976) first defined *self-care* as a layperson functioning on his or her own behalf to promote health and detect, prevent, and treat disease. The concept gained currency during the 1980s in opposition to a trend toward the biomedicalization of common health and illness events (De Friese, Woomert, Guild, Steckler, & Konrad, 1989). It has since evolved to refer to the participative roles that laypersons play in shaping the processes and outcomes of professional care—roles that extend to self-management of chronic health conditions (Ory, DeFriese, & Duncker, 1998). An inclusive definition is offered by a special working group of the World Health Organization (as cited in Ory et al., 1998):

> Self-care in health refers to the activities individuals, families, and communities undertake with the intention of enhancing health, preventing disease, limiting illness, and restoring health. These activities are derived from knowledge and skills from the pool of both professional and lay experience. They are undertaken by lay people on their own behalf, either separately or in participative collaboration with professionals. (p. xvii)

Rapid growth in the prevalence of chronic diseases, coupled with major structural changes in health care delivery—most notably managed care—has fostered a wealth of social science and health services research on the behavioral aspects of disease management. Much of this work has focused on understanding the processes and outcomes of self-care. Drawing on knowledge from multiple disciplines, intervention models to enhance self-care have proliferated. Theoretical developments in the field have lagged, although most interventions aim to help individuals develop and maintain appropriate self-care behaviors through cognitive-behavioral and rational decision-making processes.

Leventhal, Leventhal, and Robitaille (1998) offer a compelling argument for theoretical approaches to knowledge development, particularly for understanding replication failures and reconciling contradictory findings (e.g., identifying personal and sociocultural factors such as ethnicity and age that moderate self-care outcomes) and for developing effective educational and therapeutic interventions for behavioral change. These authors critically review the two main types of psychological models: (a) those based on risk perception, for example, the health beliefs model (Rosenstock, 1966) and the theory of reasoned action (Ajzen & Fishbein, 1980); and (b) those based on behavioral change and skill acquisition, for example, social learning theory (Bandura, 1977) and cognitive behavior therapy (Meichenbaum, 1977).

Concluding that these models ignore significant dimensions of self-care and fail to account for individual differences, Leventhal and colleagues (1998) propose a self-care model based on self-regulation that incorporates motivation and integrates risk perception with response performance. This model, which has shown promise in empirical research, posits that self-care is an ongoing problem-solving process that (a) accounts for disease change over time, (b) relies on emotional processes that directly inhibit and motivate self-care, and (c) occurs in the context of individual personal characteristics and sociocultural factors.

Prohaska and colleagues (Prohaska, 1998; Prohaska & DiClemente, 1983) further posit a promising transtheoretical model of behavior change that highlights its temporal features and has been used successfully in self-care programs for older adults (Barke & Nicholas, 1990; Clark, Kviz, Prohaska, Crittenden, & Warnecke, 1995). Emphasizing that self-care is a *process of change,* this model assumes that people alter their behaviors by moving through stages of precontemplation, contemplation, preparation, action, and maintenance. Accordingly, interventions are designed to facilitate movement from one stage to the next. These and other developing theoretical approaches to self-care can effectively guide research, practice, and policy on this topic in gerontology and in social work.

SIGNIFICANCE TO GERONTOLOGY AND HEALTH CARE

Self-care is a vital component of health promotion and disease prevention and management across the life course, but it has special salience for older adults and, more broadly, for an aging population. Acute conditions abate with advancing age, and the likelihood of chronic, disabling conditions rises rapidly. Citing national health statistics, Hoffman and Rice (1996) note that four of every five older Americans have at least one chronic health condition, and 69% have multiple conditions. Twelve million, or 40%, of noninstitutionalized elders are limited by these conditions, and 3 million are unable to perform routine activities of daily living (ADLs). Furthermore, chronic diseases account for 70% of all deaths, and more than 60% of the nation's medical care costs. The individual and societal costs of lengthy, disabling illnesses thus accrue in terms of morbidity and disability, mortality, and health care expenditures.

Appropriate self-care can enhance quality of life and reduce health-related costs for persons who have these conditions by preventing or postponing progressive disablement and functional decline, the development of mental and other physical comorbidities, and the need for intensive informal and formal caregiving (Morrongiello & Gottlieb, 2000; Stearns et al., 2000). To realize these benefits, however, health planners, policy makers, and practitioners must address the social, cultural, behavioral, and economic dimensions of chronic, disabling conditions.

Of special concern are well-documented racial and ethnic disparities in the prevalence, costs, and quality of care for these conditions. The risks and burdens of chronic illnesses are borne disproportionately by low-income and ethnic minority persons, owing to both the cumulative effects of low educational attainment and underemployment over the life course and current social and economic disadvantage (National Institute on Aging, 2000). Efforts to understand the processes and outcomes of self-care in later life must attend, therefore, to the current needs and developmental histories of specific subgroups of older adults. Yet research to date on this topic has focused almost exclusively on non-Latino Whites.

Taken together, the epidemiological shift toward chronic diseases, the increasing diversity of the older population, and well-documented racial and ethnic disparities in health risks and negative outcomes of chronic diseases in later life constitute a compelling rationale to better understand and enhance the self-care practices of African American elders through applied practice and public policy.

The non-Latino White population aged 65 years and older is projected to increase by 91% between 1990 and 2030, compared to a 150% projected increase for older African Americans, who compose the largest group (8%) of ethnic minority elders. National health statistics on African American elders reveal that overall mortality ratios relative to Whites are high and that they peak in middle age, then decline in old age. A number of studies have shown a mortality crossover effect whereby Black/White mortality ratios at advanced ages decline to less than 1.0; however, this phenomenon has been questioned because of the dubious accuracy of self-reported age (Markides & Miranda, 1997).

With respect to health status and health outcomes, Clark and Gibson (1997) cite national health statistics that confirm the health disadvantages of African American elders relative to same-aged Whites for chronic conditions and disabilities in early old age. Yet with the exceptions of obesity and disability (assessed by ADLs), these relative risks tend to decline or disappear after age 80 years. The diseases most commonly related to progressive functional limitations and disability in later life are arthritis, diabetes, heart disease, hypertension, cancer, hip fracture or osteoporosis, and stroke (Guralnik et al., 1993). Diabetes and hypertension are especially problematic for African American elders.

SIGNIFICANCE TO PROFESSIONAL PRACTICE

Patient education activists and health care professionals, including nurses and physical, occupational, and speech therapists, physicians, public health workers, and social workers are increasingly incorporating knowledge and principles of self-care into their routine practice with older adults. Drawing on disciplinary and interdisciplinary knowledge and skills, they are developing, implementing, and evaluating educational and supportive self-care strategies, most often with the aim of enabling people to manage symptoms of specific chronic diseases. These activities take place across community (e.g., home health, senior centers, primary care, and supported living) and institutional (e.g., nursing homes, rehabilitation facilities) service settings.

Through activities such as the collection and analyses of data on the etiology and effects of late-life chronic health conditions, public testimonies, and legislative research and action, practitioners also help define policy issues and develop policy options to enhance the motivation, opportunity, and capacity of older adults to accomplish self-care goals. The ethical and economic aspects of health and social policies that govern behavioral health practices are of special relevance to self-care. Autonomy and choice are basic tenets of health care decision-making in the United States. Practitioners must ensure that older people have sufficient knowledge of their options and the requisite resources to realistically pursue their choices. Punitive practices and policies that treat personal responsibility for prior and current high-risk health behaviors as a justification to limit services, must be eschewed in favor of those that account for and promote such knowledge and resources.

Policies that facilitate access to culturally sensitive approaches to self-care also foster the health benefits of distributive justice (Daniels, Kennedy, & Kawachi, 1999) and, through secondary and tertiary prevention, have the potential to yield long-term cost savings (see Lorig et al., 1999). Finally, interventions and policies should account for the fundamental fact that self-care is but one component of the care continuum; as such, it should supplement rather than supplant informal and formal sources of care, particularly for persons who have complex needs and sparse resources.

SOCIAL WORK AND SELF-HEALTH CARE

In 1987, nearly 30,000 social workers worked full- or part-time with older adults. By 2020, a projected 60,000 to 70,000 social workers will be needed, with the greatest demands in health and aging (National Institute on Aging, 1987). In a recent Delphi study on setting national research priorities for geriatric social work, two expert panels—one of academic researchers, and the other of practitioners—identified chronic illness among the field's 10 most pressing concerns (Burnette, Morrow-Howell, & Chen, in press). As a core profession in the interdisciplinary fields of aging and health, social work makes a number of unique contributions to practice, policy, and research on self-care in late life.

First, social work's dual focus on person and environment provides an exceptional vantage point from which to identify and address the social, behavioral, and environmental sources of risk and resilience associated with chronic conditions. Social workers possess critical knowledge of complex psychosocial factors that can create and exacerbate risks and impede appropriate self-care, and they routinely assess informal and formal sources that can facilitate and support these practices. The profession's life-course perspective on human development also enables social workers to contribute to our understanding of the developmental nature of illness and self-care processes.

Second, because social workers are extensively involved in frontline service delivery to older adults and their families, they are optimally positioned to go beyond identifying problems to translate self-care research in applied practice and policy settings. Most social workers express a need for the knowledge and skills to work with older adults even though only a minority of them work solely in aging settings (Gibelman & Schervish, 1997). For example, in a National Association of Social Workers membership survey, more than three fifths of respondents indicated a need for aging knowledge (Peterson & Wendt, 1990). And in a Council on Social Work Education (2001) survey on practice competencies in aging, practitioner and academic respondents endorsed more than half of 65 competencies listed as needed by all social workers. Social workers thus play a key role in formulating best-practice guidelines for self-care with older adults and can implement and test these in both aging-specific and more generic health settings.

Third, many traditional functions of professional social work (e.g., assessment, information and referral, case management, patient education) and emerging consumer-informed and consumer-driven roles are highly commensurate with the basic elements of teaching, monitoring, and supporting appropriate self-care practices and identifying the need for professional care (Von Korff, Gruman, Schaefer, Curry, & Wagner, 1997). Social workers are also responsible to both employing social service agencies and funding sources for the efficient planning and delivery of cost-effective services. In considering social workers' vital role in containing spiraling health care costs, self-care can be seen as a key arena for immediate and long-term-cost containment.

Finally, social workers are exquisitely positioned to inform the development and delivery of ethnic-sensitive strategies for self-care and to inform research in this area. Professional social-work education stresses the influence of sociocultural and economic factors on social and health problems of diverse populations. Mastery of knowledge, skills, and values for effective practice with diverse individuals, families, small groups, and communities is an essential outcome of the educational process. Because social workers practice extensively with socially and economically disadvantaged elders, including members of ethnic minority groups, they are well-equipped to hone effective practice modalities with diverse clientele over time and to inform social work research on the crucial impact of social and cultural conditions and self-care practices on health status (see Pincus, Esther, De-Walt, & Callahan, 1998).

PRIOR RESEARCH AND KNOWLEDGE BASE

Epidemiological data provide information on morbidity, mortality, and disability, and social science research enhances understanding of the social and cultural aspects of illness and behavior and health service use (Dean, 1989). These knowledge bases, as they pertain to African American elders (the focus of this chapter), are reviewed next.

With respect to social science research, Clark and Gibson (1997) posit a chronic disease–disability continuum (based on Johnson & Wolinsky, 1993; Nagi, 1990; Patrick & Bergner, 1990; Vebrugge & Jette, 1994; Wilson & Clearly, 1995) that provides a useful heuristic for considering social, behavioral, and cultural influences in the disablement process. The starting point of the model is disease, the underlying pathology of which can lead to physiological impairment that can physically or emotionally limit functioning and may in turn produce disability. Each step in the continuum is also influenced by four interdependent factors—genetic endowment, culture, behavior, and social and physical environments—plus various resources. Disability is usually identified through biological and physiological evaluations and through cognitive and sensory assessments, often in the form of signs and symptoms. Once a condition is identified, a chief task for persons with a chronic condition is to minimize its progression and impact by managing symptomatic acute exacerbations and maintaining normal activities. Self-care is thus heavily influenced by perceptions of, and responses to, states of ill health as experienced and expressed through symptoms. Burnette's (2002) study, described later in this chapter, focuses on understanding how African American elders evaluate and respond to symptoms of chronic conditions and on how cultural, behavioral, and environmental factors and resources influence these processes.

Davis and Wykle (1998) note that the health attitudes, beliefs, and behaviors of African American elders stem from cultural history and from enduring social and economic inequalities in the formal health care system. In a discussion of Black folk medicine, they explain that many health beliefs and practices of older African Americans originated in West African and Caribbean cultures and in the American

South and are based on beliefs that disease and illness stem from natural (e.g., physical conditions such as adverse weather) and unnatural (e.g., evil spirits, bad luck, ill fate, or interpersonal conflict) causes. Such beliefs encourage the routine practice of self-care, including traditional folk remedies, as does limited access to high-quality formal care. Those people who have directly or vicariously experienced discriminatory practices in the health care system may be especially prone to delay or forgo seeking help from the formal health care system, even when needed.

CURRENT RESEARCH

We turn now to a study by one of the authors of this chapter (Burnette, 2002) that used a prospective health diary in conjunction with focus groups and a multidimensional health assessment interview to explore symptom-focused aspects of self-care for chronic health conditions in a sample of community-dwelling African American elders. Noting the narrow focus of most self-care research on the association of specific health behaviors and disease outcomes or on predictors of service use, Dean (1989) calls for innovative methodologies—specifically, prospective health diaries—to assess the daily complexities of illness experience and symptom management for various groups.

Health diary studies with older adults have examined preventive and symptom-related attitudes, beliefs, and behaviors and have been used fruitfully to explore correlates and patterns of self-care. Daily diaries offer an especially promising approach to underexamined questions of how non-White ethnic elders view their illnesses and manage the exigencies of these conditions in daily life (Becker, Beyene, Newsom, & Rodgers, 1998). We begin with an overview of the study, then present general findings and discuss how the project builds on and advances extant knowledge. Following Haug and colleagues (1989) and Stoller (1993), we explore self-care in terms of responses to perceived symptoms rather than preventive health behaviors.

This study explored self-care for symptoms of chronic health conditions in a nonprobability sample of 144 African American persons in the Harlem community of New York City. Respondents, who were 55 years of age or older and have at least one physician-diagnosed chronic condition, were recruited from three senior centers. Two initial focus groups comprising 6 and 8 African American elders were conducted at a fourth senior center to explore health attitudes, beliefs, and behaviors; clarify and address questions and concerns about the health assessment interview; and ensure the content and structure of the health diaries was relevant, feasible, and culturally sensitive. Four focus group members served as respondents in piloting the interview and diary instruments. Once finalized, two fully trained African American interviewers (one male and one female) who were indigenous to the community conducted the health interviews face-to-face upon study enrollment. This interview gathered information on sociodemographic characteristics and psychosocial and illness-related correlates of self-care (e.g., mental health, social support, health beliefs, service use, types and severity of conditions).

Interviewers then scheduled and administered a semistructured, symptom-focused 14-day health diary to assess participants' perceptions, interpretations, and responses to 26 symptoms of chronic conditions commonly experienced by older adults (Table 6.1; see Stoller, 1993). Of the 144 study participants, 129 (90%) completed the health diary. The interviewers collected the diary data in person during the late afternoon at senior centers on Monday through Friday. Respondents were asked to recall symptoms experienced during the previous 24 hours and to respond to a series of questions about each symptom (described later in this section). They recorded their own responses during the two weekends, then carefully reviewed these with the interviewers on Monday. The content and quality of data recorded by the interviewers and the participants were consistent. Sole reliance on self-recording would have been less expensive, but this option was rejected because the focus groups suggested that monitoring would be difficult and that issues such as vision problems and low literacy would be problematic for some respondents.

Sixty-two percent of the sample was female, their average age was 74.4 (SD = 8.3), and their average years of formal education was 11.2 (SD = 3.0). Sixty-four percent were born in the American South, and two thirds were living alone. Only 15% were married; 22% had never married, 33% were widowed, and 29% were divorced or separated. The average monthly family income was $1,024 ($MD$ = $800); 60% had annual incomes under $10,500.

Participants reported fairly good health overall, but about 40% rated their health fair or poor; about the same proportion reported functional limitations, and two thirds stated that pain interfered significantly with their usual activities. Respondents' overall mental health and

TABLE 6.1 Health Diary: Typical Frequency of Symptom Experience and Percentage of Experienced Symptom at Least 1 Day During 14-Day Diary Period

Aggregate Grid of Symptom Assessment

Symptom	Never	Occasionally	Often	Regularly	At least 1 day in 2-week diary period
1. Fever or chills	84.5	15.5	—	—	3.1
2. Runny nose	67.4	28.7	2.3	1.6	18.6
3. Sore throat	82.21	17.1	0.8	—	2.3
4. Cough	58.9	36.4	1.6	3.1	22.5
5. Shortness of breath	61.2	31.0	4.7	3.1	16.3
6. Chest pain	79.8	19.4	0.8	—	12.4
7. Heart palpitations	80.6	17.8	2.3	—	4.7
8. Swelling	72.9	18.6	2.3	6.2	19.4
9. Stomach pain	87.6	10.9	1.6	6.2	10.9
10. Nausea	87.6	12.4	—	—	2.3
11. Diarrhea	86.8	13.2	—	—	3.1
12. Constipation	63.6	28.7	3.1	4.7	11.7
13. Indigestion/gas	55.8	36.4	2.3	5.4	15.5
14. Rectal bleeding	96.1	3.9	—	—	0.8

(continued)

TABLE 6.1 (continued)

Symptom	Never	Occasionally	Often	Regularly	At least 1 day in 2-week diary period
		Aggregate Grid of Symptom Assessment			
15. Vision problems	51.9	31.8	7.0	9.3	25.6
16. Headache	76.0	21.7	1.6	0.8	11.6
17. Weakness/numbness	66.7	27.9	2.3	3.1	23.3
18. Fainting	97.7	2.3	—	—	0.8
19. Dizziness	81.4	17.8	—	0.8	11.6
20. Urination problems	67.4	20.2	7.0	3.9	15.5
21. Tiredness/fatigue	54.7	34.4	7.0	3.9	27.9
22. Falling	96.9	3.1	—	—	0.8
23. Muscle/joint pain	51.2	35.7	7.0	6.2	41.9
24. Sleep difficulties	73.4	14.8	6.3	5.5	15.5
25. Nervousness	75.2	20.9	0.8	3.1	10.9
26. Depression	73.6	20.9	3.1	2.3	7.8

Note: From "Self-care Responses to Symptoms of Older People," by E. P. Stoller, L. E. Forster, and S. Portugal, 1993, Medical Care, 31(1), pp. 40–42. Copyright 1993 by Medical Care. Adapted with permission of the author.

social supports appeared fair to good, but again, a sizeable minority reported problems in these critical domains. Health beliefs and attitudes (including health locus of control, self-reliance, and personal vulnerability in health) were all in the moderate range, and most respondents expressed a willingness to seek professional help for problems perceived to be potentially serious.

The health diary queried individuals about the daily incidence of 26 symptoms (Table 6.1) and about five specific dimensions of each symptom: perceived seriousness, pain or discomfort, interference with routine activities, causal attribution, and response to the symptom. The average number of symptoms reported over the 14-day period was three. As seen in Table 6.1, symptoms reported by at least 20% of diarists were (a) muscle and/or joint pain, (b) tiredness and/or fatigue, (c) vision problems, (d) weakness and/or numbness, and (e) cough. Few respondents interpreted their symptoms as definitely serious. However, virtually all experienced symptoms were reported to cause at least some pain or discomfort on at least 1 day of the diary period, and between two thirds and three quarters of persons who had diarrhea, dizziness, urination problems, or sleep difficulties noted that these symptoms interfered "some" or "a lot" with routine activities.

Causal attributions were conceptualized as medical or nonmedical; most respondents who had chest pain, swelling, stomach pain, vision problems, weakness and/or numbness, dizziness, urination problems, and muscle and/or joint pain attributed these to medical rather than nonmedical causes. Almost half of those with urinary difficulties attributed this problem to the aging process, as did one third of those who had constipation and tiredness and/or fatigue. With the exceptions of cough and depression, participants who sought help for symptoms appealed far more often to lay than professional sources.

Finally, behavioral responses to symptoms were categorized as (a) self-care (do nothing, or wait and see), prayer, over-the-counter medication, dietary home remedies, other home remedies, medication prescribed for others, stay in bed, cut back activities, read about symptoms, change behaviors, and pursue leisure activities); (b) medical care (medication prescribed for self, saw physician in emergency room or walk-in clinic, and saw physician in office); or (c) self-care plus medical care. Most respondents used self-care rather than professional care to manage their symptoms.

These data thus show a group of inner-city, community-dwelling African American elders who have fair to good physical, functional, and mental health and social supports. Their health attitudes and beliefs suggest a balance of internality and externality. And, consistent with literature reviewed above, the prospective health diaries show a propensity to use self-care rather than professional care, particularly for symptoms perceived as less serious, and to appeal to lay rather than medical sources for help managing their symptoms. Also noteworthy for intervention planning, diarists' perceptions, interpretations, and responses to symptoms varied considerably by symptom, and some symptoms that posed the greatest threat to daily activities (e.g., sleep and urinary difficulties) are very responsive to behavioral treatment.

This study advances knowledge about self-care in later life by providing fresh insights into how African American elders experience and respond to symptom-related illness experiences. It confirms the role of various psychosocial and illness-related facets of self-care and, through the use of a prospective health diary, it advances our knowledge of the complexities and symptom-specific features of managing the exigencies of chronic conditions in day-to-day life. It also demonstrates the feasibility and worth of combining methods of data collection to obtain a fuller picture of a phenomenon of interest.

FURTHER RESEARCH NEEDS

DeFriese, Ory, and Vickery (1998) note that although research on self-care has matured over the past quarter century, much room remains for systematic inquiry in all three domains of self-care, including health promotion and disease prevention, chronic disease and assistive care, and medical self-care. Together with findings from previous research, the current study suggests directions for future research on this topic in terms of developing more sophisticated, thoroughly integrated theories, research methodologies, and targeted interventions.

As noted in the introductory section, current interventions are based largely on psychological principles of individual change. Theoretical insights about readiness for change and processes of change could be enhanced by research on how health attitudes, beliefs, and behaviors develop over the life course and within the singular and combined contexts of family, community, and health care systems. Studies might also focus on variations in self-care across subgroups, whether in terms of setting (community, for example, home health, senior center, primary care, supported living) or institutional, for example, nursing home, rehabilitation; geographic area (rural, suburban, and urban); population subgroups (gender, ethnicity, and age cohort); or service delivery mechanism (different providers or types of health care organizations; DeFriese et al., 1998). Studies are also needed on (a) self-care for comorbid physical and mental health conditions, (b) decision-making processes (how conscious are self-care decisions? how symptom-specific? how modifiable?), and (c) pathways among changes in self-care behaviors and outcomes of interest.

DeFriese and colleagues (1998) further argue the need for a progression of research designs at multiple levels, including developmental and theory-based research, pilot and observational studies, and controlled studies and randomized clinical trials. Improved means of assessing and monitoring self-care (e.g., technological innovations such as beepers, hand-held devices, and telemetry) will improve reporting accuracy. Establishing standard measures of key variables, including outcomes, and common measuring points for self-care practices, will facilitate more systematic approaches to understanding self-care processes. Prohaska (1998) also highlights the need for increased attention to recruitment and attrition in self-care studies. Knowing who does not get recruited and who fails to go beyond the early stages of change would enable practitioners to target precise stages of self-care and to specify subgroups to target at various stages.

Intervention studies should explore variable mixes of level and types of self-care for specific conditions, symptoms, behavioral risk factors, and so forth and combinations of self-care, informal care, and professional care. Building on a growing body of knowledge on individual behavioral responses to illness and symptoms, researchers will also do well to develop and test specific interventions that enhance the acquisition and maintenance of appropriate self-care knowledge, attitudes, and skills. Additional knowledge is also needed about the development and dissemination of informational and instructional materials for self-care, which have been shown to be effective in improving functional outcomes and lowering health care utilization costs (DeFriese et al., 1998).

Finally, there is much to be learned from research on complementary and alternative medicine (CAM) and traditional healing approaches in self-care. For example, in a study to assess predictors and patterns of CAM therapy use by older adults, Astin, Pelletier, Marie, and Haskell (2000) assessed 728 Californians enrolled in a Medicare risk program that covered acupuncture and chiropractics. Forty-one percent of respondents reported using CAM therapies (chiropractic services, 20%; acupuncture, 14%; herbs, 24%; and massage, 15%); and 80% noted benefits of these therapies—yet 58% did not discuss their use with their physicians. Research is thus needed to better understand older adults' use of complementary and alternative methods of self-care, the effectiveness of such approaches, and their interface with more traditional treatment modalities.

POLICY IMPLICATIONS

Inasmuch as the main goal of self-care is to maintain functioning and independence, its potential to enhance the long-term social and health independence of older adults, and hence its national policy significance, is substantial. The quality and costs of health care associated with chronic health conditions is, of course, the most obvious policy arena relevant to issues of self-care. As DeFriese and colleagues (1998) note, apart from policies and programs directed at individual, lay decision making, there is an emerging call to incorporate self-care more broadly within organizational and societal efforts to restructure health care systems. To do so would at once acknowledge the centrality of self-care in health and further construe it as a possible means to effectively manage the ever-increasing demand for expensive health care services. Adequate reimbursement mechanisms for teaching and monitoring self-care could, for example, prevent premature morbidity and disability and inappropriate hospitalizations and emergency visits.

   A major policy question in the field of self-care is the appropriate site for education and practice (DeFriese et al., 1998). These functions might be reasonably incorporated as core services in community-based health delivery systems, such as home health and outpatient clinics. Providing these services in clinical settings means, however, that these skills must be incorporated into the professional education of providers and that policy practice research on self-care would do well to examine systematically the implications of service delivery in these and other settings.

   Managed care programs increasingly include older adults, and behavioral health has emerged as a major focus of health promotion, prevention, and disease management under managed care plans. The development and implementation of policies governing self-care for older adults must therefore be guided by empirical knowledge about correlates and patterns of self-care for various diseases and for people at different life stages and from sociocultural backgrounds. Policies that deliberately seek to reduce health disparities by targeting high-risk populations, including older African American persons, are especially critical.

Finally, Medicare coverage of prescription medications and the expansion of state and local coverage (e.g., through Medicaid and the New York City Elder Pharmaceutical Insurance Coverage) to include effective over-the-counter drugs, proven complementary and alternative treatments, and appropriate assistive devices for enhanced functioning are vital policy issues for self-care in later life.

INTEGRATING KNOWLEDGE INTO THE CURRICULUM

Evidentiary knowledge about self-care for chronic health conditions in later life is now sufficiently developed to suggest several points for inclusion in social work curricula. A first point of established knowledge is that self-care in combination with, and supported by, informal and formal sources of care is a major component of the care continuum for chronic health conditions. Second, knowledge is growing about various types and classes of correlates of self-care that can facilitate and impede older adults' acquisition of knowledge and skills for appropriate self-care. These include personal factors (e.g., gender, race and ethnicity, educational attainment); social, psychological, economic, and environmental conditions (e.g., health beliefs and attitudes, social supports, depression, income); and illness-related factors (e.g., diagnoses, severity, duration, level of related impairment). And third, behavioral change, including changes needed for appropriate self-care, occurs incrementally and can be facilitated and sustained through educational and supportive interventions.

Content on these key knowledge points about self-health care could be readily introduced and integrated into social work curricula in several ways. Organizing themes that transcend curricular areas are (a) health and illness as developmental processes over the life course, (b) family and community contexts of self-care, and (c) sociocultural influences on health and illness. And, more specific topics could be introduced in both foundational and advanced, specialized courses.

First, and perhaps most generally, fostering self-help and autonomy is a core practice concept across fields of practice and client populations. Older adults are often portrayed as frail and dependent due to multiple chronic health conditions. Enhancing students' understanding of self-care is an effective way to demonstrate that most older adults are self-directed, autonomous decision-makers who are capable of mastering even complex care regimens to stabilize and improve their own health and functional status.

Principles and methods for improving clients' self-care capacities through knowledge and skills enhancement could be taught in generic or health- or aging-specific practice courses and could focus on evidence-based interventions at the individual, group, and community levels. Client-centered psychoeducation models that facilitate and support decision making and behavioral change have a particularly strong empirical base.

Self-care as a psychological and sociocultural concept related to autonomy, independence, and empowerment might be introduced in human-behavior and social-environment courses. Developmental, risk and resilience, and systems models would be especially useful. A developmental life-course approach, for example, could further students' understanding of how epidemiological and social scientific aspects of chronic health conditions are a function of individual lives in the context of larger social forces over time and are outcomes of life-long sources of risk and resilience, including those associated with race, ethnicity, and gender (see Wykle & Haug, 1993). Students might be asked to conduct a life-history narrative of personal or family health, either their own or that of a client system.

Research on self-care could also provide instructive illustrations in research courses. Methodological issues might include sampling (community versus health-system based samples); measurement (triangulation of data types and sources, ethnic-sensitive norms and psychometrics, rapid assessment instruments, scales and indices for attitudinal and behavioral measures); and data collection (ethnographic studies, qualitative health interviews, standardized assessment instruments). Students might be assigned the task of developing a rapid assessment instrument to screen for acceptable levels of self-care for a specific condition.

Finally, knowledge about self-care might be incorporated into social policy courses in the context of health policy or long-term-care policy. Relevant topics might be costs and benefits of various service delivery models and methods of reimbursement for supporting self-care (e.g., consumer-health education programs, assistance with monitoring care); and determining the optimal balance of nonmedical and complementary and alternative supports for self-care. Exploration of appropriate venues and providers for such services would also be important, as would costs and benefits of self-care alone versus self-care and various configurations of informal and formal sources of care. Students might be asked, for example, to examine national, state, or local health statistics to assess the epidemiology of a specific chronic condition, its expected future course, and the self-care requirements for managing that condition.

CONCLUSION

As the nation ages in the coming decades, long-term, incurable conditions will continue to characterize the health problems of most Americans. Practitioners, policy makers, and researchers must collaborate across disciplines and with consumers on the planning and delivery of effective, equitable health and social services to support both the prevention and management of these conditions. There is growing attention to the need to better understand the principles and processes of self-care, which is increasingly viewed as a practical, effective, and relatively inexpensive means to improve quality of life and contain health care costs among older adults.

Social work has a pivotal role to play in the current movements toward managed health care, consumer-driven and collaborative service-delivery models, renewed emphasis on personal responsibility, and recognition of the importance of self-care as a critical adjunct of professional care. Social workers are proximal to the health experiences of older adults, particularly those at high risk for chronic illnesses and poor health outcomes across a wide range of settings. As noted, for example, health professionals know that African Americans are particularly disadvantaged in terms of chronic conditions and disabilities in early old age, that hypertension and diabetes are particularly troublesome, and that the main health concerns of this population are excessive functional impairment and disability. Professional knowledge and skills enable social workers to provide key services for initiating and monitoring self-care for these and other older adults, and social work strengths in these areas will be enhanced through active partnerships with providers from other professions.

As health professionals work collaboratively to advance theoretical knowledge, improve methodological sophistication, and develop effective practical applications of self-care in the lives of older adults with chronic disabling conditions, they will do well to aim for strategies that will maximize functional independence and health-related quality of life.

REFERENCES

Ajzen, I., & Fishbein, M. (1980). *Understanding attitudes and predicting social behavior.* Englewood Cliffs, NJ: Prentice Hall.

Astin, J. A., Pelletier, K. R., Marie, A., & Haskell, W. L. (2000). Complementary and alternative medicine use among elderly persons: One-year analysis of a Blue Shield Medicare supplement. *Journals of Gerontology, 55,* M4–M9.

Bandura, A. (1977). Self efficacy: Toward a unifying theory of behavioral change. *Psychological Review, 84,* 191–215.

Barke, C., & Nicholas, D. (1990). Physical activity in older adults: The stages of change. *Journal of Applied Gerontology, 9,* 216–223.

Becker, G., Beyene, Y., Newsom, E. M., & Rodgers, D. V. (1998). Knowledge and care of chronic illness in three ethnic minority groups. *Family Medicine, 30*(3), 173–178.

Burnette, D. (2002). *Self-care by urban, African American elders.* Unpublished manuscript. Columbia University School of Social Work, New York.

Burnette, D., Morrow-Howell, N., & Chen, L. M. (in press). Setting research priorities for gerontological social work: A national Delphi study. *Gerontologist.*

Clark, D. O., & Gibson, R. C. (1997). Race, age, chronic disease, and disability. In K. Markides & M. Miranda (Eds.), *Minorities, aging, and health* (pp. 107–126). Thousand Oaks, CA: Sage.

Clark, M., Kviz, F., Prohaska, T., Crittendon, K., & Warnecke, R. (1995). Readiness of older adults to stop smoking in a televised intervention. *Journal of Aging and Health, 7,* 119–138.

Council on Social Work Education. (2001). *Strengthening the impact of social work to improve the quality of life for older adults and their families: A blueprint for the new millennium.* Alexandria, VA: Author.

Daniels, N., Kennedy, B. P., & Kawachi, I. (1999). Why justice is good for our health: The social determinants of health inequalities. *Daedalus, 128*(4), 215–251.

Davis, L., & Wykle, M. L. (1998). Self-care in minority and ethnic populations: The experience of older black Americans. In M. G. Ory & G. H. DeFriese (Eds.), *Self-care in later life* (pp. 170–179). New York: Springer.

Dean, K. (1986a). Self-care behavior: Implications for aging. In K. Dean, T. Hickey, & B. E. Holstein (Eds.), *Self-care and health in old age* (pp. 58–93). London: Croom Helm.

Dean K. (1986b). Lay care in illness. *Social Science & Medicine, 22,* 275–284.

Dean, K. (1989). Conceptual, theoretical, and methodological issues in self-care research. *Social Science & Medicine, 29,* 117–123.

DeFriese, G. H., Ory, M., & Vickery, D. M. (1998). Toward a research agenda for addressing the potential of self-care in later life. In M. G. Ory & G. H. DeFriese (Eds.), *Self-care in later life: Research, program, and policy issues* (pp. 193–199). New York: Springer.

DeFriese, G. H., Woomert, A., Guild, P. A., Steckler, A. B., & Konrad, T. R. (1989). From activated patient to pacified activist: A study of the self-care movement in the United States. *Social Science & Medicine, 29,* 195–204.

Eisenberg, D. M., Kessler, R. C., Goster, C., Norlock, F. E., Calkins, D. R., & Delbanco, T. L. (1993). Unconventional medicine in the United States. *New England Journal of Medicine, 328,* 246–252.

Gibelman, M., & Schervish, P. (1997). *Who are we? A second look.* Washington, DC: National Association of Social Workers.

Guralnik, J. M., LaCroix, A. Z., Abbott, R. D., Berkman, L. F., Satterfield, S., Evans, D. A., et al. (1993). Maintaining mobility in late life. *American Journal of Epidemiology, 137,* 845–868.

Haug, M. R., Wykle, M. L., & Namazi, K. H. (1989). Self-care among older adults. *Social Science & Medicine, 29,* 171–183.

Hickey, T., Akiyama, H., & Rakowski, W. (1991). Daily illness characteristics and health care decisions of older people. *Journal of Applied Gerontology, 10*(2), 169–184.

Hoffman, C., & Rice, D. P. (1996). *Chronic care in America: A 21st century challenge.* Princeton, NJ: The Robert Wood Johnson Foundation.

Johnson, R. J., & Wolinsky, F. D. (1993). The structure of health status among older adults: Disease, functional limitations, and perceived health. *Journal of Health and Social Behavior, 34,* 105–121.

Leventhal, E. A., Leventhal, H., & Robitaille, C. (1998). Enhancing self-care research: Exploring the theoretical underpinnings of self-care. In M. G. Ory & G. H. DeFriese (Eds.), *Self-care in later life: Research, program, and policy issues* (pp. 118–141). New York: Springer.

Levin, L., Katz, A., & Holst, E. (1976). *Self care: Lay initiatives in health.* New York: Prodist.

Lorig, K. R., Sobel, D. S., Stewart, A. L., Brown, B. W., Jr., Bandura, A., Ritter, P., et al. (1999). Evidence suggesting that a chronic disease self-management program can improve health status while reducing hospitalization: A randomized trial. *Medical Care, 37*(1), 5–14.

Markides, K. S., & Miranda, M. R. (1997). Minorities, aging, and health: An overview. In K. S. Markides & M. R. Miranda (Eds.), *Minorities, aging and health* (pp. 1–11). Thousand Oaks, CA: Sage.

Meichenbaum, D. (1977). *Cognitive-behavior modification: An integrative approach.* New York: Plenum Press.

Morrongiello, B. A., & Gottlieb, B. H. (2000). Self-care among older adults. *Canadian Journal on Aging, 19*(Suppl. 1), 32–57.

Nagi, S. Z. (1990). Disability concepts revisited: Implications for prevention. In A. M. Pope & A. R. Tarlov (Eds.), *Disability in America: A national agenda for prevention* (Appendix A, pp. 309–327). Washington, DC: National Academy Press.

National Institute on Aging. (1987). *Personnel for health needs of the elderly through the year 2020.* Bethesda, MD: Department of Health and Human Services, Public Health Service.

National Institute on Aging. (2000, August). *Strategic plan to address health disparities: Fiscal years 2000–2005.* Washington, DC: Author.

Ory, M. G., DeFriese, G. H., & Duncker, A. P. (1998). Introduction: The nature, extent, and modifiability of self-care behaviors in later life. In M. G. Ory & G. H. DeFriese (Eds.), *Self-care in later life: Research, program, and policy issues* (pp. xv–xviii). New York: Springer.

Patrick, D. L., & Bergner, M. (1990). Measurement of health status in the 1990s. *Annual Review of Public Health, 11,* 165–183.

Peterson, D. A., & Wendt, P. F. (1990). Employment in the field of aging: A survey of professionals in four fields. *Gerontologist, 30,* 679–684.

Pincus, T., Esther, R., DeWalt, D. A., & Callahan, L. F. (1998). Social conditions and self-management are more powerful determinants of health than access to care. *Annals of Internal Medicine, 129,* 406–411.

Prohaska, T. (1998). The research basis for the design and implementation of self-care programs. In M. G. Ory & G. H. DeFriese (Eds.), *Self-care in later life: Research, program, and policy issues* (pp. 62–84). New York: Springer.

Prohaska, T., & DiClemente, C. (1983). Stages and processes of self-change in smoking: Toward an integrative model of change. *Journal of Consulting and Clinical Psychology, 5,* 390–395.

Rosenstock, I. M. (1966). Why people use health services. *Milbank Memorial Fund Quarterly, 44,* 94ff.

Stearns, S. C., Bernard, S. L., Fasick, S. B., Schwartz, R., Konrad, R., Ory, M. G., et al. (2000). Economic implications of self-care: The effect of lifestyle, functional adaptations, and medical self-care among a national sample of Medicare beneficiaries. *American Journal of Public Health, 90,* 1608–1612.

Stoller, E. P. (1993). Interpretations of symptoms by older people: A health diary study of illness behavior. *Journal of Aging and Health, 5*(1), 58–81.

Verbrugge, L. M., & Jette, A. M. (1994). The disablement process. *Social Science & Medicine, 38,* 1–14.

Von Korff, M., Gruman, J., Schaefer, J., Curry, S. J., & Wagner, E. H. (1997). Collaborative management of chronic illness. *Annals of Internal Medicine, 127,* 1097–1102.

Wilson, I. B., & Cleary, P. D. (1995). Linking clinical variables with health related quality of life. *Journal of the American Medical Association, 273,* 59–65.

Wykle, M. L., & Haug, M. R. (1993). Multicultural and social-class aspects of self-care. *Generations, Fall,* 25–28.

APPENDIX A

Selected Bibliography for Self-Care

Backett, K. C., & Davison, C. (1995). Lifecourse and lifestyle: The social and cultural location of health behaviors. *Social Science & Medicine, 49,* 629–638.

Becker, G., Beyene, Y., Newsom, E. M., & Rodgers, D. V. (1998). Knowledge and care of chronic illness in three ethnic minority groups. *Family Medicine, 30*(3), 173–178.

Belgrave, L. (1990). The relevance of chronic illness in the everyday lives of elderly women. *Journal of Aging and Health, 2,* 475–500.

Bernard, M. (2000). *Promoting health in old age: Critical issues in self-care.* Buckingham, England: Open University Press.

Center for the Advancement of Health. (1999). *How managed care can help older persons live well with chronic conditions.* Washington, DC: Author.

Clark, N. M., Becker, M. H., Janz, N. K., Lorig, K., Rakowski, W., & Anderson, L. (1991). Self-management of chronic disease by older adults: A review and questions for research. *Journal of Aging and Health, 3*(1), 3–27.

Clark, M. C., & Lester, J. (2000). The effect of video-based interventions on self-care. *Western Journal of Nursing Research, 22,* 895–911.

Coulton, C. J. (1990). Ethnicity, self-care, and use of medical care among the elderly with joint symptoms. *Arthritis Care and Research, 3*(1), 19–28.

Dean, K. (1986). Self-care behavior: Implications for aging. In K. Dean, T. Hickey, & B. E. Holstein (Eds.), *Self-care and health in old age* (pp. 58–93). London: Croom Helm.

Dean, K. (1986). Lay care in illness. *Social Science and Medicine, 22,* 275–284.

Dean, K. (1989). Conceptual, theoretical, and methodological issues in self-care research. *Social Science and Medicine, 29,* 117–123.

Dean, K., Hickey, T., & Holstein, B. E. (1986). *Self-care and health in old age: Health behaviour implications for policy and practice.* London: Croom Helm.

DeFriese, G. H., & Konrad, T. (1993). The self-care movement and the gerontological health care professional. *Generations, 20,* 37–40.

DeFriese, G. H., Woomert, A., Guild, P. A., Steckler, A. B., & Konrad, T. R. (1989). From activated patient to pacified activist: A study of the self-care movement in the United States. *Social Science and Medicine, 29,* 195–204.

Dill, A., Brown, P., Ciambrone, D., & Rakowski, W. (1995). The meaning and practice of self-care by older adults: A qualitative assessment. *Research on Aging, 17*(1), 8–41.

Edwardson, S. R., & Dean, K. (1999). Appropriateness of self-care responses to symptoms among elders: Identifying pathways of influence. *Research in Nursing and Health, 22,* 329–339.

Edwardson, S. R., Dean, K., & Brauer, D. (1995). Symptom consultation in lay networks in an elderly population. *Journal of Aging and Health, 7,* 402–416.

Haug, M. R., Wykle, M. L., & Namazi, K. H. (1989). Self-care among older adults. *Social Science and Medicine, 29*, 171–183.

Health Canada, Health Promotion and Programs Branch. (1998). *Supporting self-care: The contribution of nurses and physicians: An exploratory study*. Ottawa, Canada: Minister of Public Workers and Government Services.

Health Canada, Health Promotion and Programs Branch. (1998). *Supporting self-care: Perspectives of nurse and physician educators: An exploratory study*. Ottawa, Canada: Minister of Public Workers and Government Services.

Hickey, T., Akiyama, H., & Rakowski, W. (1991). Daily illness characteristics and health care decisions of older people. *Journal of Applied Gerontology, 10*(2), 169–184.

Holtzman, J. M., Akiyama, H., & Maxwell, A. J. (1986). Symptoms and self-care in old age. *Journal of Applied Gerontology, 5*, 183–200.

Kart, C. S., & Dunkle, R. E. (1989). Assessing capacity for self-care among the aged. *Journal of Aging and Health, 1*, 430–450.

Kart, C. S., & Engler, C. A. (1994). Predisposition to self-health care: Who does what for themselves and why? *Journal of Gerontology: Social Sciences, 49*, S301–S308.

Kart, C. S., & Engler, C. A. (1995). Self-health care among the elderly: A test of the health behavior model. *Research on Aging, 17*, 434–458.

Kemper, D., Lorig, K., & Mettler, M. (1993). The effectiveness of medical self-care interventions: A focus on self-initiated responses to symptoms. *Patient Education and Counseling, 21*, 29–39.

Klonoff, E., & Landrine, H. (1994). Culture and gender diversity in commonsense beliefs about the causes of six illnesses. *Journal of Behavioral Medicine, 17*, 407–418.

McDonald-Miszczak, L., Wister, A. V., & Gutman, G. M. (2001). Self-care among older adults: An analysis of the objective and subjective illness contexts. *Journal of Aging and Health, 13*(1), 120–145.

Morrongiello, B. A., & Gottlieb, B. H. (2000). Self-care among older adults. *Canadian Journal on Aging, 19*(Suppl. 1), 32–57.

Musil, C. M., Ahn, S., Haug, M., Warner, C., Morris, D., & Duffy, E. (1998). Health problems and health actions among community-dwelling older adults: Results of a health diary study. *Applied Nursing Research, 11*(3), 138–147.

Norburn, J. E. K., Bernard, S. L., Konrad, R. R., Woomert, A., DeFriese, G. H., Kalsbeek, W. D., et al. (1995). Self-care and assistance from others in coping with functional status limitations among a national sample of older adults. *Journal of Gerontology: Social Sciences, 50B*, S101–S109.

Ory, M. G., & DeFriese, G. H. (Eds.). (1998). *Self-care in later life: Research, program, and policy issues*. New York: Springer.

Penning, M., & Chappell, N. (1990). Self-care in relation to informal and formal care. *Ageing and Society, 10*(1), 41–59.

Rakowski, W., Julius, M., Hickey, T., Verbrugge, L. M., & Halter, J. B. (1988). Daily symptoms and behavioral responses: Results of a health diary with older adults. *Medical Care, 26*, 278–297.

Roelands, M., Van Oost, P., Depoorter, A., & Buysse, A. (2002). A social-cognitive model to predict the use of assistive devices for mobility and self-care in elderly people. *Gerontologist, 42*, 39–50.

Stearns, S. C., Bernard, S. L., Fasick, S. B., Schwartz, R., Konrad, R., Ory, M. G., et al. (2000). Economic implications of self-care: The effect of lifestyle, functional adaptations, and medical self-care among a national sample of Medicare beneficiaries. *American Journal of Public Health, 90,* 1608–1612.

Stoller, E. P. (1993). Interpretations of symptoms by older people: A health diary study of illness behavior. *Journal of Aging and Health, 5*(1), 58–81.

Stoller, E. P., Forster, L. E., & Portugal, S. (1993). Self-care responses to symptoms by older people: A health diary study of illness behavior. *Medical Care, 31*(1), 24–42.

Stoller, E., Kart, C., & Portugal, S. (1997). Explaining pathways of care taken by elderly people: An analysis of responses to illness symptoms. *Sociological Focus, 30*(2), 147–165.

Strain, L. A. (1996). Lay explanations of chronic illness in later life. *Journal of Aging and Health, 8*(1), 3–26.

Verbrugge, L. M. (1985). Triggers of symptoms and health care. *Social Science & Medicine, 20,* 855–876.

Woomert, A. (1998). Appendix: Self-care in later life—An annotated bibliography of research findings and policy issues. In M. G. Ory & G. H. DeFriese (Eds.), *Self-care in later life: Research, program, and policy issues* (pp. 200–257). New York: Springer.

World Health Organization. (1983, November 21–25). *Health education in self-care: Possibilities and limitations.* Report of a scientific consultation, Geneva, Switzerland.

Wykle, M. L., & Haug, M. R. (1993, Fall). Multicultural and social-class aspects of self-care. *Generations,* 25–28.

Chapter 7

PHYSICAL HEALTH AND ECONOMIC WELL-BEING OF OLDER AFRICAN AMERICAN WOMEN: TOWARD STRATEGIES OF EMPOWERMENT

Letha A. Chadiha and Portia Adams

The physical health status and economic well-being of older Black women are complex interwoven issues of substantial import to gerontology and social work, because a disproportionate number of older Black women will live most of their aged years with a chronic illness and in poverty. *Health* has been defined by the World Health Organization as a "complex state of physical, mental, and social well-being" and not just disease absence (Johnson & Misra, 2001, p. 104). It also has been defined as "a complex and multi-determined issue, influenced by a wide variety of factors," both internal and external to people (Rodin & Ickovics, 1990, p. 1018). This chapter will provide empirical evidence supporting both definitions of health. For example, improved physical health of older Black women may depend, in part, upon their self-empowerment to prevent disease or delay its onset. Or improved health may depend on governmental support through policies for better health services, flexibility of hours, economic issues of pay equity, and expanded health insurance coverage. Our discussion is guided by the work of Grason, Minkovitz, Misra, and Strobino (2001). These researchers have expanded the biomedical model of health, which focuses on prevention, detection, and treatment of disease, to include social factors such as age, race and ethnicity, women's status, social class, and caregiving roles.

SIGNIFICANCE TO GERONTOLOGY, HEALTH CARE, AND HEALTH PROFESSIONALS

The minority elderly population (aged 65 years and older)—designated as Black or African American, Asian and Pacific Islander, Hispanic, and American Indians/Alaskan Native—is 16.4% of all elderly people (U.S. Bureau of the Census, 2001). (The words Black and African American are used interchangeably.) According to this estimate, older Blacks comprised one half (8.2%) of the minority elderly population (Administration on Aging, 2001). Women comprised the largest share of the Black elderly population. The gender ratio is an indicator of the greater number of older women in the Black population. In 1995, for example, there were 71 Black men per 100 Black women for the young-old group, those aged 65 to 74 years (Siegel, 1994). There were only 40 Black men per 100 Black women for the older Black age group, those aged 85 years and older. The low ratio of men to women in old age is due, in part, to a lower life expectancy rate among Black men (Siegel, 1994). Also, older Black women, like older women in the general population, owe their greater representation in the elderly Black population, in part, to a dramatic leap in life expectancy over the past century (Ephraim, Misra, Nguyen, & Vahratian, 2001). In 1900, the life expectancy at birth for Black women, Black men, White women, and White men was 33.5 years, 32.5 years, 48.7 years, and 46.6 years respectively (Ephraim, Misra, Nguyen, et al., 2001). Fifty years later, all four groups showed significant gains in life expectancy—Black women at 62.7 years, Black men at 58.9 years, White women at 72.2 years, and White men at 66.5 years. Toward the end of the twentieth century, there were even greater gains in life expectancy for all groups: Black women at 74.8 years, Black men at 67.6 years, White women at 80.8 years, and White men at 74.5 years.

Although the gap in life expectancy had closed between Black women and White men, Black women's life expectancy lagged 6 years behind White women's (Mouton, 1997). Despite improvements in overall health and socioeconomic status (SES) of older Black women over the past century, the quality of their physical health and SES has yet to achieve parity with non-Hispanic White women's physical health and SES (Grason et al., 2001). Because of inadequate research on mental health conditions in the Black elderly population, particularly at the national level (Johnson & Misra, 2001), we have not included these conditions in this chapter.

There is growing evidence that the physical health of older Black women depends upon a complex set of interrelated social factors such as age, race, gender, class, and social roles (e.g., caregiving). Empowerment literature suggests that improving the health status of older Black women will require social workers to not only use a multilevel practice approach that targets individual needs, but also to seek to empower these women through sociopolitical change (Gutierrez, 1990; Lee, 2001). *Empowerment,* according to Cox and Parsons (1996), is "a process through which individuals and groups become strong enough to participate within, share in the control of, and influence events and institutions affecting their lives" (p. 130). Critical elements in the empowerment process include education, mutual support, self-help, consciousness raising, collective action, coalition building, and resource mobilization (Cox & Parsons, 1996; Gutierrez, 1990; Lee, 2001; Solomon, 1976). In addition to building people's capacity through mobilizing resources to change deleterious environments, empowerment practice that builds coalitions with clients and other health professions may facilitate both practice and policy with older Black women.

Social work, as a field of study, considers both prevention and intervention to be of import to clients' well-being. Fried (1996) has noted that "clinical preventive health care is highly revelant to the health status and care needs of older adults" (p. 176). As clinicians and service providers, social workers are able to influence the physical health of older Black women through services offered in both the social service and health sectors. It is well established that social workers play a major role in providing services to older people (Rosen & Zlotnik, 2001). As helping professionals, social workers are involved with older adults on multiple levels of practice (e.g., with elders and their families, agencies, government). Thus, social workers are placed in an ideal position to help facilitate effective prevention and intervention strategies that will enhance the physical health and SES in older Black women.

PRIOR RESEARCH AND KNOWLEDGE BASE

Ephraim, Misra, Nguyen, et al. (2001) have defined a *chronic condition* as one requiring periodic medical attention or medication or both. Chronic physical health conditions are the major cause of illness, disability, and mortality in the U.S. population (Ephraim, Misra, Nguyen, et al., 2001; National Academy on an Aging Society [NAAS], 1999). In ranked order, a list of chronic conditions for Black women between the ages of 45 and 74 included hypertension, arthritis, sinusitis, orthopedic impairments, and diabetes (NAAS, 1999).

An assessment of a person's physical health over the life span involves the rate of mortality, prevalence of chronic disease and illness, and life expectancy. The *Women's Health Data Book* (Ephraim, Misra, Nguyen, et al., 2001) documented the death rate for women from the 10 leading causes of death in 1998 and reported that the mortality rate for women varied by race and ethnicity, as well as by age. The death rate per 100,000 for older women aged 65 or older, in the categories of "all causes" and for some specific causes of death (i.e., malignant neoplasms, heart diseases, cerebrovascular diseases, and diabetes), was higher for older Black women than for older non-Hispanic White women or Hispanic women. In contrast, death rates for accidents and adverse effects, pulmonary diseases and allied conditions, and pneumonia and influenza were lower for older Black women than they were for older non-Hispanic White women.

Among older Black women aged 65 and older, heart disease was the number one cause of death in the United States in 1998 (Ephraim, Misra, Nguyen, et al., 2001). Older Black women were more likely than White or Hispanic women to die from heart disease. Statistically, older Black women had a death rate from heart disease of 1,799.1 per 100,000 compared to 1,671.9 and 959.8 per 100,000 for White and Hispanic women, respectively.

Hypertension, a major risk factor for heart disease for women, is the most common chronic condition for Black women. Chronic conditions vary more by gender than race across the life span, although certain chronic conditions are more associated with race and age than others. According to the NAAS (2000e), more elderly women than elderly men have hypertension: 63% of the elderly population with hypertension are women. More Blacks than Whites across the age span have hypertension. The greatest race divergence on the prevalence of hypertension is found in persons aged 55 to 64 years old, where twice as many Blacks as Whites have hypertension. The rate of hypertension for Blacks decreases for 65- to 74-year olds and rises again for those 75 years old and older. Because the Black elderly population is composed of women disproportionately and more women than men will live to be 75 years old, hypertension is of considerable import for older Black women.

Besides hypertension, other known risk factors for heart disease include menopause, diabetes, high cholesterol, overweight, lack of physical activity, and smoking cigarettes. Black women through the course of life are at high risk for heart disease, in part because of a high rate of hypertension, diabetes, and obesity and a low level of physical activity (Leigh & Lindquist, 1998). Older persons tend to engage in lower levels of physical activity (Brownson et al., 2000; Crespo, Smit, Andersen, Carter-Pokras, & Ainsworth, 2000; Young, Miller, Wilder, Yanek, & Becker, 1998). Evidence indicates that older Black, Hispanic, and Asian American women may engage in less physical exercise than older White women (Ephraim, Misra, Strobino, & Vahratian, 2001). Physical activity can reduce not only a woman's risk of heart disease but also her risk of osteoporosis and obesity (Ephraim, Misra, Strobino, et al., 2001). However, osteoporosis, a preventable condition in old age, may be affecting older Black women because of the lack of knowledge, the misinformation about risk factors (Huff & Sadler, 1997), and the failure to engage in high levels of physical activity (Ephraim, Misra, Strobino, et al., 2001; Wilcox, Castro, King, Housemann, & Brownson, 2000). Young and older Black women are less likely than young and older White women to report smoking cigarettes; consequently, cigarette smoking is not considered a high risk factor for older Black women (Ephraim, Misra, Strobino, et al., 2001). The role that genetic or biological factors may play in heart disease among older Black women has been neither confirmed nor refuted (Landrine & Klonoff, 1992).

Diabetes mellitus is more common among older women of color than among older White women (Ephraim, Misra, Nguyen, et al., 2001), and more older Black than older White women will die from diabetes or related diabetes complications (McNabb, Quinn, & Tobian,

1997). Statistically, among women aged 60 to 74, Black (32.4%) and Hispanic women (32.5%) are twice as likely to have diabetes as White women are (16.0%) (Ephraim, Misra, Nguyen, et al., 2001). According to McNabb and colleagues (1997), Black women older than age 50 are more likely to have non-insulin-dependent diabetes, by far the most common type of diabetes affecting Black women in their late adult years. Risk factors for diabetes in Black women include race, gender, age, genetics, obesity, low physical inactivity, SES, urban residence, and institutional racism in disease diagnosis. Diabetes can lead to other health complications such as kidney disease, eye disease, lower extremity vascular disease, and heart or coronary artery disease (McNabb et al., 1997). Diabetes, according to McNabb and colleagues, is a serious public health issue for African Americans because of late diagnosis and high treatment costs. Screening for diabetes and developing "community-based lifestyle modification programs" may prevent or delay the early onset of the disease (McNabb et al., 1997, p. 290).

Breast cancer is the most frequently occurring female malignancy among U.S. women (Dignam, 2000). National data show that breast cancer incidence is greater among White women than Black women; however, more Black women than White women die from breast cancer (Chu, Tarone, & Brawley, 1999). Breast cancer mortality rates decreased in the last decade for White women but not for Black women (Chu et al., 1999; Dignam, 2000). During a time when early detection through mammography screening and advances in treatment have contributed to improved survival rates of breast cancer, Black women, particularly those aged 70 or older, have lower survival rates (Chu et al., 1999). Since the early 1980s, decreasing age-specific breast cancer mortality rates were reported by Chu and colleagues for Black and White women across two age groups: those younger (aged 30–39) and those older (aged 40–69). However, for Black women aged 70+, cancer mortality rates began to increase around 1987 and this trend continued through the 1990s, the latest time period for which breast cancer data was reported. Older Black women are less likely to report having a mammogram, as compared with relatively younger Black women or White women of any age group (Leigh & Lindquist, 1998). Thus, older Black women may be less likely to benefit from increased early detection of breast cancer by mammography and improved breast cancer treatment therapy, factors contributing to higher breast cancer survival rates among White women.

Although research has documented continuing racial disparities in health and mortality rates from heart disease for Black and White women, evidence by Chu and colleagues (1999) has indicated a narrowing of the race gap for deaths from breast cancer. These researchers found that Black and White women baby-boomers (those born after 1946) had similar breast cancer mortality rates, thus suggesting a convergence in declining mortality from breast cancer among this birth cohort. Despite a narrowing of the gap in breast cancer mortality among baby boomers, the overall situation with high breast cancer mortality for Black women has not reversed. Chu and colleagues (1999) have noted: "The racial disparity in breast cancer mortality rates has grown despite indications that the percentage of black women from 1990 through 1994 having mammography is close to that of white women" (p. 526). Dignam (2000) provides a brighter picture on Black women's breast-cancer mortality and the equal treatment of Black and White women. Through a review of data from key national studies, he concluded that "black women, diagnosed at comparable disease stage as white women and treated appropriately, tend to experience similar breast cancer prognoses and survival" (p. 50).

To reiterate, health is "a complex and multi-determined issue, influenced by a wide variety of factors," both internal and external to people (Rodin & Ickovics, 1990, p. 1018). Older Black women's experience with chronic disease is complicated by greater disease morbidity associated with aging (Ephraim, Misra, Nguyen, et al., 2001). Older Black women relative to younger Black women are at greater risk of having multiple diseases including hypertension, heart disease, stroke (a complication of hypertension), end-stage renal disease, arthritis, and dementia (Leigh & Lindquist, 1998; NAAS, 2000a, 2000d, 2000e). A growing amount of literature suggests that structural factors such as institutional racism may affect the quality of health care services offered to older Black women. For example, older Black women with chronic conditions may receive poorer quality health care than older White women, even when medical services are being delivered to patients covered by government insurance and critical demographic variables are controlled (Ayanian, Udvarhelyi, Gatsonis, Pashos, & Epstein, 1993; Gornick et al., 1996; Schneider, Zaslavsky, & Epstein, 2002). In a study of Medicare enrollees in managed health care plans, Schneider and colleagues (2002) found that Blacks were significantly less likely than Whites to receive mammograms, eye examinations in the case of diabetes, beta-blocker drugs after heart attack, and post-hospital treatment for mental illness. Racial disparities remained statistically significant among Medicare enrollees even when controlling for age, sex, Medicaid status, income, education, and rural residence. Consequences of these findings for older Black women's health are found in the words of Schneider and colleagues: "To the extent that (Blacks) fail to receive quality care, they may be at risk for complications that could otherwise have been ameliorated or prevented altogether" (2002, p. 1288).

It is important to note inconsistent findings about the role that race may play in determining services received. For example, a study on medical services received found no race differences between Whites and Blacks (Miller et al., 1997). Inconsistent findings among studies may be a result of different outcome measures (e.g., services versus treatments versus mortality) and the type of samples used. Despite data inconsistencies, an abundant literature implicates race as a structural factor in poor quality health care of Blacks (Hummer, 1996; Jackson et al., 1996; Krieger, 1990; Krieger, Rowley, Herman, Avery, & Phillips, 1993; Leigh & Lindquist, 1998; National Institute on Aging, 2001; Williams, 1992a, 1992b, 1999; Williams, Lavizzo-Mourey, & Warren, 1994).

In conclusion, the physical health status of older Black women is a complex issue requiring attention not only to individual factors but also to the role that structural factors play in predisposing these women to poor health status and health care. The role of different factors directs social workers and health professionals to multiple rather than single strategies of prevention and intervention in older Black women's physical health care.

PRIOR RESEARCH AND KNOWLEDGE BASE

On the basis of extant literature, we have identified three salient economic indicators of older Black women's economic well-being: employment, income, and poverty. Despite noticeable improvements in economic well-being of both the Black and elderly populations over the last three decades, economic inequalities persist. Employment and income inequalities, as well as poverty, provide compelling evidence that women of color—especially Black women—are highly disadvantaged in old age.

With regard to employment, Black women historically have participated in the labor market at a higher rate and for longer periods than

White women have. Using Social Security Administration data, Ozawa (1995) found that older Black women, defined as aged 62 and older, had longer adult working lives than either White or Hispanic women of similar age. However, their higher rate of labor market participation has not yielded rewards similar to those of older White and, to some degree, older Hispanic women. Black women averaged the lowest social security benefit—53% of White men's average as compared with Hispanic and White women, 56% and 62% of White men's average, respectively (Ozawa, 1995).

Oliver and Shapiro's (1995) work suggests that a history of low wages and individual and institutional discrimination, coupled with unequal and restricted asset accumulation, may help explain the cumulative effect of older Black women's economic disadvantage. The income and earning disadvantage of elderly people increases with age, in part because of a drop in labor market participation (U.S. Bureau of the Census, 1999). Older Black women are among the most vulnerable groups of older workers for having low income and low earnings in old age, again because of a lifetime of employment in low-wage and low-skill jobs before and after retirement (NAAS, 2000c).

Marital status, a social factor, intersects with age to further increase women's economic disadvantage in old age (Collins, Estes, & Bradsher, 2001). Older nonmarried Black women are highly vulnerable to income disadvantage in old age, in part because of nonmarital status over the life span but in old age in particular (Ozawa, 1995). Collins and colleagues provide data showing that older nonmarried women and men across five age groups (65–69, 70–74, 75–79, 80–84, 85 or older) are more likely to have lower median incomes than married couples, and nonmarried women's median income is the lowest of all three groups. In short, marriage may be a protective factor serving to shield older Black women from not only isolation and loneliness but also from economic disadvantage (Tucker, Taylor, & Mitchell-Kernan, 1993). Older Black women's economic disadvantage associated with nonmarital status may derive from a decline in marriage among African Americans in general over the last four decades (Tucker & Mitchell-Kernan, 1995). Poverty is a known risk factor for older adults (Rank & Hirschl, 1999a, 1999b), especially for unmarried older women who fare the worse in terms of poverty (Ozawa, 1995). Statistically, in Ozawa's study, 62% of unmarried Black women in the age group of 62 to 64 fell below 125% of the poverty line, as compared with 24% and 32% of White and Hispanic women, respectively. For unmarried women in the age group of 65+ and below 125% of the poverty line, there were 62% of Black women, as compared with 31% of White women and 45% of Hispanic women (Ozawa, 1995).

Not only do older Black women have lower incomes and earnings than older White women, but they also have fewer sources of income, less wealth, and fewer assets than White women have. In a study by Ozawa (1995), white women's income sources were more likely to include private pensions, annuities, and assets whereas Black and Hispanic women's income sources were more likely to include public aid. On the basis of a study by Oliver and Shapiro (1995), Collins and colleagues (2001) concluded that the net worth of Whites in old age is nearly five times the net worth of Blacks in old age. In a profile of young retirees and older workers, the NAAS (2000f) reported that "net household wealth for black retirees is approximately $18,000 compared to $120,000 for white retirees, and blacks comprise only 2 percent of retirees in the top wealth quintile" (p. 5). Income and wealth disparity by race and gender in old age is highly relevant for older Black women because they comprise a disproportionate number of the Black elderly population. For the most part, a person's income and wealth in old age has accumulated in prior years; both income and wealth are related to the opportunities and life chances that a person has had prior to old age. Older African American women may have had less opportunity to accumulate substantial income and wealth largely because of structural barriers such as institutional discrimination in the labor market (Ozawa, 1995).

In sum, older Black women have longer work histories, less income, greater poverty, fewer income sources, fewer assets, and less wealth than their White counterparts have. A life-course perspective suggests that Black women's greater economic disadvantage and poorer health in old age represents a lifetime of social and economic disadvantage (Jackson, 1996). A life-course perspective assumes that prior life experiences and events shape current life events; prior life experiences are cumulative over the life course (Hareven, 2000).

CURRENT RESEARCH ON OLDER BLACK FEMALE CAREGIVERS

Taken together, prior discussion provides considerable evidence about the poor physical health and economic well-being of older Black women. However, there is a critical piece missing from this discussion because prior evidence is heavily focused on across-race comparisons. Such comparisons, as Stoller and Gibson (2000) have argued, portray a partial reality of older Black women. These researchers also argue that "To fully comprehend the situation of any group of older people, we also need to consider differences within that group" (p. 80). On the basis of this argument, we provide data from current research on chronic health conditions, health behaviors, and economic factors in a sample of Black rural and urban women caregivers. The significance of caregiving as a known risk factor for women's poor health and economic status is well established (Arno, Levine, & Memmott, 1999; Grason et al., 2001). This research adds to the knowledge base of our discussion on older Black women's chronic health conditions and health behaviors, as the findings yield insights into the intersection of older Black women's aging, caregiving role, health, and economic status as well as addressing within-group heterogeneity.

An aging population portends a larger share of older caregivers assisting elderly family members (NAAS, 2000b). More than three out of four caregivers of older Blacks are Black women (National Alliance for Caregiving and American Association of Retired Persons, 1997). Although prior literature documents the economic well-being of caregivers (see Arno et al., 1999), little is known about the chronic health conditions, preventive health behaviors, and economic well-being of older Black women caregivers. Thus, the data presented herein represents a step toward closing this knowledge gap. We analyzed data for physical health (chronic conditions and health behaviors) and socioeconomic variables (household income and education) using frequency distributions, chi-square (categorical variables), and t-test (continuous variables) statistical analyses.

The sample of 93 rural and 103 urban caregivers was a subgroup of 521 Black women, aged 18 and older who cared for a dependent Black elder (aged 65 years and older) living in the community.[1] We chose the lower limit of age 60 rather than age 65 because evidence shows that chronic diseases such as hypertension and diabetes tend to occur much earlier than 65 years of age among Black women (Ephraim, Misra, Nguyen, et al., 2001; Leigh & Lindquist, 1998).

---

[1]This cross section study of urban–rural Black women caregivers' mental health, social functioning, and service use was funded by the National Institute on Aging and Office of Research on Women's Health (Grant AG15962). More information about the study can be obtained from L. Chadiha.

With regard to chronic conditions, the highest percentage of caregivers reported that a doctor had told them they had hypertension (74%), and the lowest percentage of caregivers reported that a doctor had told them they had cancer or stroke (5%, respectively). The next highest percentage of caregivers, 56%, reported that a doctor had told them they had arthritis or rheumatism. Almost one quarter (23%) of older Black women caregivers reported that a doctor had told them they had diabetes. Slightly less than one third of caregivers (31%) reported that a doctor had told them they had high blood cholesterol and slightly more than one third of caregivers (35%) reported that a doctor had told them they were overweight.

Caregivers ranked their overall subjective health as good to excellent on a scale that ranged from poor, fair, good, very good, to excellent. Regarding health-enhancing behaviors, 86% of women caregivers reported that they did not smoke cigarettes. A majority of caregivers reported good preventive health behaviors. Specifically, on average, caregivers reported having an annual physician checkup, a mammogram, and a clinical breast examination within the past 12 months. Caregivers also reported doing breast self-exams averaging once a month.

A within-group comparison between rural and urban caregivers revealed that urban caregivers were significantly more likely than rural caregivers to report that a doctor had told them they were overweight ($\chi^2 = 4.29$, $df = 1$, $p = .04$). Rural caregivers reported significantly lower levels of educational attainment in years of schooling completed than urban caregivers did ($t = 4.83$, $M = 9.47$, $SD = 2.92$; $t = 4.88$, $M = 11.76$, $SD = 2.50$, $p < .0001$, respectively). Rural caregivers reported significantly lower levels of annual household incomes than urban caregivers did. For example, 69% of rural caregivers reported annual household incomes under $18,000 compared with 43% of urban caregivers who reported annual household incomes under $18,000 ($\chi^2 = 13.35$, $df = 3$, $p < .0004$).

In conclusion, hypertension results in this subgroup of older Black rural and urban women caregivers are highly consistent with national data on older women in the general population. Hypertension is a leading risk factor for heart disease and a contributing factor to older Black women's relatively higher mortality rate (Ephraim, Misra, Nguyen, et al., 2001). Although relatively fewer older Black women caregivers reported that a doctor had told them they had high blood cholesterol, diabetes, and were overweight, all three conditions when combined with hypertension form a constellation of risk factors for heart disease. Arthritis or rheumatism, chronic conditions affecting the joints, is the second most frequently mentioned chronic condition by older Black women caregivers. Current research findings on older Black women caregivers coincide with reports about arthritis being prevalent among women in general (NAAS, 2000b). The National Academy on an Aging Society has reported arthritis as a "a leading cause of disability in the United States" (p. 1). An aging population portends more women with arthritis and disability, as a disproportion- ate number of women across all age groups have degenerative arthritis, osteoporosis, or inflammatory arthritis. Additionally, people with ar- thritis experience more functional limitations, financial difficulties, and occupational difficulties, and have lower levels of life satisfaction and optimism than people without arthritis (NAAS, 2000b). Caution is warranted because current findings are descriptive and not predictive. Nonetheless, findings on significant urban-rural differences of caregiv- ers' being told by a doctor that they were overweight, caregivers' education in years, and caregivers' annual household incomes support the claim of group differences within older Black women, as suggested by Stoller and Gibson (2000).

FURTHER RESEARCH NEEDS

Progress has been made in documenting the physical health status, and to some extent the health care, as well as the economic well-being of older Black women. More research is needed on the physical health status and economic well-being of older Black women, particularly in social work research where these women are largely invisible. Social work researchers have a great deal to offer to a research agenda on older women inasmuch as social workers integrate knowledge from a variety of sources and apply this knowledge in ways that facilitate both practice and policy. We have adopted nine recommendations from the *Women of Color Health Data Book* for further research needed (Leigh & Lindquist, 1998). Recommendations are consistent with the aforementioned review of literature and the empowerment approach to social work practice presented in this chapter.

1. Develop intervention research programs to empower older Black women in their use of health care, including preventive health

behaviors such as mammograms, cervical pap smears, and breast self-exams.

2.   Increase health promotion and disease-prevention research programs by facilitating older Black women's participation in clinical trials and disseminating results to these women. Additionally, identify barriers from the participant's point of view that prevent older Black women from participating in clinical trials.

3.   Encourage research on the impact of managed care on the quality and equity of care received by older Black women.

4.   Involve older Black women at the community level on research projects as participants in the research process. This will empower older Black women as consumers of their right to seek quality health care.

5.   Develop culturally and ethnically appropriate outcome measures.

6.   Design more within-race or gender studies to tap the heterogeneity within older Black women, particularly rural-urban differences.

7.   Develop effective outreach strategies when conducting clinical trial research to identify older Black women who never seek health care or who do so only during crisis.

8.   Collaborate with Black women on a community level by locating research centers within the community and by collaborating with Black churches or other community-based organizations.

9.   Use research to give back to the community by providing health care, education, training, and employment to older Black women, using a life-course approach and both qualitative and quantitative methods to examine the economic opportunities and inequalities in different age cohorts of older Black women.

In summary, research is needed to determine the effects of chronic illness caused by physical health conditions and the effects of poor economic well-being on quality of life for older Black women. Such research should consider both risk and protective factors in the physical health and economic well-being of older Black women.

POLICY IMPLICATIONS

Evidence unveiled in this chapter about older African American women's physical health and economic well-being has policy implications. One policy implication is the need for affordable health insurance prior to age 65 to cover preventive health and critical gaps in women's health insurance coverage. Women of color are highly vulnerable to lack of insurance and gaps in insurance coverage. For example, the *Women of Color Health Data Book* (Leigh & Lindquist, 1998) highlighted health insurance as a critical issue in a discussion on the health status of women of color. These women were more than half of the 19 million uninsured women in the U.S. in 1995 even though they were only about a quarter of all U.S. women. Lillie-Blanton, Bowie, and Ro (1996) noted that the inclusion of preventive health-care services for Black women will facilitate access to their health care, given that a disproportionate number are poor or near-poor and cannot afford to pay out-of-pocket. Fried (1996) stated that "improved health care coverage could make a substantial difference in the use of needed care by older women" (p. 198). Beckerman, Hawkins, Misra, Salganicoff, and Wyn (2001) noted that women of color are disproportionately disadvantaged economically while they also "have a disproportionate share of morbidity and mortality across a wide range of health conditions" (p. 174). Using data from the Commonwealth Fund Survey, Fried (1996) concluded that not having insurance was a "significant, independent factor" in whether an older woman had a primary care physician, had an annual well-woman physical, or used preventive services prescribed for her age group (p. 198). After age 64, health insurance issues for older women are less about coverage because a majority of older persons benefit from Medicare or supplemental health insurance coverage (Beckerman et al., 2001). Rather, health insurance coverage for older women after age 64 is more about their increasing need for good quality health care, prescribed medications, and coverage gaps that engender problems of health care access.

Second, educating the public about women's health is warranted and the link between it and women's economic disadvantage, particularly for participants in the labor market, on a local, state, and national level (Fried, 1996; Wyn, Brown, & Yu, 1996). Public education is needed to inform older Black women about the importance of disease prevention with aging, as Fried (1996) has noted that prevention is essential to curtailing both disease and disability among older women. Additionally, public education about risk factors and preventive health behaviors should target the current and future generations of older Black women, and young and old Black women who have not completed high school. Women with less than a high school education appear to be at greatest risk of poor physical health and low levels of preventive health than women who complete high school and beyond (Lillie-Blanton et al., 1996).

Third, evidence about race and health disparities in the U.S. health care system in this chapter suggests that social and political factors influence the physical health status of older women. Health care services may be available, but older Black women may not use services because they feel powerless—they may not feel an ability to influence control over their health care. Racism and sexism may not only impede access to health services for older Black women: they may also influence the quality of care received. Policies are needed to eliminate access problems to health services and to equalize services received. Furthermore, policies are needed to build professional capacity by increasing the number of minority professionals (social workers, physicians, and researchers) and to educate White care service providers to reduce service system biases.

TOWARD STRATEGIES OF EMPOWERMENT

An important goal of this chapter was to recommend strategies of empowerment and ways to enhance knowledge in social work practice and policy about the physical health and economic well-being of older African American women. Empowerment is a process in which social workers work with clients to help them define their problems, make decisions to solve problems through individual and collective actions, and to build on clients' strengths in order to help clients access critical environmental resources (Gutierrez, 1990; Lee, 2001). Social workers help facilitate empowerment strategies to increase life quality in areas of health and SES.

An empowerment approach embraces collaboration and teamwork. Working with multidisciplinary teams of providers on different practice levels, social workers can help facilitate older Black women's capacity building by providing accurate and timely knowledge about risk factors predisposing all women to certain diseases and disease complications. Social workers can help empower older Black women in their physical health by raising their awareness of the role they may play in controlling their own health. Along with raising awareness of older Black women, social workers can foster older Black women's self-care in terms of putting themselves first before they care for other people.

Empowerment literature suggests that issues of economic disadvantage warrant collective actions that seek to raise older Black women's awareness of economic deficits and to increase political solutions to such deficits. On empowering impoverished older Black women, social workers can take note of the *National Association of Social Workers Code of Ethics.* The code states that "The primary mission of the social work profession is to enhance human well-being and help meet the basic human needs of all people, with particular attention to the needs and empowerment of people who are vulnerable, oppressed, and living in poverty" (as cited in Rank & Hirschl, 1999a, p. 212). As Rank and Hirschl have concluded about poverty and policy, social workers can facilitate the empowerment of vulnerable people by working for policies that ameliorate poverty. We think that social workers will want to go beyond ameliorating poverty to protecting current national policies that greatly benefit older Black women, particularly Medicare and Social Security. In its action plan for aging research, the National Institute on Aging (2001) has asserted that as a group, minority elderly depend more heavily on Social Security and have fewer economic assets than their White counterparts.

Social workers may facilitate the empowerment of older Black women in the area of physical health by working to eradicate both individual and institutionalized racism in the health care delivery system. To reiterate the point of Schneider and colleagues (2002), when Blacks do not receive quality care, they are placed at risk of disease and illness complications that may have been avoided. Many older Black women may delay seeking help or not seek it altogether for disease and illness because of past experiences in discrimination from service providers. The evidence we have presented about racial disparity in the health care delivery system would justify older Black women's fear of discrimination. Whether older Black women's fear of discrimination is real or perceived, social workers need to work to reform and transform a health care system that may play a role in older Black women's delay in seeking help or failure to seek help at all.

An important challenge to the physical health and economic well-being of older Black women is their family role responsibilities as caretakers or caregivers. Research suggests that older Black women who engage in multiple caregiving roles (e.g., caring for grandchildren and others) may be predisposed to physical health risks as a result of juggling multiple roles (Casper & Bryson, 1998; Chadiha, Adams, Biegel, Auslander, & Gutierrez, 2002; Grason et al., 2001; Whitley,

Kelley, & Sipe, 2001). When older Black women allow caregiving responsibilities to take priority over their health, then caregiving may interfere with their ability to practice preventive health behaviors and to avoid poor health. Social workers might consider an empowerment approach to help older Black women take better care of themselves through engagement in small group interactions with similar caregivers (Cox & Parsons, 1996; Gutierrez, 1990). Neither the self-care of older Black women nor their strong coping will eradicate the panoply of social and individual factors associated with their poor health status, health care, and economic well-being. Research, practice, and policy can go a long way, however, to eliminate such factors.

INTEGRATING KNOWLEDGE INTO THE CURRICULUM: AN ILLUSTRATED COURSE OUTLINE

Older women, especially Black women, represent an invisible stream in social work curriculum. To gain a comprehensive understanding of older women, social workers must be familiar with their heterogeneity—age, race, ethnicity, nationality, culture, sexual orientation, place of residence, and so on. Understanding older Black women's heterogeneity especially is essential to developing and implementing ethnically and culturally sensitive practice with regard to their physical health and economic well-being. Given the lack of content about older women in social work curriculum, we have developed an illustrative course outline on this topic (see Appendix A). Although the focus is on older women in general, we pay special attention to women of color because of their health and economic vulnerability. Though we have identified that there is enough information to require a specific course on older women, nonetheless we think it is also important to infuse content about older women, particularly older Black women, into direct practice, human behavior and social environment, and social policy courses.

CONCLUSION

Although older Black women experience many rewards in old age, these women face prodigious challenges in both their physical health status, health care, and economic well-being. Their SES (e.g., employment, income, poverty, and occupation) is a strong determinant of their mortality and morbidity across the life course. On the whole, evidence presented in this chapter implies a nexus between the social factors, physical health, and economic well-being of older Black women. In comparing the health and SES of older Black women with that of White women, the experience and outcomes of systematic race- and gender-related inequalities are evident. Thus, it may be easy to portray older Black women as victims of such inequalities (Hughes & Mtezuka, 1992). We are reminded that older Black women have spent much of their lives having to confront race and gender stereotypes (Stoller & Gibson, 2000). The statistical comparisons that researchers make between older Black women and White women, although accurate in numbers, may engender stereotypical images of older Black women (Stoller & Gibson, 2000). Older Black women are survivors of a lifetime of gender and race inequalities that have adversely impacted their lives in similar ways to other women of color. In a treatise on older women, Hughes and Mtezuka (1992) have noted that older women are survivors as much as victims of oppression. For example, older women's personal biographies "are endowed with resources and experiences which are not sufficiently acknowledged" (p. 232). A comprehensive understanding of older Black women involves knowing their challenges, survival strategies, and social supports.

We would be remiss if we failed to acknowledge older Black women's strength in very old age. Despite poor physical health and economic well-being, many older Black women, after years of hard work, engage in paid work and family caregiving roles. Their work and caregiving roles serve as a testament to their resiliency in old age. Further evidence of the resiliency of older Black women is also observed in what Gibson (2000) labels their age-by-race advantage around and after 75 years old. Specifically, after age 65 and prior to age 75, Blacks appear to be more disadvantaged in mortality than Whites do, whereas after age 75, Blacks appear to gain the advantage in mortality over Whites. The question for social workers is how to use the knowledge about older African American women's poor physical health status, economic disadvantage, multiple role vulnerabilities, and resiliency to increase the quality of their lives. A full discussion of older Black women's survival strategies and social supports was beyond the scope of this chapter. Instead, we highlighted these women's vulnerabilities in physical health and SES as a way of challenging rather than validating their image as victim.

ACKNOWLEDGMENT

David E. Biegel, national mentor for the Hartford Geriatric Social Work Faculty Scholars Program, provided mentoring to L. Chadiha while writing this chapter. Emmanuel Akuamoah, Alice Ansah-Koi, Swapna Kommidi, Jane Rafferty, and Marcia Schnittger provided technical assistance.

REFERENCES

Administration on Aging. (2001). *A profile of older Americans.* Washington, DC: U.S. Department of Health and Human Services.

Arno, P. S., Levine, C., & Memmott, M. M. (1999). The economic value of informal caregiving. *Health Affairs, 18,* 182–188.

Ayanian, J. Z., Udvarhelyi, I. S., Gatsonis, C. A., Pashos, C. L., & Epstein, A. M. (1993). Racial differences in the use of revascularization procedures after coronary angiography. *Journal of the American Medical Association, 269,* 2642–2646.

Beckerman, Z., Hawkins, M., Misra, D., Salganicoff, A., & Wyn, R. (2001). Access, utilization and quality of health care. In D. Misra (Ed.), *The women's health data book* (3rd ed., pp. 168–186). Menlo Park, CA: Jacobs Institute of Women's Health and the Henry J. Kaiser Family Foundation.

Brownson, R. C., Eyler, A. A., King, A. C., Brown, D. R., Shyu, Y., & Sallis, J. F. (2000). Patterns and correlates of physical activity among US women 40 years and older. *American Journal of Public Health, 90,* 264–271.

Casper, L. M., & Bryson, K. R. (1998). Co-resident grandparents and their grand-children: Grandparent maintained families. *Population division working paper, No. 26,* U.S. Bureau of Census (pp. 1–19). Washington, DC: Government Printing Office.

Chadiha, L. A., Adams, P., Biegel, D. E., Auslander, W., & Gutierrez, L. (2002). *Empowering African American women caregivers: A literature synthesis and practice recommendations.* Unpublished manuscript.

Chu, K. C., Tarone, R. E., & Brawley, O. W. (1999). Breast cancer trends of Black women compared with White women. *Archives of Family Medicine, 8,* 521–528.

Collins, C. A., Estes, C. L., & Bradsher, J. E. (2001). Inequality and aging. In C. L. Estes & Associates (Eds.), *Social policy and aging* (pp. 137–163). Thousand Oaks, CA: Sage.

Cox, E. A., & Parsons, R. R. (1996). Empowerment-oriented social work practice: Impact on late life relationships of women. *Journal of Women and Aging, 8,* 129–143.

Crespo, C. J., Smit, E., Andersen, R. E., Carter-Pokras, O., & Ainsworth, B. E. (2000). Race/ethnicity, social class and their relation to physical inactivity during leisure time: Results from the Third National Health and Nutrition

Examination Survey, 1988–1994. *American Journal of Preventive Medicine, 18,* 46–53.

Dignam, J. J. (2000). Differences in breast cancer prognosis among African-American and Caucasian women. *Cancer Journal for Clinicians, 50,* 50–64.

Ephraim, P., Misra, D., Nguyen, R., & Vahratian, A. (2001). Chronic conditions. In D. Misra (Ed.), *The women's health data book* (3rd ed., pp. 64–103). Menlo Park, CA: Jacobs Institute of Women's Health and the Henry J. Kaiser Family Foundation.

Ephraim, P., Misra, D., Strobino, D., & Vahratian, A. (2001). Health behaviors. In D. Misra (Ed.), *The women's health data book* (3rd ed., pp. 118–149). Menlo Park, CA: Jacobs Institute of Women's Health and the Henry J. Kaiser Family Foundation.

Fried, L. P. (1996). Older women: Health status, knowledge, and behavior. In M. M. Falik & K. S. Collins (Eds.), *Women's health. The Commonwealth Fund Survey* (pp. 175–204). Baltimore: Johns Hopkins University Press.

Gibson, R. C. (2000). The age-by-race gap in health and mortality in the older population: A social science research agenda. In E. P. Stoller & R. C. Gibson (Eds.), *Worlds of difference: Inequality in the aging experience* (pp. 312–324). Thousand Oaks, CA: Pine Forge Press.

Gornick, M., Eggers, P. W., Reilly, T. W., Mentnech, R. M., Fitterman, L. K., Kucken, L. E., et al. (1996). Effects of race and income on mortality and use of services among Medicare beneficiaries. *New England Journal of Medicine, 335,* 791–799.

Grason, H., Minkovitz, C., Misra, D., & Strobino, D. (2001). Impact of social and economic factors on women's health. In D. Misra (Ed.), *The women's health data book* (3rd ed., pp. 2–3). Menlo Park, CA: Jacobs Institute of Women's Health and the Henry J. Kaiser Family Foundation.

Gutierrez, L. (1990). Working with women of color: An empowerment perspective. *Social Work, 35,* 149–154.

Hareven, T. K. (2000). *Families, history, and social change.* Boulder, CO: Westview Press.

Huff, M., & Sadler, C. (1997). African American women and osteoporosis. *Association of Black Nursing Faculty Journal, 8,* 48–50.

Hughes, B., & Mtezuka, M. (1992). Social work and older women: Where have older women gone? In M. Langan & L. Day (Eds.), *Women, oppression and social work* (pp. 220–241). London: Routledge.

Hummer, R. A. (1996). Black-white differences in health and mortality: A review and conceptual model. *Sociological Quarterly, 37,* 105–125.

Jackson, J. S. (1996). A life-course perspective on physical and psychological health. In R. J. Resnick & R. H. Rozensky (Eds.), *Health psychology through the life span* (pp. 39–57). Washington, DC: American Psychological Association.

Jackson, J. S., Brown, T. N., Williams, D. R., Torres, M., Sellers, S., & Brown, K. (1996). Racism and the physical and mental health status of African Americans: A thirteen-year National Panel Study. *Ethnicity and Disease, 6,* 132–147.

Johnson, C. D., & Misra, D. (2001). Mental health. In D. Misra (Ed.), *The women's health data book* (3rd ed., pp. 104–115). Menlo Park, CA: Jacobs Institute of Women's Health and the Henry J. Kaiser Family Foundation.

Krieger, N. (1990). Racial and gender discrimination: Risk factors for high blood pressure. *Social Science and Medicine, 30,* 1273–1281.

Krieger, N., Rowley, D. L., Herman, A. A., Avery, B., & Phillips, M. T. (1993). Racism, sexism, and social class: Implications for studies of health, disease, and well-being. *American Journal of Preventive Medicine, 2,* 82–122.

Landrine, H., & Klonoff, E. A. (1992). Culture diversity and health psychology. In A. Baum, T. A. Revenson, & J. E. Singer (Eds.), *Handbook of health psychology* (pp. 851–891). Mahwah, NJ: Erlbaum.

Lee, J. A. B. (2001). *The empowerment approach to social work practice. Building the beloved community* (2nd ed.). New York: Columbia University Press.

Leigh, W. A., & Lindquist, M. A. (Eds.). (1998). *Women of color health data book.* Bethesda, MD: Office of Research on Women's Health.

Lillie-Blanton, M., Bowie, J., & Ro, M. (1996). African American women: Social factors and the use of preventive health services. In M. M. Falik & K. S. Collins (Eds.), *Women's health. The Commonwealth Fund survey* (pp. 99–122). Baltimore: Johns Hopkins University Press.

McNabb, W., Quinn, M., & Tobian, J. (1997). Diabetes in African American women: The silent killer. *Women's Health: Research on Gender, Behavior, and Policy, 3,* 275–300.

Miller, B., Campbell, R. T., Furner, S., Kaufman, J. E., Li, M., Muramastu, N., et al. (1997). Use of medical care by African American and White older persons: Comparative analysis of three national data sets. *Journal of Gerontology: Social Sciences, 52B,* S325–S335.

Mouton, C. P. (1997). Special health considerations in African-American elders. *American Family Physician, 55,* 1243–1253.

National Academy on an Aging Society. (1999, November). *Chronic conditions.* Washington, DC: Author.

National Academy on an Aging Society. (2000a, March). *Arthritis.* Washington, DC: Author.

National Academy on an Aging Society. (2000b, May). *Caregiving.* Washington, DC: Author.

National Academy on an Aging Society. (2000c, August). *How financially secure are young retirees and older workers?* Washington, DC: Author.

National Academy on an Aging Society. (2000d, September). *Alzheimer's disease and dementia.* Washington, DC: Author.

National Academy on an Aging Society. (2000e, October). *Hypertension.* Washington, DC: Author.

National Academy on an Aging Society. (2000f, December). *Do young retirees and older workers differ by race?* Washington, DC: Author.

National Alliance for Caregiving and American Association of Retired Persons. (1997). *Family caregiving in the U.S.: Findings from a national survey.* Bethesda, MD: Author.

National Institute on Aging. (2001). *Action plan for aging research: Strategic plan for fiscal years 2001–2003.* Bethesda, MD: Author.

Oliver, M., & Shapiro, T. M. (1995). *Black wealth/white wealth: A new perspective on racial inequality.* New York: Routledge.

Ozawa, M. (1995). The economic status of vulnerable older women. *Social Work,* *40,* 323–331.

Rank, M. R., & Hirschl, T. A. (1999a). The likelihood of poverty across the American adult life span. *Social Work, 44,* 201–216.

Rank, M. R., & Hirschl, T. A. (1999b). Estimating the proportion of Americans ever experiencing poverty during their elderly years. *Journal of Gerontology: Social Sciences, 54B,* S184–S193.

Rodin, J., & Ickovics, J. R. (1990). Women's health. *American Psychologist, 45,* 1018–1034.

Rosen, A. L., & Zlotnik, J. L. (2001). Social work's response to the growing older population. *Generations, 25,* 69–71.

Schneider, E. C., Zaslavsky, A. M., & Epstein, A. M. (2002). Racial disparities in the quality of care for enrollees in Medicare managed care. *Journal of the American Medical Association, 287,* 1288–1294.

Siegel, J. S. (1994). Demographic introduction to racial/Hispanic elderly populations. In T. Miles (Ed.), *Full color aging* (pp. 1–20). Washington, DC: Gerontological Society of America.

Solomon, B. (1976). *Black empowerment: Social work in oppressed communities.* New York: Colombia University Press.

Stoller, E. P., & Gibson, R. C. (2000). Cultural images of old age. In E. P. Stoller & R. C. Gibson (Eds.), *Worlds of difference: Inequality in the aging experience* (pp. 75–88). Thousand Oaks, CA: Pine Forge Press.

Tucker, M. B., & Mitchell-Kernan, C. (Eds.). (1995). *The decline in marriage among African Americans.* New York: Russell Sage Foundation.

Tucker, M. B., Taylor, R. J., & Mitchell-Kernan, C. (1993). Marriage and romantic involvement among aged African Americans. *Journal of Gerontology: Social Sciences, 48,* S123–S132.

U.S. Bureau of the Census. (1999). *The Black population in the United States.* Washington, DC: U.S. Department of Commerce.

U.S. Bureau of the Census. (2001). *Census bureau facts for features* (U.S. Bureau of the Census Publication No. CB01-FF.02). [On-line]. Available: http://www.census.gov/Press-Release/www/2001/cb01ff02.html. Retrieved March 22, 2002.

Whitley, D. M., Kelley, S. J., & Sipe, T. A. (2001). Grandmothers raising grandchildren: Are they at increased risk of health problems? *Health and Social Work, 26,* 105–114.

Wilcox, S., Castro, C., King, A. C., Housemann, R., & Brownson, R. C. (2000). Determinants of leisure time physical activity in rural compared with urban older and ethnically diverse women in the United States. *Journal of Epidemiology Community Health, 54,* 667–672.

Williams, D. (1992a). Black-White differences in blood pressure: The role of social factors. *Ethnicity and Disease, 2,* 126–141.

Williams, D. (1992b). Racism and health: A research agenda. *Ethnicity and Disease, 6,* 1–6.

Williams, D. (1999). Race, socioeconomic status, and health: The added effects of racism and discrimination. *Annals of the New York Academy of Sciences, 896,* 173–188.

Williams, D., Lavizzo-Mourey, R., & Warren, R. (1994). The concept of race and health status in America. *Public Health Reports, 109,* 26–41.

Wyn, R., Brown, R., & Yu, H. (1996). Women's use of preventive health services. In M. M. Falik & K. S. Collins (Eds.), *Women's health: The Commonwealth Fund survey* (pp. 49–75). Baltimore: Johns Hopkins University Press.

Young, D. R., Miller, K. W., Wilder, L. B., Yanek, L. R., & Becker, D. M. (1998). Physical activity of urban African Americans. *Journal of Community Health, 23,* 99–112.

APPENDIX A: ILLUSTRATIVE COURSE SYLLABUS IMPACT OF THE SOCIAL CONTEXT ON OLDER WOMEN'S PHYSICAL HEALTH CREDIT HOURS: 3

I.   Course Domain and Boundaries

In the *Women's Health Data Book* (Misra, 2001), Grason, Minkovitz, Misra, and Strobino report a substantial increase in the number of older women (aged 65 or older), tripling from 6.5 million in 1950 to more than 20 million in 1998. The U.S. population of older women is ethnically and racially diverse with women of color (e.g., Black, Hispanic, Asian and Pacific Islander, American Indian and Alaskan Native) comprising a larger share of the population. This course considers the impact of race, ethnicity, gender, culture, age, social class, and family and household characteristics on both poor and good health of older women. Special attention will be paid to the vulnerability and strengths of women of color. This course will use the stress and coping, life course, and empowerment frameworks to facilitate examination of how social and cultural factors are interconnected to one another and related to the physical health of older women. Students will evaluate practice and policy recommendations to address the empowerment and capacity-building preventive interventions for addressing older women's physical health.

II.   Course Objectives

1.   To enable students to know and understand demographic trends in the older female population and the relationship be-

tween such trends and the physical health status and health care of older women

2. To provide students with specific theoretical frameworks for understanding older women's physical health status and care

3. To enable students to develop an understanding of the impact of race, gender, ethnicity, culture, age, social class, and family and household characteristics on both good and poor physical health of older women

4. To enable students to develop an understanding of the interconnectedness of race, gender, ethnicity, age, and social class to social and economic justice in relation to the physical health status and health care of older women, particularly older women of color

5. To enable students to develop knowledge of, and skills in, identifying and assessing evidence-based prevention and intervention capacity-building programs with older women, particularly with older women of color

6. To enable students to develop knowledge of, and skills in, using social work values, and recognizing and responding appropriately to ethical dilemmas that may arise within the social and cultural context of social work practice with older women

7. To enable students to translate knowledge about older women's physical health into practice and policy recommendations that facilitate the empowerment of older women

III. Educational Outcomes

Upon completion of this course, students are expected to

1. know and understand demographic trends in the older female population and the relationship between such trends and the physical health status and health care of older women;

2. know specific theoretical frameworks for understanding older women's physical health status and care;

3. demonstrate understanding of the impact of race, gender, ethnicity, culture, age, social class, and family and household characteristics on both good and poor physical health of older women;

4. demonstrate understanding of the interconnectedness of race, gender, ethnicity, age, and social class to social and economic

justice in relation to the physical health status and health care of older women, particularly older women of color;

5. demonstrate knowledge of, and skills in, identifying and assessing evidence-based prevention and intervention capacity-building programs with older women, particularly with older women of color;

6. demonstrate knowledge of, and skills in, using social work values, and recognizing and responding appropriately to ethical dilemmas that may arise within the social and cultural context of social work practice with older women;

7. demonstrate ability to translate knowledge about older women's physical health into practice and policy recommendations that facilitate the empowerment of older women.

IV.   Selected Suggested Textbooks and Readings

Calasanti, T. M., & Slevin, K. F. (2001). *Gender, social inequalities, and aging*. Walnut Creek, CA: Altamira Press.

Estes, C. L. (2001). Sex and gender in the political economy of aging. In C. L. Estes and Associates (Eds.), *Social policy and aging* (pp. 119–135). Thousand Oaks, CA: Sage.

Falik, M. M., & Collins, K. S. (Eds.). (1996). *Women's health: The Commonwealth Fund survey*. Baltimore: Johns Hopkins University Press.

Hughes, B., & Mtezuka, M. (1992). Social work and older women: Where have older women gone? In M. Langan & L. Day (Eds.), *Women, oppression and social work* (pp. 220–241). London: Routledge.

Jackson, J. S. (1996). A life course perspective on physical and psychological health. In R. J. Resnick & R. H. Rozensky (Eds.), *Health psychology through the life span* (pp. 39–57). Washington, DC: American Psychological Association.

Krieger, N., Rowley, D. L., Herman, A. A., Avery, B., & Phillips, M. T. (1993). Racism, sexism, and social class: Implications for studies of health, disease, and well-being. *American Journal of Preventive Medicine, 2*, 82–122.

Landrine, H., & Klonoff, E. A. (1992). Culture diversity and health psychology. In A. Baum, T. A. Revenson, & J. E. Singer (Eds.), *Handbook of health psychology* (pp. 851–891). Mahwah, NJ: Erlbaum.

Lee, J. A. B. (2001). *The empowerment approach to social work practice. Building the beloved community* (2nd ed.). New York: Columbia University Press.

Leigh, L., & Lindquist, M. A. (1998). *Women of color health data book*. Bethesda, MD: Office of Research on Women's Health, Office of the Director and National Institutes of Health.

Misra, D. (Ed.). (2001). *Women's health data book: A profile of women's health in the United States* (3rd ed.). Washington, DC: Jacobs Institute of Women's Health and the Henry J. Kaiser Family Foundation.

National Institute on Aging. (2001). *Action plan for aging research: Strategic plan for fiscal years 2001–2003.* Bethesda, MD: National Institute on Aging.

Ozawa, M. (1995). The economic status of vulnerable older women. *Social Work, 40,* 323–331.

Pearlin, L. I., & Skaff, M. M. (1998). Perspectives on the family and stress in late life. In J. Lomranz (Ed.), *Handbook of aging and mental health* (pp. 323–340). New York: Plenum Press.

Rosen, A. L., & Zlotnik, J. L. (2001). Social work's response to the growing older population. *Generations, 25,* 69–71.

Stoller, E. P., & Gibson, R.C. (Eds.). (2000). *Worlds of difference: Inequality in the aging experience.* Thousand Oaks, CA: Pine Forge Press.

Whitley, D. M., Kelley, S. J., & Sipe, T. A. (2001). Grandmothers raising grandchildren: Are they at increased risk of health problems? *Health and Social Work, 26,* 105–114.

V. Organization of Course

Lectures, class discussion, audiovisual materials, small group exercises, and older women guest speakers.

VI. Course Assignments

A short critique on the strengths and weaknesses of one of three theoretical frameworks (stress and coping, life-course perspective, empowerment) used to frame the physical health and health care experiences of older women (8–10 pages). A midterm take-home examination; a term paper on an issue relating to older women's physical health or health care with practice and policy strategies (20–25 pages).

VII. Course Outline (Possible Topics)

1. Demographic trends in the general and older female population
2. Health status, disability, and health care of older women
3. Stress and coping, life course, and empowerment frameworks as theoretical lenses
4. The social context of older women's health: impact of race, gender, ethnicity and culture
5. The social context of older women's health: impact of social class, family characteristics, household characteristics, and multiple roles

6. Social and economic justice issues in delivering health care to older women
7. Evidence-based and capacity-building preventive health programs for older women
8. Evidence-based and capacity-building intervention health programs for older women
9. Policy considerations: coverage, access to services, and public education needs for older women

ACKNOWLEDGMENT

This course outline was adapted from a course syllabus by Dr. Tonya Edmond entitled "Intervention Approaches With Women," and a course syllabus by Dr. Lisa Morris entitled "Feminization of Poverty," both syllabi from the George Warren Brown School of Social Work, Washington University, St. Louis, MO.

Chapter 8

GRANDPARENTS RAISING GRANDCHILDREN

Nancy P. Kropf and Scott Wilks

Over recent decades, the number of grandparents who are raising grandchildren has increased dramatically. This family form, termed *custodial grandparenting* or *skipped generation parenting*, has become more common within various social welfare and health care contexts. The latest U.S. Census reports that there are about 2.4 million grandparent caregivers in the United States with about 75% who have taken care of grandchildren for more than 1 year (Bryson, 2001). On the basis of numbers of grandchildren, estimates indicate that about 3.9 million children live in households with grandparents (Lugalia, 1998). Taken together, these figures indicate that intergenerational families are numerous and are involved in multiple service networks, and social workers across a variety of contexts and practice roles will have involvement with clients within these family systems.

Although grandparents have historically been involved in family life and have served as supports for child care, the reasons for caregiving have become more complex. The major factor for coresidence of grandchildren and grandparents is the drug addiction of a parent, especially crack cocaine (Burton, 1992; Minkler, Roe, & Price, 1992; Minkler, Roe, & Robertson-Beckley, 1994; Roe, Minkler, & Barnwell, 1994; Roe, Minkler, Saunders, & Thomson, 1996). Concomitantly, social problems associated with drug addiction are also precipitating factors, such as incarceration and child maltreatment (Barnhill, 1996; Dressel & Barnhill, 1994; Grant, Gordon, & Cohen, 1997). In addition, HIV/AIDS has also been a significant factor as children whose parents have died or are physically incapacitated frequently are raised by their grandparents (Caliandro & Hughes, 1998; Poindexter & Linsk, 1999; Whetten-Goldstein & Nguyen, 2001).

Because of the significance of this issue for social work, this chapter will highlight several of the social, physical, and emotional issues of raising grandchildren. Practice and policy implications will be summarized to help motivate social workers and allied professionals to be more responsive to the needs within these families. In addition, an individualized intervention approach will be highlighted that has specific use with grandparents who are outside of existing support services. Finally, educational strategies will be presented to help educate future social workers about this family form.

SIGNIFICANCE TO GERONTOLOGY, HEALTH CARE, AND HEALTH PROFESSIONALS

Because custodial grandparenting is an intergenerational issue, there is significance for a number of professions. Specifically, social workers may become involved with a number of health providers around issues of the health and well-being of the grandparents. In addition, this issue is significant to child welfare as personnel may work with more older adults in kinship care roles. This section provides an overview of the various issues associated with custodial grandparents across a variety of professional areas.

Fairly recently, the field of aging has become more involved in research and practice on grandparents raising grandchildren. Examples are recent issues of the *Journal of Aging and Mental Health* and the *Journal of Gerontological Social Work* that are entirely devoted to this family form (Burnette, 2000; McCallion & Janicki, 2000). Because of the changing demographics, the field of aging has developed a literature on older adults who have responsibility to care for younger generations. Besides custodial grandparents, other late-life caregiving roles include parents of adults with developmental, psychiatric, or physical disabilities (e.g., see chapter 9 in this volume). Attention to late life caregivers has expanded the way that caregiving has been conceptualized within the field of aging.

From a gerontological perspective, the research on these intergenerational families has focused on the experience of the grandparents. Like other caregiving roles, the care of grandchildren includes both stress and reward (Pruchno, 1999). The various responsibilities that accompany caregiving tasks can compromise physical and social functioning in late life. Examples of particular problems include a sense of isolation, economic vulnerability, and depression, yet the experience of raising grandchildren also includes positive aspects. In research on rewarding experiences, grandparents report having a sense of companionship, holding an important social role, and being able to keep the care of their grandchildren within the family system (Morrow-Kondos, Weber, Cooper, & Hesser, 1997; Poindexter & Linsk, 1999).

A great deal of research has been conducted on the health and well-being of custodial grandparents. Raising children is a physically demanding task, and grandparents who are in mid or late life may experience health problems as a result of performing within this role. For example, research that compared caregiving and noncaregiving grandparents found that those who were raising their grandchildren had poorer physical and mental health outcomes than grandparents in noncustodial roles (Bowers & Myers, 1999; Jendrek, 1993; Morrow-Kondos et al., 1997; Musil, 1998; Poindexter & Linsk, 1999; Szinovacz, DeViney, & Atkinson, 1999). In addition, when custodial grandparents were compared with other types of care providers, such as spouses and adult children, grandparents experienced more health problems and stressful life events (Strawbridge, Wallhagen, Shema, & Kaplan, 1997). Although grandparents who assume care have been termed *silent saviors* for many children (Creighton, 1991), the experience of care provision may compromise their overall health and well-being.

Social well-being also may suffer when grandparents have caregiving responsibility for grandchildren. The demands of caregiving can potentially decrease the degree of contact between the grandparent and his or her established social network (Burnette, 1999b; Jendrek, 1993; Minkler et al., 1994; Strawbridge et al., 1997). Social isolation may also be the result of managing stigmatizing situations, such as the HIV status of a grandchildren (Caliandro & Hughes, 1998; Linsk & Poindexter, 2000). As grandparents spend time raising their grandchildren, they have less energy, time, and motivation to connect with family, friends, and other relationships within their communities.

Because of the intergenerational nature of this family form, several service networks may be involved with grandparents who are raising grandchildren. One service sector that has contact with many grandparents is child welfare, as kinship care has become a primary method to increase stability and permanency of care for children. Within child welfare, personnel work frequently with grandparents who are in either formalized or informal kinship care arrangements (Kolomer, 2000). The primary focus is on child well-being, yet attention to the entire family system must be considered to assure permanency of care.

The school setting is another child-related institution that is involved with custodial grandparents. School social workers, teachers, and other personnel are becoming more aware of the numbers of grandparents who are raising grandchildren. If grandchildren have special needs, grandparents may be involved in constructing individual education plans, managing behavioral challenges, and handling other school-related issues. In addition, grandparents may have to initiate a school change if their grandchildren had to relocate to reside with them.

Grandparents may also need the services of professionals in the health care system. In addition to their own health issues, grandparents may also be in the role of managing severe and chronic emotional and physical conditions of their grandchildren (cf. McCallion & Janicki, 2000). As stated, precipitating factors for co-residence may include parental addiction, abuse, or HIV. In these situations, there are associated health, behavioral, and emotional risks for the children.

Legal professionals are also commonly involved with intergenerational families. Attorneys may be involved with grandparents in securing formal custody or adoption. In addition, numerous other issues may require legal attention such as drafting wills or more extensive estate planning. These families may also need the assistance of attorneys if they experience problems as a result of raising grandchildren such as housing or entitlement programs.

SOCIAL WORK CONTRIBUTION

Because of the person-in-environment orientation of social work, the profession holds a leadership role in promoting the health and well-being of custodial grandparents. As a broad profession, social workers practice in a wide context of areas and fields of practice. Social work's investment in this area will be presented from an ecological framework, that is, spanning practice with individuals to a transformation of social policy.

At the micro system level, social work practitioners assess and intervene with the individual and family system. In practice with custodial grandparents, several areas are potential issues for intervention. One is with the family system, as intergenerational families often confront challenging issues within family subsystems and boundaries (Bartram, 1996; Goldberg-Glen, Sands, Cole, & Cristofalo, 1998). For example, grandchildren often struggle with what name to call their grandparent—is it grandma or mama? This semantic question opens the larger issue of the confusion that many grandchildren feel about the role of the grandparent in their lives. In addition, grandparents struggle with ways to move from a traditional grandparenting role to assuming parenting, including dealing with discipline issues and boundary setting. In addition, other subsystems within the family may be affected by the child-raising role, including the marital partnership and relationships to other children or grandchildren within the family. These family level challenges may be issues that social workers experience in their practice with intergenerational families.

Micro system issues also include the experiences of individuals within the family, for both the grandparents and grandchildren. For grandparents, the experience often involves feelings of grief and loss. If the precipitating factor for caregiving is due to the death of their son or daughter, the experience of raising their grandchildren is combined with the "off-time" loss of losing their own child. In other situations, losses are associated with their disappointment in their child's ability to parent and their management of the tension between retaining hope that the child's parent may be able to assume care at some point. This experience of holding divided loyalties between their son or daughter and grandchildren can be extremely confusing and complicated for grandparents. The grandchildren in intergenerational families may also benefit from social interventions. Often, these children perceive that they are different from peers and may feel stigmatized about living with grandparents. In addition, role relationships may be extremely confusing for grandchildren, especially in situations where they have contact with their biological parent. Brief periods of reconnection, such as times when a parent is drug free, may lead to renewed feelings of abandonment when the parent leaves again. This period is often a time for the child to exhibit hostile or angry behavior toward the grandparent.

Social work interventions are also appropriate at the mezzo system, which involves the relationships between the family and other systems within the environment. At this level of practice, social workers can work to transform community organizations and networks to be more responsive to the needs of this family form. Examples of initiatives include helping child welfare and aging services to work in a coordinated manner, as often the needs of intergenerational families span both of these service networks. In addition, social work case-management services are important at the mezzo system. Frequently, grandparents may feel confused or isolated from services that do exist in the community because often they have been out of the child-raising role for several years. Case managers can assist families to receive services including public welfare, Supplemental Security Income (SSI), and children's recreational programs. Unfortunately, grandparents may be unaware of the types of resources that may be available to them and their grandchildren.

At the macro level, social workers can serve as advocates to change policies that impact intergenerational families. These typically include child custody, family leave, and tax credits that can support families and provide economic resources. In addition, many intergenerational families live in communities that have limited resources that are available to assist them with caregiving (Myers, Kropf, & Robinson, 2002). Other macro-level practice roles include promoting effective and efficacious programs and interventions within areas that currently underserve this family form.

PRIOR RESEARCH AND KNOWLEDGE BASE

Research on intergenerational families has been conducted in several disciplines including gerontology, child welfare, and family studies. Although studies of intergenerational families may be based upon various theoretical frameworks, several themes have emerged in the type of research that has been conducted. Descriptive research provided a profile of custodial grandparents across a variety of contexts. Other studies have estimated the impact of care provision upon the grandparent, specifically in the areas of health, social functioning, and well-being. Research at the family system level has identified precipitating factors for caregiving and the impact of raising grandchildren upon the family unit. Finally, a limited body of outcome literature is emerging to assess the impact of interventions with custodial grandparents.

Descriptive Research

In descriptive research, studies have described the population of inter-generational families from an individual and family system perspective. The average age of grandparents who are raising grandchildren is 59 years (Fuller-Thomson, Minkler, & Driver, 1997) with an age range between mid 30s and upper 80s (Caputo, 1999). In addition, other research has focused on the racial and ethnic proportions of intergenerational families (Chalfie, 1994). Although the greatest number of intergenerational families is White, African American and Hispanic families are disproportionately represented. Gender issues of caregiving have also been investigated. Similar to other caregiving roles, the majority of grandparents who are raising grandchildren are female (Fuller-Thompson et al., 1997). Geographically, families have also been found to live largely in urban areas (74%), yet a significant percentage (26%) live in nonurban settings (Pebley & Rudkin, 1999).

Health and Well-Being

The impact of the child-raising experience on health and well-being has also been a focus of research on grandparents. These studies investigate the outcomes of the caregiving experience on grandparents. In comparisons of various types of caregiving roles, custodial grandparents have been found to experience poorer health than either non-custodial grandparents or caregivers in other roles (e.g., adult children, spouses) (Bowers & Myers, 1999; Strawbridge et al., 1997; Szinovacz et al., 1999). Social issues have also been addressed and indicate that grandparents who are raising grandchildren report feelings of isolation, loneliness, and disconnection from friends (Kelley, 1993; Musil, 1998). In addition, grandparents also report negative psychosocial outcomes including anxiety, depression, and feelings of disempowerment (Burnette, 1999a; Minkler, Fuller-Thompson, Miller, & Driver, 1997; Robinson, Kropf, & Myers, 2000; Sands & Goldberg-Glen, 1998).

Other health research has investigated the ability of custodial grandparents to care for their own health needs. Research on health promoting activities (e.g., exercise, good diet) indicates that grandparents neglect these positive practices in their own lives. In addition, grandparents also report engaging in lifestyle behaviors that negatively impact health and functioning such as skipping medical appointments and alcohol or tobacco use (Emick & Hayslip, 1999; Minkler et al., 1992).

Family-Level Research

In addition to research on individual members, studies have been conducted at the family system level. Qualitative research into caregiving has identified various pathways that grandparents take into the caregiving role (Jendrek, 1993; Kropf & Robinson, 2002). These include immediately assuming care (as in the case of sudden parental death), the dissolution of a multigenerational family system where the parent generation moves from the household and the children stay with the grandparents, and an incremental pathway where the grandparents assume care after attempting remediation strategies with the children's parents. Depending on the pathway into care, the grandparents may have different experiences in child-rearing and service needs.

Other research has focused on subsystems within the family, such as the marital dyad. Some research indicates that raising grandchildren impacts marital quality negatively (Jendrek, 1993). Other research, however, suggests that the quality of the marriage may not suffer, yet the tasks associated with raising the grandchildren are primarily assumed by the grandmother (Minkler et al., 1994).

Using an ecological perspective, the linkage between family and community has been studied. In research on rural grandparents, findings indicated that grandparents felt a sense of disempowerment within their communities (Robinson et al., 2000). Other research in this area has found that there is limited knowledge about resources that are available within community settings (Whitley, White, Kelley, & Yorker, 1999). Taken together, these studies indicate that grandparents may not be linked to resources that potentially could be sources of support within their caregiving role.

Intervention Approaches

Although various intervention strategies have been described, a limited body of outcome literature exists with custodial grandparents. Burnette (1998) measured the impact of a psychoeducational group for Latino grandparents. The intervention, based upon a stress and coping framework, reduced caregiver depressive symptomology and enhanced their coping repertoire. In addition, the participants reported high levels of satisfaction with the group experience. In addition, an empowerment group with African American custodial grandparents has also reported positive outcomes such as increased self-efficacy and problem solving skills (Cox, 2001).

The predominant intervention model for custodial grandparents is a support or psychoeducational group (Minkler, Driver, Roe, & Bedeian, 1993). Typically, these groups have the goals of providing an avenue to increase social networks of custodial grandparents, assist with skill development to enhance the caregiving role, and provide a mutual aid context for shared problem-solving. Often these groups are the sole intervention that is provided for grandparents within a community.

Even though these groups may be effective for participants, disadvantages exist in providing interventions within a group format. Although a large number of groups exist, there are still not groups available within every community, for example, in rural or isolated geographical areas. Unfortunately, many grandparents may not benefit from resources even when they are available within community settings, as barriers to participation may still exist. These include the grandparents' lack of transportation, lack of child care options, or inability to attend during established meeting times.

Case management projects have also been implemented with intergenerational families, with goals of providing linkages to community resources (cf. Whitley et al., 1999). Within case management models, interventions may benefit the entire family system or be structured to assist either grandparents or the grandchildren. In both cases, the intended outcome is to enhance the goodness of fit between the family and their environment.

An evaluation of a multidisciplinary case-management model has also been conducted. In a study on grandparents in a large urban area, a multidisciplinary intervention that consisted of case managers, nurses, legal assistance, and support groups was evaluated (Kelley, Yorker, Whitley, & Sipe, 2001). After participating in this program, custodial grandparents reported lower stress and higher levels of social support than prior to the intervention. Although the outcomes may be beneficial, several potential disadvantages are associated with a case management model as well. These projects tend to be labor-intensive as the case managers carry a caseload of families that are seen on a regular basis. In addition, case management programs tend to be demonstration projects that are not owned by any service network.

Because the needs of intergenerational families span diverse service sectors (e.g., aging, child welfare, health, and mental health, etc.), a lack of ownership may exist where the family is not considered a client of any service system. Unfortunately, this perception may lead to a lack of responsiveness on the part of service providers.

CURRENT RESEARCH—LET'S TALK: AN AUDIO INTERVENTION FOR CUSTODIAL GRANDPARENTS

The intervention reported now, developed by one of the authors of this chapter (Kropf, 2001), was based upon a unique, individualized intervention approach with custodial grandparents. The intervention was structured to reach grandparents across geographic areas and those individuals who may be outside of current services to grandparents. In addition, the goal was to provide information and support across various behavioral and functional domains.

Let's Talk is an audio-based curriculum that was developed and produced specifically for custodial grandparents (Kropf, 2001). Using a theoretical framework of self-efficacy (Bandura, 1977, 1978), the intervention promotes health, well-being, and caregiving competence. The series consists of eight audiotapes and employs a dialogue format that simulates conversations between grandparents and various service providers (hence the title of the series, *Let's Talk*). Through the discussions on the tapes, grandparents are encouraged to construct individualized plans to enhance functioning within their own lives.

The intervention was constructed using both theoretical and empirical methods. As an initial step, the literature on intergenerational families was reviewed across gerontology, child welfare, and family studies. An analysis of the major themes about the role of custodial grandparents was performed and substantive issues were identified. From a list of the major areas that emerged within the literature, a list of topics was constructed that was pilot tested with a sample ($n = 14$) of custodial grandparents. These grandparents were asked to rate each of the topics on a Likert scale of *very important* to *unimportant* in their role of raising grandchildren. In addition, the grandparents were asked to identify particular areas within the themes that were most relevant to them. For example, the theme that achieved the highest rating was their health, with all of the grandparents agreeing that this topic was very important or important to them. Making time to care for themselves and methods to preserve energy in the context of raising grandchildren were some of the areas that grandparents identified as important in the area of health.

After completing the pilot test phase, the topics were combined into eight categories and scripts were written. Each script was constructed to meet the following three objectives: (a) provide basic information on the topic's content, (b) identify risk situations that potentially could escalate into major problems or crises, and (c) promote behavioral change in the lives of grandparents. The length of each tape ranges from about 12 to 23 minutes. The content areas that constitute the series are health issues, child behavior issues, identifying and using community resources, legal questions and concerns, school issues, self-care, and social support issues.

To evaluate the impact of this intervention, the tape series was administered using a prescribed protocol to ensure treatment fidelity. After completing a pretest, grandparents received the first tape in the series, "Let's Talk About Raising Grandchildren." This tape provides a context for understanding themselves as custodial grandparent, including demographics of this family form, various pathways into care, and typical concerns and experiences within their caregiving role. In addition, this first tape gives a descriptive summary of the remaining tapes in the series. Afterwards, grandparents receive two tapes twice a month and can individualize the order in which they listen to the remaining tapes. In this way, participants can prioritize the topics that have the most relevance within their own lives. During each 2-week period, every grandparent receives a phone call from a member of the project staff. The purpose of this contact is to encourage the participants to listen to the tapes, if they have not done so already, and specify the selection for the next round of tapes. The purpose of this structured format for the intervention is to increase compliance with the intervention (e.g., to determine that they listen to all the tapes within the series), as well as to provide an empirical way to determine the priorities in topical areas across the participant sample. The final tape in the series, "Let's Talk Again," provides a recap of the other topics and leaves the grandparent with a final message of hope for the caregiving role.

The evaluation of the intervention tape series is currently being conducted. The study hypothesizes that after listening to the *Let's Talk* tape series, grandparents will be more effective in their role as caregivers for their grandchildren and take better care of themselves both physically and socially. Grandparents who are not involved in grandparent support programs have been recruited. The instruments that are used in a pre- and posttest design are Ways of Coping Scale (Folkman, Lazarus, Pimley, & Novacek, 1987), Grandparent Burden and Reward Scale (Pruchno, 1999), Parental Locus of Control (Campis, Lyman, & Prentice-Dunn, 1986), and the Brief Symptom Inventory (Derogatis & Melisaratos, 1983).

FURTHER RESEARCH NEEDS

The *Let's Talk* tape series is an innovative intervention that provides an individualized method of providing information and support to custodial grandparents. Although this method is one way of expanding the service options to these grandparents, additional outcome research is necessary to determine particular interventions that have beneficial effects. In addition, researchers also must conduct studies with intergenerational families to promote a more comprehensive understanding of the dynamics of these caregiving relationships.

Research Evaluating Interventions

Interventions for custodial grandparents have increased, yet there is a lack of outcome research on the efficacy of these programs to determine whether, and under what conditions, participation promotes positive change within the lives of these caregivers. Research needs to further the outcome literature on custodial grandparent programs. Outcome studies need to determine which program models have potential to make the greatest degree of change with different constellations of interventions. Case management may produce a greater degree of change than participation in a support group, for example, but the labor and resource intensity may limit this program model to narrow geographic areas.

In addition, researchers need to undertake studies using various subpopulations of grandparent caregivers. Great diversity exists within the custodial grandparent population on many variables including race and ethnicity, age of grandparent, age of grandchildren, geographic location (urban or rural), and gender. Program interventions that benefit a certain profile of grandparent may be ineffective with another. Clearly, additional data on the effect of various intervention approaches is warranted.

Research on Risk Situations and Junctures

Using a life-course perspective, the experience of being part of an intergenerational family is dynamic and changing. Anecdotally, service providers may develop practice wisdom about types of situations that can precipitate problems. However, theoretical models of life-course transitions have not been developed specifically to address issues within these family systems. Where are the points that hold particular risks within the family? In the absence of valid assessment models, practitioners may miss opportunities to intervene prior to a crisis situation.

Thus, one area of needed research is on the various junctures that create stress within the family system. Because most grandparents raise grandchildren in informal kinship arrangements, one stressful juncture may be at the point where the family establishes linkages with external systems. Problems may occur around decision-making authority on the part of the grandparents if a child requires medical care or other services, for example. In addition, institutions may have changed tremendously from the time when grandparents were raising their own child (e.g., schools), which can cause confusion about roles and procedures. These types of linkages with external systems may be confusing, intimidating, and overwhelming for some grandparents.

Another risk situation is when a grandchild's behavior mirrors the problems experienced by his or her own parent. Experimentation with alcohol or drugs is not unusual in adolescence, but these behaviors may be intolerable if the teen has a parent with an addiction. Sexual experimentation may create the same level of tension if the child's parent was infected with the HIV virus as a result of a sexual relationship. In these situations, the grandparent may fear that the grandchild is following in the path of the parent and may feel overwhelmed and unable to cope.

Similar to other off-time caregiving relationships, another stressful juncture is the point at which the care provider experiences a health care problem. Since the national average age for custodial grandparents is 59 years, many of these adults are beginning to experience health-related changes. In addition, the demands of child care may exacerbate an existing health problem and precipitate a medical crisis. In these situations, family homeostasis and stability may be threatened. Another threat to stability is the pattern of *sometimes parenting* that happens within the context of some family systems. Especially if addiction is present, the child's parent may reenter the family for brief periods (e.g., come over when high, or move back into the household during a period of sobriety). This situation can be traumatic for all members, as roles and subsystems need to rebalance. For example, does the grandparent retreat into a nonparenting role when a mother spends the weekend? This experience can also be extremely confusing for the grandchildren who are uncertain of the role relationships between themselves, their parents, and their grandparents. In addition, the children may reexperience a sense of abandonment after the parent leaves the household (e.g., goes back to drinking or drugging) and act out anger and hostility in behaviorally challenging ways.

Longitudinal Studies

The research on intergenerational families is largely cross-sectional. Although this type of analysis provides a description of the families' experiences at a given point in time, this design lacks a dynamic perspective. Longitudinal research has the potential to identify changes and experiences across the life course of a family.

One area for longitudinal research is determining how grandparents and grandchildren fare within an intergenerational family system. The concomitant aging process of the children and grandparents may change the family experience over time. For example, limited data indicates that the constellation of the older grandparents raising older grandchildren fares more poorly on functioning and well-being measures than younger grandparents and grandchildren (Robinson et al., 2000). The empirical question is whether this change is a result of the concurrent aging process or poorer initial outcomes that were present within these families initially. Using a longitudinal design, researchers would track functioning within families over time to address this and related questions.

An additional area for longitudinal research is to assess the changes if the grandchild and parent are reunited. In some caregiving situations, a parent does reassume caregiving for the child upon being released from prison or achieving sobriety. How do grandparents reorganize their lives after grandchildren leave the household? How do the parents and grandparents renegotiate their changed roles and their role with the child? Although grandparents may welcome the opportunity to have the parent regain the caregiving role, there are also losses that are experienced, such as companionship. In addition, the grandparent may question the permanency of the caregiving and worry that the child will reenter their household at some later point. These questions would be answered with longitudinal research about changes when a parent reenters as care provider of the child.

POLICY IMPLICATIONS

Numerous policy changes need to be implemented to support custodial grandparents. These initiatives call for social workers to serve in a variety of roles to promote more comprehensive policies at the state and federal level. One role is to function as an advocate to change social welfare policy to be more responsive to intergenerational families. Because many custodial grandparents are raising grandchildren in informal care arrangements, they may lack entitlement to financial and social support. In addition, laws and policies vary geographically. For example, 26% of custodial grandparents live in rural areas (Pebley & Rudkin, 1999). Traditionally, these locations have minimal resources to assist grandparents, who then face economic and social problems without support.

In addition, social workers need to participate in research to determine the efficacy of various demonstration projects for intergenerational families. There is no comprehensive service system for these families, and various small, idiosyncratic programs are found across diverse locations. Research can determine the outcomes of various types of interventions at the family level and for grandparents. These outcome data can be used to make sound decisions about expanding successful programs to serve greater numbers of families.

To provide a more comprehensive system to support intergenerational families, various issues that have particular relevance to these families need to be considered and evaluated within policy arenas. Particular issues include establishing eligibility for social programs, guardianship and custody, and flexibility with labor force options. Policy changes that allow intergenerational families options to meet the needs of their particular situation would enhance functioning and well-being for the grandparents and grandchildren.

Eligibility for Social Programs

Social welfare programs are provided in an array of fragmented and uncoordinated services. One area of confusion and frustration for grandparents is the assortment of programs that exists, specifically in the area of economic support such as Temporary Assistance for Needy Families (TANF) or the SSI program (Flint & Perez-Porter, 1997). Some programs, such as SSI, are based upon the particular situation of the child (e.g., parents are dead or disabled). Other programs, such as TANF, involve calculation of household resources. These various approaches to social programs are confusing for many families, and too often these families do not qualify for resources that could potentially support their functioning and well-being.

Guardianship and Custody

A major legal issue that grandparents confront involves custody decisions. Formalizing a child-care arrangement may bring certain advantages, such as additional financial support. However, most grandparents are informal kinship-care providers and often resist moving to a more formal arrangement such as legal custody or adoption. Various options and decision-making capacities also create confusion within the family (Karp, 1996).

There are numerous reasons why most family caregiving remains at the informal level. First, grandparents may fear that their grandchildren will be placed in foster care. This sentiment translates into a lack of trust in formal systems, with the typical outcome of remaining outside of formal child welfare services. Second, cultural norms and values may be at odds with public policy that seeks to reconfigure authority and relationships within the family system (Burnette, 1997). In addition, the movement toward a formal custody arrangement also has clinical meaning for grandparents. Even in cases where there are significant rewards (e.g., financial, decision making), grandparents may feel that formalizing the relationship with their grandchildren sends a message that they have given up on their own child. The tension of divided loyalties between their own son or daughter and their grandchild can be very emotional for the grandparent.

Because of these issues, custody needs to have a more fluid and flexible structure for grandparents. Although the structure and process for legal custody vary by state, most have fairly restrictive procedures for grandparents to receive services and entitlements that involve formalized custody arrangements. Additional analysis of more fluid structures needs to be performed, such as grandparents who care for grandchildren for shorter periods of time (e.g., less than 1 year) or with irregular circumstances.

Labor Force Policy

Raising grandchildren may also impact labor force participation of grandparents. Like other caregivers, grandparents may need to alter employment because of child care demands (Sands & Goldberg-Glen, 1998). Because of economic stresses, some grandparents need to retain jobs past their expected time of retirement. Other grandparents may need to leave their jobs or forego advancements such as promotions, in order to be available to their grandchildren. These care providers have to juggle child care and work and may lose the opportunity for enhancing their income.

Several changes in labor force policy may create an environment that is friendlier to custodial grandparents. Raising a child is expensive, and adequate child tax credits may help families preserve income for basic necessities. In addition, policies that promote family-centered employment situations (such as on-site day care or adequate family leave policy) may relieve the stress in handling multiple demands of work and family.

The structure of the typical work pattern is another area that is problematic for families with children. The most common employment pattern is the 40-hours-plus position. Unfortunately, part-time jobs may be rare and lack fringe benefits such as insurance or pension plans. Policy changes that make part-time employment or job-sharing strategies more attractive to businesses may provide families with greater labor force options. If a grandparent is able to work less than a 40-hour week, it might promote time to be in the household when the children are home and allow older grandparents to reserve some physical and emotional energy for childcare demands.

INTEGRATING KNOWLEDGE INTO THE CURRICULUM

Because of the nature and prevalence of this family form, students need to be exposed to practice and policy issues of intergenerational families. However, discussion of custodial grandparents should not be confined to gerontology courses, especially when one considers that being a *grandparent* is certainly not restricted to the older population. Content regarding life experiences of grandparents raising grandchildren can be infused into various required and elective courses (c.f. Kropf & Burnette, 2003). Samples of ways to present content on intergenerational families are offered.

Cultural Diversity

The impetus for social work education to implement a course on cultural diversity begins with the values and ethics of the profession. One has to look no further than the National Association of Social Workers Code of Ethics to see social work's commitment to cultural diversity (NASW, 1996). Specifically, section 1.05 of the Code (Cultural Competence and Social Diversity) recognizes social workers' obligation to understanding the nature of social diversity and strengths within all cultures and populations. In terms of grandparents raising grandchildren, there are at least two themes that are germane within the curricula of cultural diversity coursework: (a) acknowledging and understanding the prevalence of custodial grandparents as a distinct culture, and (b) understanding and affirming the ethnic diversity within this culture, particularly in African American and Hispanic families.

Persell (1987, p. 47) defined culture as "the accumulation of customs, values, and artifacts shared by a people." In this fashion, the population of custodial grandparents is indeed a social culture. In a society where a parent is deemed the natural custodian of the child, grandparents share a characteristic of assuming time-disordered roles as caregivers. Other shared characteristics of many within this culture include relatively small household incomes (compared to the median household income), a feeling of empowerment in raising grandchildren, and the belief that their primary caregiving role is permanent (Heywood, 1999).

How predominant is this culture? Roughly 10% of American grandparents are raising their grandchildren in the absence of the parents (Fuller-Thomson et al., 1997). Compared with only 4% of White families in America, the prevalence of custodial grandparents in African American and Hispanic families is more pronounced (Pinson-Millburn, Fabian, Schlossberg, & Pyle, 1996). More than 13% of African American children and 6% of Hispanic children are being raised by their grandparents. For both the custodial grandparent population as a whole and within ethnic cultures, the numbers are eye-opening, certainly enough to merit attention within the cultural diversity curricula.

Human Behavior and the Social Environment (HBSE)

Human behavior and the social environment courses usually cover broad themes in content, expounding upon theories of human behavior that influence a variety of paradigms in social work practice. General elements of HBSE coursework include traditional and alternative perspectives of individuals (e.g., developmental theories and identity development), families (e.g., family-centered practice and feminist perspectives), groups (e.g., group theory and ecological perspectives), and communities (e.g., social systems and social justice). HBSE provides a forum for readdressing and redefining the concept of family to include the diversity of modern American families. The concept of kinship care (Schriver, 1998), which emerged from African American scholars, is currently noted in literature as an alternative definition of family. Referring to any relative (by blood or by marriage) who may care for children who may otherwise be placed in out-of-home care, the kinship care family certainly includes households with custodial grandparents. In fact, Schriver noted in his HBSE text that kinship care may be responsible for preserving the African American family.

Advanced Practice and Intervention

There are a number of issues within the life experiences of custodial grandparents and their grandchildren that could be addressed in practice courses. In conducting family-centered practice with this population, it is important to examine factors that lead to grandparents' assumption of caregiving, such as drug addiction, HIV/AIDS, incarceration, or death of the birthparents (Kelley et al., 2001). Additionally, these factors may lead to potential physical problems (e.g., neurological disorders and developmental delays) or psychological problems (e.g., depression or anxiety) in the grandchildren.

There are a number of assessment and intervention strategies that foster healthy custodial grandparent-grandchild relationships, as well as empower grandparents so that they may confidently make decisions regarding their grandchildren (Kelley et al., 2001). Examples include strengths assessment, support groups for these grandparents, individual and group counseling, narrative therapy, and legal intervention (to improve the legal status of custodial arrangements). Advanced practice and intervention curricula provide opportunities for social work students to understand various techniques in improving the psychological and social well-being of custodial grandparents.

Religion and Spirituality Courses

Places of worship (churches, synagogues, mosques, temples) are fixtures in the lives of many custodial grandparents. In seeking and maintaining cultural connectedness, particularly in African American families, support groups for these grandparents often convene in churches (Roe & Minkler, 1998–99). Jendrek (1993) mentioned the church's significant impact on the caregiving lifestyle of grandparents raising their grandchildren.

Religious faith is an institution that is a source of resilience, courage, and togetherness in many American homes. Numerous studies have shown that a person's relationship with a Higher Power is a key source of strength in a number of ways: defeating loneliness, promoting a sense of purpose, instilling a sense of self-worth, and providing hope for the future (Ellison & Levin, 1998; Hodge, 2001; Pargament, 1997). If it is determined that a client's (in this case, the custodial grandparent and family) strength includes religious beliefs, the relationship with his or her God can be explored and nourished—the same process that therapists use to explore other client relationships.

The previous four examples are a brief illustration of the need to integrate the issues of grandparents raising grandchildren across the continuum of social work education. The numbers for this population continue to rise. For social work educators, addressing the strengths and concerns of custodial grandparents complies with the Council on Social Work Education's ethical tenet to understand, affirm, and respect persons of all cultures.

CONCLUSION

The numbers of grandparents and grandchildren who are members of intergenerational families have increased dramatically over recent years. Although aging services is one area where social workers and allied professionals will work with custodial grandparents, service providers in diverse service sectors—health care, school settings, mental health, juvenile justice, family service agencies—will also have clients who are part of these family systems. Clearly, there is a need for formal service professionals to understand the complex issues that exist within these family systems.

A number of issues related to custodial grandparents have been summarized in this chapter. A profile of intergenerational families was presented, with particular emphasis on health and social functioning. In addition, current intervention approaches were highlighted and critiqued. Specifically, the research project conducted as part of the John A. Hartford Geriatric Social Work Faculty Scholars Program was summarized. Titled *Let's Talk*, this intervention has specific utility with a large population of custodial grandparents who typically may be outside of existing service networks. In addition, content on intergenerational families was presented within the framework of the social work curriculum. Because this family form has increased dramatically, students within social work and related disciplines will need to learn content and skill development to work effectively with these families.

REFERENCES

Bandura, A. (1977). Self efficacy: Toward a unifying theory of behavioral change. *Psychological Review, 84,* 191–215.

Bandura, A. (1978). Reflections on self-efficacy. *Advances in Behaviour Research and Therapy, 37,* 139–161.

Barnhill, S. (1996, Spring). Three generations at risk: Imprisoned women, their children, and grandmother caregivers. *Generations,* 39–40.

Bartram, M. H. (1996). Clarifying subsystem boundaries in grandfamilies. *Contemporary Family Therapy, 18,* 267–277.

Bowers, B. F., & Myers, B. J. (1999). Grandmothers providing care for grandchildren: Consequences of various levels of caregiving. *Family Relations, 48,* 303–311.

Bryson, K. R. (2001, November). *New Census Bureau data on grandparents raising grandchildren.* Paper presented at the 54th Annual Scientific Meeting of the Gerontological Society of America, Chicago, IL.

Burnette, D. (1997). Grandparents raising grandchildren in the inner city. *Families in Society: Journal of Contemporary Human Services, 78,* 489–499.

Burnette, D. (1998). Grandparents rearing grandchildren: A school-based small group intervention. *Research on Social Work Practice, 8,* 10–27.

Burnette, D. (1999a). Social relationships of Latino grandparent caregivers: A role theory perspective. *Gerontologist, 39,* 49–58.

Burnette, D. (1999b). Physical and emotional well-being of custodial grandparents in Latino families. *American Journal of Orthopsychiatry, 69*, 305–318.

Burnette, D. (Ed.). (2000). Mental health of grandparent caregivers [Special issue]. *Journal of Mental Health and Aging, 6*(4).

Burton, L. M. (1992). Black grandparents rearing children of drug-addicted parents: Stressors, outcomes, and social service needs. *Gerontologist, 32*, 744–751.

Caliandro, G., & Hughes, C. (1998). The experience of being a grandmother who is the primary caregiver for her HIV-positive grandchild. *Nursing Research, 47*, 107–113.

Campis, L. K., Lyman, R. D., & Prentice-Dunn, S. (1986). The Parental Locus of Control Scale: Development and validation. *Journal of Clinical Child Psychiatry, 15*, 260–267.

Caputo, R. K. (1999). Grandmothers and coresident grandchildren. *Families in Society: Journal of Contemporary Human Services, 80*, 120–126.

Chalfie, D. (1994). *Going it alone: A closer look at grandparents parenting grandchildren.* Washington, DC: American Association of Retired Persons.

Cox, C. B. (2001). Empowering African American custodial grandparents. *Social Work, 47*, 45–54.

Creighton, R. (1991, December 16). "Silent saviors": Grandparents raising grandchildren. *U.S. News & World Report*, 83–89.

Derogatis, L. R., & Melisaratos, N. (1983). The Brief Symptom Inventory: An introductory report. *Psychological Medicine, 13*, 595–605.

Dressel, P. L., & Barnhill, S. K. (1994). Reframing gerontological thought and practice: The case of grandmothers with daughters in prison. *Gerontologist, 34*, 685–691.

Ellison, C. G., & Levin, J. S. (1998). The religion-health connection: Evidence, theory, and future directions. *Health Education and Behavior, 25*, 700–720.

Emick, M. A., & Hayslip, B. (1999). Custodial grandparenting: Stress, coping skills, and relationships with grandchildren. *International Journal of Aging and Human Development, 48*, 35–61.

Flint, M. M., & Perez-Porter, M. (1997). Grandparent caregivers: Legal and economic issues. *Journal of Gerontological Social Work, 28*, 63–76.

Folkman, S., Lazarus, R. S., Pimley, S., & Novacek, J. (1987). Age differences in stress and coping processes. *Psychology and Aging, 2*, 171–184.

Fuller-Thomson, E., Minkler, M., & Driver, D. (1997). A profile of grandparents raising grandchildren in the United States. *Gerontologist, 37*, 406–411.

Goldberg-Glen, R., Sands, R. G., Cole, R. D., & Cristofalo, C. (1998). Multigenerational patterns and internal structures in families in which grandparents raise grandchildren. *Families in Society: Journal of Contemporary Human Services, 79*, 477–489.

Grant, R., Gordon, S. G., & Cohen, S. T. (1997). An innovative school-based intergenerational model to serve grandparent caregivers. *Journal of Gerontological Social Work, 28*, 47–60.

Heywood, E. M. (1999). Custodial grandparents and their grandchildren. *Family Journal, 7*, 367–373.

Hodge, D. (2001). Spiritual assessment: A review of major qualitative methods and a new framework for assessing spirituality. *Social Work, 46,* 203–215.

Jendrek, M. P. (1993). Grandparents who parent their grandchildren: Effects on lifestyle. *Journal of Marriage and the Family, 55,* 609–621.

Karp, N. (1996, Spring). Legal problems of grandparents and other kinship caregivers. *Generations,* 57–60.

Kelley, S. J. (1993). Caregiver stress in grandparents raising grandchildren. *IMAGE: Journal of Nursing Scholarship, 25,* 331–337.

Kelley, S. J., Yorker, B. C., Whitley, D., & Sipe, T. A. (2001). A multi-modal intervention for grandparents raising grandchildren: Results of a pilot study. *Child Welfare, 53,* 27–50.

Kolomer, S. (2000). Kinship foster care and its impact on grandmother caregivers. *Journal of Gerontological Social Work, 33,* 85–102.

Kropf, N. P. (2001). *Let's Talk: An audio tape series for grandparents raising grandchildren.* Athens: University of Georgia, Office of Instructional Development.

Kropf, N. P., & Burnette, D. (2003). Grandparents as family caregivers: Lessons for intergenerational education. *Educational Gerontology, 29*(1), 1–11.

Kropf, N. P., & Robinson, M. M. (2002, February). *Pathways into caregiving for rural custodial grandparents.* Paper presented at the Annual Program Meeting, Council on Social Work Education, Nashville, TN.

Linsk, N. L., & Poindexter, C. C. (2000). Older caregivers for family members with HIV or AIDS: Reasons for caring. *Journal of Applied Gerontology, 19,* 181–202.

Lugalia, T. (1998). *Marital status and living arrangements: March 1998.* Washington, DC: U.S. Bureau of the Census.

McCallion, P., & Janicki, M. P. (Eds.). (2000). Grandparent carers of children with disabilities: Facing the challenge [Special issue]. *Journal of Gerontological Social Work, 33*(3).

Minkler, M., Driver, D., Roe, K. M., & Bedeian, K. (1993). Community interventions to support grandparent caregivers. *Gerontologist, 33,* 807–811.

Minkler, M., Fuller-Thompson, E., Miller, D., & Driver, D. (1997). Depression in grandparents raising grandchildren: Results of a national longitudinal study. *Archives of Family Medicine, 6,* 445–452.

Minkler, M., Roe, K. M., & Price, M. (1992). The physical and emotional health of grandmothers raising grandchildren in the crack cocaine epidemic. *Gerontologist, 32,* 752–761.

Minkler, M., Roe, K. M., & Robertson-Beckley, R. J. (1994). Raising grandchildren from crack-cocaine households: Effects on family and friendship ties of African-American women. *American Journal of Orthopsychiatry, 64,* 20–29.

Morrow-Kondos, D., Weber, J. A., Cooper, K., & Hesser, J. L. (1997). Becoming parents again: Grandparents raising grandchildren. *Journal of Gerontological Social Work, 28,* 35–46.

Musil, C. M. (1998). Health, stress, coping, and social support in grandmother caregivers. *Health Care for Women International, 19,* 441–455.

Myers, L., Kropf, N. P., & Robinson, M. M. (2002). Grandparents raising grandchildren: Case management in a rural setting. *Journal of Human Behavior in the Social Environment, 5,* 53–71.

National Association of Social Workers. (1996). *Code of Ethics of the National Association of Social Workers*. Washington, DC: NASW.

Pargament, K. I. (1997). *The psychology of religion and coping*. New York: Guilford Press.

Pebley, A. R., & Rudkin, L. L. (1999). Grandparents caring for grandchildren: What do we know? *Journal of Family Issues, 20*, 218–242.

Persell, C. H. (1987). *Understanding society: An introduction to sociology*. New York: Harper and Row.

Pinson-Millburn, N. M., Fabian, E. S., Schlossberg, N. K., & Pyle, M. (1996). Grandparents raising grandchildren. *Journal of Counseling and Development, 74*, 548–554.

Poindexter, C. P., & Linsk, N. L. (1999). I'm just glad that I'm here: Stories of seven African American HIV-affected grandmothers. *Journal of Gerontological Social Work, 32*, 63–81.

Pruchno, R. (1999). Raising grandchildren: The experience of Black and White grandmothers. *Gerontologist, 39*, 209–221.

Robinson, M. M., Kropf, N. P., & Myers, L. (2000). Grandparents raising grandchildren in rural communities. *Journal of Aging and Mental Health, 6*, 1–13.

Roe, K. M., & Minkler, M. (1998–99, Winter). Grandparents raising grandchildren: Challenges and responses. *Generations*, 25–32.

Roe, K. M., Minkler, M., & Barnwell, R. S. (1994). The assumption of caregiving: Grandmothers raising the children of the crack cocaine epidemic. *Qualitative Health Research, 4*, 281–303.

Roe, K. M., Minkler, M., Saunders, F., & Thomson, G. E. (1996). Health of grandmothers raising children of the crack cocaine epidemic. *Medical Care, 34*, 1072–1084.

Sands, R. G., & Goldberg-Glen, R. S. (1998). The impact of employment and serious illness on grandmothers who are raising their grandchildren. *Journal of Women and Aging, 10*, 41–58.

Schriver, J. M. (1998). *Human behavior and the social environment: Shifting paradigms in essential knowledge for social work practice* (2nd ed.). Boston: Allyn and Bacon.

Strawbridge, W. M., Wallhagen, J. I., Shema, S. J., & Kaplan, G. A. (1997). New burdens or more of the same? Comparing grandparent, spouse, and adult-child caregivers. *Gerontologist, 37*, 505–510.

Szinovacz, M. E., DeViney, S., & Atkinson, M. P. (1999). Effects of surrogate parenting on grandparents' well-being. *Journal of Gerontology: Social Sciences, 54B*, S376–S388.

Whetten-Goldstein, K., & Nguyen, T. Q. (2001). Characteristics of individuals infected with the human immunodeficiency virus and provider interaction in the predominantly rural southeast. *Southern Medical Journal, 94*, 212–222.

Whitley, D. M., White, K. R., Kelley, S. J., & Yorker, B. (1999). Strengths-based case management: The application to grandparents raising grandchildren. *Families in Society: Journal of Contemporary Human Services, 80*, 110–119.

Chapter **9**

AGING PERSONS
WITH DEVELOPMENTAL
DISABILITIES AND
THEIR CAREGIVERS

Philip McCallion and Stacey R. Kolomer

Adults with developmental disabilities are living longer, which raises concerns about a growing need for caregivers and a demand for services and special attention that many states and localities are ill-prepared to address (Braddock, 1999; Seltzer & Krauss, 1994). In addition, social workers and other professionals have little training in meeting the special needs of this population group (McCallion, 1993).

Historically, state disability systems gave more attention to developing educational and vocational services for children and work-age adults with developmental disabilities than to the needs of those persons who reach old age (Braddock, 1999; McCallion, 1993). Disagreements over how to proceed have also slowed the development of needed services. For example, which service system should be responsible—aging or developmental disabilities? Is the primary client the aging caregiver, the person with a developmental disability, or the family? Finally, what are appropriate service models—maintaining the family living situation, planning for transitions to out-of-home placement, or promoting the independence of the person with a developmental disability (McCallion & Janicki, 1997)? A further complication is the well-documented conflictual relationship between older caregivers who provide long-term care and formal service providers (McCallion & Tobin, 1995; Smith & Tobin, 1993).

The pressing need for attention to this population arises in part because until recently, few people with developmental disabilities lived to old age. Those who did reach later adulthood were often invisible because family members provided lifetime care (Roberto, 1993). In recent decades, the likelihood has increased of aging persons with developmental disabilities living into retirement years and outliving family caregivers has increased (Fujiura, 1998). Hence, there is a growing and pressing need to address the aging years.

The aging of persons with developmental disabilities is frequently not a part of discourse on the graying of society. This has significant implications for the health care system, the roles of social workers and other professionals, the operation of public-funded services, and for policy assumptions. Limited attention also has been given to lifelong caregiving by the parents of these individuals. The literature has primarily focused on child care in young-adult and middle-adult years, parent care in late middle-adult years, and spouse care in older-adult years. The more recent discovery of "sandwich" caregivers—those caring for multiple generations—and of grandparents caring for their grandchildren also challenges the initial assumptions of that literature. A better understanding of older caregivers of persons with developmental disabilities may provide further insights into the needs and resilience of all caregivers. Similarly, understanding how the developmental disabilities service system is working within the community to accommodate the needs of aging persons, particularly those with symptoms of dementia, may suggest alternatives for the care of all persons with dementia.

This chapter will present some recent developments on the aging of this population and their caregivers and will review both prior knowledge and research, relating this information to policy and curriculum implications. Cultural differences and recent work on grandparent caregivers also will be included. Some definitions are offered here to guide the review.

As defined in the Developmental Disabilities and Bill of Rights Act of 2000 (Public Law 106-904), a developmental disability is a severe, chronic disability that (a) is attributable to a mental or physical impairment or combination of mental and physical impairments; (b) is manifest before age 22; (c) is likely to continue indefinitely; (d) results in substantial functional limitations in three or more areas of major life activity such as abilities in self care, receptive and expressive language, learning, mobility and self-direction, capacity for independent living, and economic self-sufficiency; and (e) reflects the need for a combination and sequence of special, interdisciplinary, or generic care, treatment, or other services that are of lifelong or extended duration and are individually planned and coordinated.

Traditionally, services have been primarily targeted to people with mental retardation (persons with Down's syndrome would be considered a subgroup of persons with mental retardation; Janicki & Dalton, 2000). The historic focus on this group also is reflected in the labels used to describe such individuals, "persons with mental retardation" currently being the most common. However, there are efforts to change this to "persons with intellectual disabilities." Regardless, publicly funded formal services continue to be largely concentrated on persons with mental retardation.

Permanency (or futures) planning also is an important aspect of developmental disabilities services and is related to the later stages of life of both the family member with a developmental disability and his or her parents. It refers to establishing future life arrangements for the person with a developmental disability, generally outside the parent-child household, in the areas of residential living, legal protection, and financial well-being (Smith & Tobin, 1989). Examples of residential-living permanency planning include consideration of independent living; of shared households with siblings, other relatives, or family friends; and of transitions into supervised apartment, adult foster care, and group home programs. Legal protection issues include consideration of legal guardianship, trusteeship, and conservatorship of person and property issues, including the drafting of wills and other documents. Financial issues include arrangements to ensure continued financial eligibility for needed services for the person with a developmental disability, while providing a safety net should those services be unavailable or insufficient (McCallion, 1993). As persons with developmental disabilities age, future living arrangements and the associated legal and financial concerns become major issues, either because older caregiving parents are no longer able or available to provide care or because prior out-of-home placements no longer seem suitable for age-related needs. These are often primary concerns for social workers who come in contact with aging individuals who have developmental disabilities.

SIGNIFICANCE TO GERONTOLOGY, HEALTH CARE, AND HEALTH PROFESSIONALS

There are no accurate and complete counts of people in the United States who are aging with developmental disabilities. Estimates suggest that their life expectancy has increased from an average 18.5 years in 1930 to 59.1 years in 1970 to an estimated 66.2 years in 1993 (Braddock, 1999). Based upon analyses of New York State data, Janicki and colleagues go further, projecting continued increases that more closely match the life expectancy of the general population (Janicki, Dalton, Henderson, & Davidson, 1999). Indeed, there are estimates that by 2020 the number of persons with developmental disabilities older than age 65 will have doubled (Janicki & Dalton, 2000).

When persons with developmental disabilities were not expected to live into old age, there was a reasonable expectation that parents would outlive their offspring and offer a lifetime of care. Because most care was provided in the home, services for old age were not developed or provided. As can be seen in Figure 9.1, a majority of persons with developmental disabilities still live at home. Approximately 10% are in out-of-home placements. Some individuals live with spouses; they and those who live independently represent small percentages and tend to have less profound impairments than do those who live with caregivers. For the first time, there are sizeable groups of individuals with developmental disabilities who are aging and needing related services.

As shown in Figure 9.2, many individuals are already in households where the caregiver is older. By 2020, a majority of those who are being cared for by older caregivers will themselves be older than 60 and will likely be cared for by the same but much older caregiver. Caregivers currently in their 40s and 50s will be in their 60s and 70s in 2020. Therefore, the growth of the aging population for this group of individuals has double the implications. There are aging needs for both the person with a developmental disability and his or her caregiver, and a likelihood that greater demands will be placed on limited out-of-home services because the caregiver is no longer able or available to provide care (Braddock, 1999).

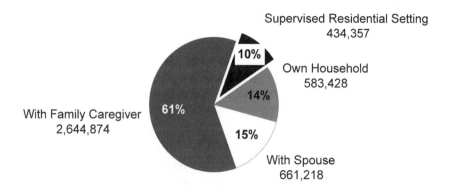

**Total Estimated Population with a
Developmental Disability: 4,323,877**

FIGURE 9.1   United States: Distribution of individuals with a developmental disability by living arrangement, 2000.

Note: Adapted from Braddock, Emerson, Felce, & Stancliffe (2001), and Fujiura (1998).

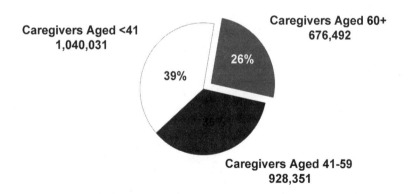

**Total Estimated Population of Persons with a
Developmental Disability Living with Family Caregivers: 2,644,874**

FIGURE 9.2   United States: Distribution of individuals with a developmental disability living with family caregivers, 2000.

Note: Adapted from Braddock et al. (2001), and Fujiura (1998).

Health Issues

A recently completed systematic study of the health needs of persons with developmental disabilities aged 40 and older, living in group homes in two catchment areas of New York State, found them to be similar to other adults of the same age in terms of overall health status (outside of expected disability-related conditions and physical conditioning). For example, psychiatric and behavioral disorders tended to decline in frequency with increasing age, whereas cardiovascular diseases and sensory impairments increased with age (Janicki et al., 2002). However, low rates of exercise and high rates of diet-related conditions were evident. More than half the cohort was classified as obese according to their body mass index (BMI) (Flegal, 1999). Obesity among these individuals, however, was not often noted by their physicians as a concern. Other researchers also have observed this. The discrepancy raises concerns that health practitioners may accept obesity as normal among adults with developmental disabilities and not address as aggressively the health consequences. Similarly, although cardiovascular and respiratory diseases and cancers have been reported as causes for death for these individuals as frequently as for the general population (Evenhuis, 1997), there was a relatively low reported rate of these diseases in the two catchment areas. This may be due to the relatively younger age of this group of adults (mean age, 54), but given the risk status of this population for these diseases due to high BMIs and infrequent exercise, these results were considered surprising and may reflect underrecognition of health conditions (Janicki et al., 2002).

Findings of low-quality health care delivery is fueling an ongoing concern within the developmental disabilities field about the relationship between the health care provided and the mortality of persons with developmental disabilities (for a review, see Hayden, 1998). Some argue that those receiving institutional care actually have greater longevity as opposed to community-based care, and that this may be due to better access to specialized and consistent health care (Strauss & Kastner, 1996). Yet there is a need to ensure that community-based care is pursued as the preferred option for persons with a developmental disability who are aging (Hayden, 1998).

Dementia

Like the population at large, persons with developmental disabilities are at greater risk of Alzheimer's disease and other dementias (ADD) as they age (Brookmeyer, Gray, & Kawas, 1998). Responding to this risk has become a major concern of the developmental-disabilities services system in the United States and elsewhere (University of Stirling, 2001). It has been estimated that in the United States there may be as many as 140,000 such older adults who are affected by ADD, and that this number will triple within the next 20 years (Janicki & Dalton, 2000). Because existing disabilities often mask symptoms of dementia, concerns noted earlier about the quality of health care available to these individuals are magnified. It also makes assessment more difficult, and concerns about the absence of treatment alternatives discourage diagnosis and active treatment (Janicki, McCallion, & Dalton, in press). Yet diagnosis and active responses are possible and available (Dalton, Tsiouris, & Patti, 2000; McCallion & Janicki, 2002; McCarron, 1999).

Among persons with developmental disabilities, adults with Down's syndrome are generally at higher risk of ADD (Holland, Karlinsky, & Berg, 1993). In a secondary analysis of out-of-home-care data maintained by state agencies in New York, Janicki and Dalton (1999) observed that the prevalence of ADD in adults with developmental disabilities was about 3% of adults aged 40 years and older and 6% of adults aged 60 years and older. For adults with Down's syndrome, the rates were 22% and 56%, respectively, for these two age groups. No data are available on families who are caring for individuals with developmental disabilities at home. Yet, as was noted earlier, the population cared for at home is larger than those participating in developmental-disabilities service systems (Braddock, 1999), and there is every reason to believe that ADD is as prevalent among this group. The first recognition of ADD symptoms usually occurs in the mid-60s for adults with other developmental disabilities and in the early 50s for adults with Down's syndrome. With respect to the course ADD takes, it appears to mirror that of the general population among adults with other developmental disabilities. However, for adults with Down's syndrome, the course tends to be compressed, the duration short, and the decline precipitous (Janicki & Dalton, 1999).

SOCIAL WORK AND CAREGIVING IN DEVELOPMENTAL DISABILITIES

As noted earlier, family caregiving is the most prevalent care of adults with developmental disabilities and many of those caregivers are themselves aging (Braddock, 1999; Fujiura, 1998). It is estimated that the length of time older parents provide care can extend to four and five decades (Essex, Seltzer, & Krauss, 1999; Walsh, Conliffe, & Birkbeck, 1993). Caring for an individual at home includes the following: shopping, personal care, food preparation, financial support, and decision making. In addition, the severity of disability has an impact on the quantity of instrumental care a parent provides. Even when the adult is not living with a parent, there are still many caretaking tasks that can consume an older parent's time. For example, one task is ensuring sufficient financial resources in ways that do not reduce a person's eligibility for governmental benefits (Bigby, 1997; Essex et al., 1999). In addition to the burden of caring for an adult with a developmental disability, aging parents must cope with their own impending health problems and eventual death. Questions and concerns about who will be responsible for their dependent adult child can become overwhelming. Conversely, social workers and other professionals often do not recognize the caregiving strength of these family members, even as they cope with their own diminishing health (McCallion & Toseland, 1993). Further, social workers may view the mutual emotional and financial support they often encounter as not in the best interest of the individual with a developmental disability (McCallion & Tobin, 1995).

One priority for social workers is to assist these families with putting formal arrangements in place for the adult child should the parent become incapacitated or die. Survey responses from administrators and practitioners suggest that many times when these plans are not in place, the illness or death of a caregiver requires a crisis response (McCallion & Tobin, 1995). This often precludes choosing the best options for the person with a developmental disability. However, it has been found that social workers need to carefully consider the timing of transitions and be sensitive to gender-based, cultural, and family values when assisting families with permanency care plans (McCallion & Grant-Griffin, 2000).

PRIOR RESEARCH AND KNOWLEDGE BASE

Traditionally, women have been the primary caregivers in families, and this is also true when there is a person with developmental disabilities. The lifelong nature of caregiving that begins in younger years increases the likelihood that two parents are or have been involved. However, in families with a child who is disabled, parent roles have been found to be even more traditional than in homes with a child who does not have an identified disability (Heller, Hsieh, & Rowitz, 1997). Most often in these homes, fathers work to support the family, while mothers stay at home to take care of the person with a developmental disability. Because they are less likely to provide hands-on care, fathers are often found to be less familiar with the support network and services (Essex et al., 1999, 2002). In the aging years, there is evidence that these patterns continue. Even after retirement, fathers are unlikely to take on additional responsibilities within the home (Essex et al., 1999; Heller, Hsieh, et al., 1997). However, it is important for social workers not to stereotype families and fathers. There is evidence that a small number of men are the primary caregivers for adults with developmental disabilities and they often feel isolated and judged by assumptions that it is a mother's role (McCallion & Kolomer, 2001).

Coping Strategies

Coping can be defined as the different ways in which people respond to stressful events (Essex et al., 1999). Providing care to an adult with an intellectual disability is likely to be perceived as both rewarding and stressful (Heller, Miller, & Factor, 1997; McCallion & Toseland, 1993). Mothers have been found to use a variety of coping strategies as they provide care for their adult child, which include acceptance, positive reinterpretation and growth, turning to religion, and planning (Hayden & Heller, 1997). In a longitudinal study, Essex and colleagues (1999) found that mothers were significantly more likely than fathers to use problem-focused coping strategies as a means of addressing stress with their dependent children who have intellectual disabilities. Problem-focused coping includes using cognitive and behavioral problem-solving efforts as a technique for reducing stress (Essex et al., 1999). In analyzing whether significant differences exist between younger and older caregivers, Hayden and Heller (1997) found that older caregivers sought spiritual support more often than their younger counterparts, and younger caregivers more often experienced greater personal burden than older caregivers. Understanding the different ways mothers versus fathers and older versus younger caregivers cope is important for social workers in designing interventions.

Rewards of Caregiving

Despite the demands of caring for an adult with a developmental disability, there are several associated rewards. Older mothers caring for adults with mental retardation have been reported as having high morale and as rating their health as good or excellent (Seltzer, Greenberg, Krauss, & Hong, 1997). Mothers who cared for adults with chronic disabilities reported more caregiving satisfaction than did fathers (Heller, Hsieh, et al., 1997). In contrast with mothers caring for an adult child with a mental illness, mothers caring for an adult child with an intellectual disability reported more social support, less subjective burden, and more effective coping strategies (Greenberg, Seltzer, Krauss, & Kim, 1997; Seltzer, Greenberg, & Krauss, 1995; Seltzer et al., 1997).

Long-Term Planning for Adults With Developmental Disabilities

Parents are often averse to creating detailed future care (permanency) plans for their adult children with developmental disabilities (Bigby, 1996). Stress, concerns for safety, and anxiety all contribute to parents' reluctance to make concrete plans (Freedman, Krauss, & Seltzer, 1997; Heller & Factor, 1991; Kaufman, Adams, & Campbell, 1991; Seltzer & Krauss, 1994). For example, Heller and Factor (1991) found that almost 75% of family care providers for persons older than 30 years of age who have a developmental disability did not make plans for future living arrangements for their family member. Often, too, there was a reluctance to speak of future living arrangements with other family members. Therefore, the expectations that other family members would assume care responsibilities were often implied rather than formally documented (Bigby, 1996). In a sample of 340 mothers, fewer than half had a specific long-term-care plan in place should the parent no longer be able to provide care (Freedman et al., 1997).

In a qualitative study of 62 adults with a developmental disability, Bigby (1996) identified four types of planning by parents. The first two are explicit and implicit key-person succession plans, which transfer the responsibility of overseeing to an appointed person. Key-person succession plans ranged from formal documented plans (explicit) to open-ended and vague plans (implicit). Family members who have been designated the implicit key person are usually aware of their designation and are usually unsure of the exact expectations that accompany the role.

The third type is a financial plan. These are decisions about income and monies for future care. Often, well-intentioned plans have been found to have unintended consequences, as families do not understand the implications of their financial arrangements for future eligibility for services.

The fourth type is a residential plan. This concerns planning where the person with a developmental disability will reside following the parent's death or inability to continue to provide care. Again, these may be marked by unrealistic expectations of what the service system can provide or may be based on outdated information. Among 62 adults with a developmental disability living in a family home, Bigby (1996) found that plans were most often implicit and much of the emphasis was placed on informal network supports. Residential care plans were least likely to have been discussed or put into place by families. Indeed, Bigby found that parents who designated a key person for succession of care often felt relieved of the responsibility to make emotionally charged decisions, such as future residential planning.

Siblings of Adults Who Have Developmental Disabilities

When parents are no longer available, siblings have been found most often to be the caregivers to adults who have developmental disabilities (Bigby, 1997). Most available literature identifies a positive connection between persons with developmental disabilities and their siblings. However, there are limited data on sibling relationships in later life. Zitlin (1986) characterized five different types of sibling relationships based on a study of 35 adults with mental retardation. Relationships ranged from intensely close to having no contact with the sibling at all. Relationships were often influenced by parental expectations, were hierarchical, and rarely offered opportunities for reciprocity. Yet the person with a developmental disability often had a strong emotional attachment to his or her brother or sister (Krauss, Seltzer, Gordon, & Friedman, 1996; Seltzer, Begun, Seltzer, & Krauss, 1991).

Research to date suggests that support by siblings is expressed in a variety of ways. Most often siblings provide emotional, affective support, for example, through telephone calls and visits (Seltzer et al., 1991). Siblings are less likely to provide hands-on or instrumental care. Parents are more likely to expect that their other children will take on the role of overseer, rather than as the hands-on care provider to their sibling (Seltzer, Begun, Magan, & Luchterhand, 1993). When one sibling is unmarried and childless, there is a greater likelihood of instrumental support as the siblings age (Bigby, 1997). In addition, siblings who identify themselves as the future care providers of their adult brothers or sisters are more likely to be older than the person with a developmental disability, and more likely to be sisters rather than brothers. Persons with developmental disabilities who have fewer behavior problems were most likely to have a plan to live with a sibling (Krauss et al., 1996; Seltzer et al., 1991). Without stereotyping families and siblings, this is important information for social workers concerned with helping families plan for the future.

Caregiving Across Cultures

Disabilities can and do occur in all cultural groups. However, persons of diverse cultures with a developmental disability and their families have been found to be underrepresented among those enrolled for services with public developmental disabilities agencies (Grant-Griffin, 1995). The cultural background of a family contributes to decisions about caregiving. One's culture—the values, beliefs, customs, behaviors, structures, and identity by which a group of people define themselves (Axelson, 1993)—does appear to influence one's willingness to use services.

Three sets of assumptions appear to be used to inappropriately justify not targeting services to persons with developmental disabilities who are from a minority group and their families. The assumptions are that (a) they prefer to use family, cultural, and community-based supports rather than formal services; (b) the role of culture in their day-to-day lives has diminished and does not need to be considered; and (c) they can be accommodated by existing formal agencies and services (McCallion & Grant-Griffin, 2000). The existence of mediators of culture, such as migration and assimilation, does mean that there is no single cultural profile for families from diverse cultures. This often causes practitioners, administrators, and policy makers to miss the significance of culture, or to argue that its impact is overrated or of declining significance over time. Culture does affect caregiving and the use of services, but its effects may be difficult to discern and may vary across families. Findings from focus groups suggest that, rather than being dismissed, the impact of culture should be assessed, family by family, if culturally competent interventions are to be initiated (McCallion, Janicki, & Grant-Griffin, 1997).

Indeed, findings from research with inner-city African American, Latino, Haitian, and Chinese American caregiving families refute the assumption that they can be accommodated by traditional agencies and existing services. The findings suggest that social workers and others must recognize and harness the strengths offered by local multicultural agencies and involve them in the expansion of services to underserved populations (McCallion et al., 1997; McCallion, Janicki, Grant-Griffin, & Kolomer, 2000). Such agencies have always existed; some are church-based, others are fraternal in nature. Many offer a combination of social, cultural, and human services, and most of their funding is raised within the community they serve. These agencies serve locally based cultural communities that do not have services, or where existing services are not appropriate, or when a cultural community's language and customs make accessing formal services difficult. They are also (a) easily accessed, do not require appointments, and have longer hours of operation than other agencies; (b) are seen by families as more likely to understand cultural concerns; (c) are more likely to see culture as an intervention facilitator rather than an intervention barrier; and (d) are likely to help families change their environment, rather than looking at families for the source of the presenting problems (Iglehart & Becerra, 1996; McCallion et al., 1997).

Interviews with families also yielded other areas for culturally competent practice. Social workers are often surprised when their help is rejected, or when families are fearful or suspicious of their intentions. Families often attribute much of the conflict to social workers' insensitivity of cultural concerns and to a lack of recognition of the need to build up trust sufficiently so that families feel comfortable discussing cultural and family issues with them. They argue that social workers are rarely open to family structures and ways of caring that are different from their own. Given this, social workers need to recognize that they are working with families, not just the presenting family members. Just as important, social workers should avoid stereotyping family members by virtue of gender, or by society's or the social worker's own cultural expectations. Social workers also must be open to recognizing that different values and structures may mean different services are called for. These findings emphasize the critical need for culturally competent practice (McCallion & Grant-Griffin, 2000).

CURRENT RESEARCH

Current work by the authors and their colleagues addresses dementia care for persons with developmental disabilities and interventions with a newly considered group of caregivers: grandparents.

Dementia Care

A recent survey of 54 group homes (Janicki et al., in press) caring for at least one person with a developmental disability and ADD found that a range of factors influenced agency decision-making about maintaining individuals in the community. These factors include the presentation of ADD symptoms, the staff and home capabilities, and the resources that the agency had available to provide ADD-related care on a continuing (or long-term) basis. Yet the survey also found that when attention was given to these issues, some service providers did adapt their current approaches to provide ADD care in small-group living or family-situation settings, irrespective of long-term disability. Several strategies proved important: (a) modifying the physical plant (to increase safety, access, and independence); (b) increasing administrative preparation in terms of planning, fiscal management, and resource allocations (to provide a supportive administrative environment for clinical services); (c) adapting best practice models for staff training (to ensure staff readiness and capability); and (d) recruiting and training staff for ADD-capable environments (to maintain a workforce familiar with ADD-related care). Conversely, lack of attention to symptoms, inappropriate staffing, training and programming, and poor connections to service systems meant that decisions about the person with a developmental disability and ADD were made in response to crises in care, and often resulted in placement in more restrictive settings. These finding have informed the development of several training packages (McCallion & Janicki, 2002; McCallion, Janicki, & Dalton, 2001).

Grandparent Caregivers

A more recent caregiving phenomenon is grandparents caring for children with developmental disabilities (Janicki, McCallion, Grant-Griffin, & Kolomer, 2000). The scant data previously available were drawn from data from kinship foster-care systems. Kinship foster care is formal care of a child that is provided by family members other than the child's biological parent under the supervision and legal custody of the child welfare system. Compared with their peers, these children have been found to have a higher incidence of health problems, more frequent difficulties in school, and more serious emotional challenges (Berrick, Barth, & Needles, 1994). These children were also found to have higher occurrences of visual and hearing problems, asthma, arrested growth, obesity, anemia, developmental disabilities, psychosomatic complaints, and dental problems (for a review, see Kolomer, 2000). Given that the most frequent reasons for placement of a child with a grandparent are parental substance abuse and child abuse and neglect, it should not be surprising that children are likely to have emotional difficulties and disabilities, as substance abuse and child abuse are also risk factors for these conditions.

Data collected in New York City on more than 600 caregiving grandparent families with and without children who have developmental disabilities both confirmed earlier findings and shed further light on their unique experiences. Grandparents caring for a child with a disability were found to receive less social support than other family caregivers, and they experienced high levels of role strain, financial strain, and life disruption (McCallion et al., 2000). Caregiving for children with disabilities in less formal grandparent caregiving arrangements was equally challenging, and there were often even fewer formal resources available (Kolomer, 2000; McCallion et al., 2000). There were individual reports of grandparents caring for adult grandchildren with developmental disabilities. These grandparents indicated that they had fewer permanency planning options than the older parents previously discussed. For all grandparent caregivers, the unexpected need to provide care appeared to be associated with heightened symptoms of depression (Janicki, McCallion, Grant-Griffin, et al., 2000; Kolomer, McCallion, & Janicki, in press).

A more focused intervention study, using a randomized experimental design, also has been undertaken, involving 97 grandparents caring for children with developmental disabilities. The study found that intensive case management and support-group interventions significantly increased a sense of caregiving mastery and reduced symptoms of depression (McCallion et al., 2000).

FURTHER RESEARCH NEEDS

Research should continue to document the current and growing needs of aging persons with developmental disabilities and to test model programs for addressing the health and dementia care needs for these individuals and supports for their family caregivers. For example, more work is needed in testing and refining the training packages being developed for dementia care and interventions for grandparent caregivers as reported in this chapter's section on current research. The goal of maintaining people who have developmental disabilities in the community faces new challenges as this population ages. Too often service responses for this population are made in response to crises and are not carefully planned out (McCallion & Tobin, 1995). Knowing that the population of aging persons will continue to increase, research has an important role to play in defining and testing the effectiveness of options to prepare for, rather than merely respond to, this challenge. A related challenge is to offer insight into more family-oriented responses and service options rather than the current approach, where funding and services are targeted on an individual basis. This has important implications for greater outreach to families of diverse cultures and grandparents, and the likelihood of an increase in the mutual support needs of older persons with developmental disabilities and their aging family caregivers.

POLICY IMPLICATIONS

To date, care of aging persons with developmental disabilities has remained largely within the purview of developmental disabilities service providers. There also have been efforts to include these persons in generic services such as senior centers. Indeed, the National Family Caregiver Support Program funded under the Older American Act Amendments of 2000 (Public Law 106-501) has identified this group and its family caregivers as a targeted population for area agencies on aging. This will represent an important bridging role for social workers and an area where they may be involved in addressing barriers. Some of the barriers have been identified and include the following: (a) two service systems, aging and developmental disabilities, which have different languages, philosophies, and priorities; (b) lack of knowledge about the specific needs of older families caring for adults with developmental disabilities, which makes it difficult to plan for their inclusion in services; (c) major differences in how services are funded and organized within each system; (d) lack of clear-cut goals in both systems, which makes joint planning more difficult; (e) the time expended on meetings, training sessions, and consultations, which is often perceived by workers in both service systems as an additional hindrance to their efforts to meet needs they poorly understand; (f) resistance by other aging constituencies to including persons with developmental disabilities in aging services planning and spending; (g) those brokering cooperative efforts are rarely seen as impartial by either service system; and (h) lack of personnel who are trained in both service systems, although such training seems critical to cooperative efforts (McCallion & Janicki, 1997). New solutions and genuine integration of persons with developmental disabilities as they age will also require sustained advocacy by social workers and others for health care, dementia care, grandparent support, and culturally competent practice.

Health Care

At the very least, it does appear that access to quality and aggressive health care in the community for aging persons with developmental disabilities is impaired by communication difficulties, a low priority given to their health care needs, inadequate physician preparation, low reimbursement, and a failure to recognize that prolonged life is becoming more normative for this population (Carlsen, Galliuzzi, Forman, & Cavalieri, 1994; Evenhuis, 1997; Evenhuis et al., 2000; Harper & Wadsworth, 1992; Henderson & Davidson, 2000; Janicki et al., 2002). Here is a critical arena where social workers must play a role in raising awareness of these concerns, locating physicians who understand and are interested in this population, and advocating for adequate levels of reimbursement so that complete and appropriate assessment and care of health conditions are provided.

Dementia Care

The developmental disabilities service system and its group homes were designed to serve a young-adult and middle-adult population.

Existing programming and staffing models were not designed to meet the unique needs of persons with developmental disabilities and symptoms of ADD. With the aging of adults who have developmental disabilities, providers of community services are being challenged to provide a new range of in-home and other community-based supports (Janicki et al., in press). Because the occurrence of ADD is expected to rise due to increases in longevity, agencies and agency social workers must raise the "index of suspicion" among care staff and families, advocate for the adaptation of services to become "ADD-capable," help address environmental barriers in family homes and group homes to promote staying in the community, work to improve diagnostic and technical resources, convince families to connect with providers, and locate services critical to maintaining persons in the community, including clinical services and end-of-life care supports (Janicki et al., in press; McCallion, 1999; McCarron, 1999; Udell, 1999; University of Stirling, 2001).

Lessons from the experiences of caring and adapting care in family homes and in small out-of-home placements for persons with developmental disabilities may be transferred to the care of the general population of persons with dementia, reducing the reliance on nursing home care. Social workers potentially can play important roles in documenting these opportunities and in disseminating useful findings and information to generic service networks for persons with dementia. Similarly, there are service models and best practices in generic dementia services that may be of value to the developmental disabilities service system. Social workers may be key conduits for gathering and translating this information. One example is in the area of program modification. The policy framework for the developmental disabilities service system places great value on programming to ensure continued acquisition of skills and has emphasized work and day program availability. In one state this had an unintended consequence. A program evaluator required a provider to obtain a doctor's prescription so that a 75-year-old individual could take a nap each afternoon. Advocacy by a social worker resulted in training for all evaluation staff on dementia issues and the development of more age-appropriate and dementia-sensitive programming expectations.

Grandparent Caregivers

Grandparents form a group that genuinely falls between service systems. As one grandparent stated, "I need a case manager for my case managers." There is no single responsible service system or gateway, and grandparents must balance conflicting regulations and expectations. Indeed, grandparents' acceptance of needed services from one system (e.g., a subsidy from the foster care system) may exclude them from seeking needed services from another (e.g., disability-related services for the child from the developmental disabilities service system) (Kolomer, 2000). This needs to be addressed along with concerns about the consequences of welfare reform for grandparents seeking to provide full-time care at home, difficulties with guardianship and conservatorship, and access to special education services.

Culturally Sensitive Services

The emphasis in contemporary developmental-disabilities service systems on person-centered permanency planning—a technique that was developed with little input from diverse communities—is an area needing the attention of social workers. This technique needs reexamination as developmental disabilities agencies begin to expand services to include more culturally varied communities. Person-centered planning focuses on the individual's development of personal relationships, positive roles in the community, and skills for self-empowerment. Six principles underpin this approach:

1. Services based upon the person's choices rather than fitting the person into existing services
2. Services that are meaningful, functional, and build upon the person's strengths and abilities
3. Client access to community resources such as jobs, housing, and friends and movement away from segregated services
4. Services coordinated around the life of the person instead of the needs of staff and programs
5. Recognition of the abilities of neighbors, coworkers, families, and other citizens to teach skills, form relationships, and support participation
6. Formation of a diverse group of people willing to know, value, and support the person (McCallion & Grant-Griffin, 2000)

Current policy applications of these principles emphasize the needs of individuals over families, and even differentiate between individual and family needs, which sets up conflicts among members of diverse communities who place high value on the family and unity of the family structure. Cultural variations in family orientation and decision making should receive more serious consideration (McCallion & Grant-Griffin, 2000). Yet this approach, for other and often good reasons, has become institutionalized in policy and practice. Changes to this approach, or at least reorienting it to be more inclusive of family care will require intervention and advocacy at multiple levels.

INTEGRATING KNOWLEDGE INTO THE CURRICULUM

To ensure that social workers are able to lead policy-based and practice-change efforts, there is a need for coursework on developmental disabilities and aging. In specialized aging courses, such training should address the health and dementia issues described here, and all coursework should offer social workers intensive training in culturally sensitive approaches. Other specific, evidence-based content, offered in specifically designed courses or as modules in existing courses, should address permanency and futures planning (Heller & Factor, 1991); dementia care (McCallion & Janicki, 2002); and community outreach, cross-agency approaches, and service delivery (McCallion et al., 2000). Contacts with state developmental-disabilities planning councils; the federal Administration on Developmental Disabilities; university-affiliated programs at universities in each state; the Rehabilitation Research and Training Center on Aging with a Developmental Disability at the University of Illinois at Chicago; the ARC of the United States; and the American Association on Mental Retardation (which includes a social work membership division) will yield curriculum materials, Web sites, listservs, model courses, and potential guest speakers.

Intensive work on understanding the roles of families, reducing family-professional conflict, and delivering support groups and other helpful interventions also can be addressed through practice courses and continuing education. Such endeavors will be enriched by additional research on changing family forms, supports needed to maintain persons with developmental disabilities in the community despite advancing age and health concerns, and sustainable retirement activities.

CONCLUSION

Persons with developmental disabilities will continue to grow older, and in their old age they will be a more diverse group of individuals who are interested in accessing services. Whereas in the past their family caregivers were almost exclusively their mothers, in the years ahead we are likely to see greater roles for siblings and grandparents. There also may be an increase in the number of fathers who assume primary responsibility. Out-of-home providers also face important challenges. More complex and aging-related health needs, the presence in some of symptoms of dementia, and the need for programming models that respect aging and reflect growing diversity will require innovative responses if persons with developmental disabilities are to remain in the community and enjoy quality lives. Social workers will be called upon to be advocates and facilitators of these innovations. The introduction by social workers of best practices from generic aging services can contribute to our success in addressing the aging needs of persons with developmental disabilities as they age. Those generic services also will benefit from social work's translation and advocacy for what is best in the developmental disabilities service system. Of particular interest will be how well dementia care is managed in small, community-based homes.

REFERENCES

Axelson, J. A. (1993). *Counseling and development in a multicultural society* (2nd ed.). Pacific Grove, CA: Brooks/Cole.

Berrick, J. D., Barth, R. P., & Needles, B. (1994). A comparison of kinship foster homes and family foster homes: Implications for kinship foster care as family preservation. *Children and Youth Services Review, 16*(1–2), 33–63.

Bigby, C. (1996). Transferring responsibility: The nature and effectiveness of parental planning for the future of adults with intellectual disability who remain at home until mid-life. *Australian Society for the Study of Intellectual Disability, 21*(4), 295–312.

Bigby, C. (1997). Parental substitutes? The role of siblings in the lives of older people with intellectual disability. *Journal of Gerontological Social Work, 29*(1), 3–21.

Braddock, D. (1999). Aging and Developmental Disabilities: Demographic and policy issues affecting American families. *Mental Retardation, 37*(2), 155–161.

Braddock, D., Emerson, E., Felce, D., & Stancliffe, R. J. (2001). Living with circumstances of children and adults with mental retardation and developmental disabilities in the United States, Canada, England, and Wales. *Mental Retardation and Developmental Disabilities Research Reviews, 7*(2), 115–121.

Brookmeyer, R., Gray, S., & Kawas, C. (1998). Projections of Alzheimer's disease in the United States and the public health impact of delaying disease onset. *American Journal of Public Health, 88,* 1337–1342.

Carlsen, W. R., Galliuzzi, K. E., Forman, L. F., & Cavalieri, T. A. (1994). Comprehensive geriatric assessment: Applications for community-residing, elderly people with mental retardation/developmental disabilities. *Mental Retardation, 32,* 334–340.

Dalton, A. J., Tsiouris, J., & Patti, P. (2000, August). *Geriatric training program for the management of age-associated conditions in persons with intellectual disabilities.* Paper presented at the 11th World Congress of the International Association for the Scientific Study of Intellectual Disabilities, Seattle, Washington.

Essex, E. L., Seltzer, M. M., & Krauss, M. W. (1999). Differences in coping effectiveness and well-being among aging mothers and fathers of adults with mental retardation. *American Journal on Mental Retardation, 104,* 545–563.

Essex, E. L., Seltzer, M. M., & Krauss, M. W. (2002). Fathers as caregivers for adult children with mental retardation. In B. J. Kramer & E. H. Thompson (Eds.), *Men as caregivers: Theory, research, and service implications.* New York: Springer.

Evenhuis, H. M. (1997). Medical aspects of ageing in a population with intellectual disabilities: III. Mobility, internal conditions and cancer. *Journal of Intellectual Disability Research, 41,* 8–18.

Evenhuis, H., Henderson, C. M., Beange, H., Lennox, N., Chicoine, B., & Working Group. (2000). *Healthy ageing—Adults with intellectual disabilities: Physical health issues.* Geneva, Switzerland: World Health Organization.

Flegal, K. (1999). The obesity epidemic in children and adults: Current evidence and research issues. *Medicine and Science in Sports and Exercise,* [Suppl.], S509–S514.

Freedman, R. I., Krauss, M. W., & Seltzer, M. M. (1997). Aging parents' residential plans for adults children with mental retardation. *Mental Retardation, 35,* 114–123.

Fujiura, G. T. (1998). Demography of family households. *American Journal of Mental Retardation, 103,* 225–235.

Grant-Griffin, L. (1995). *Best practices: Outreach strategies in multicultural communities.* Albany: New York State Office of Mental Retardation and Developmental Disabilities.

Greenberg, J. S., Seltzer, M. M., Krauss, M. W., & Kim, H. (1997). The differential effects of social support on the psychological well-being of aging mothers of adults with mental illness or mental retardation. *Family Relations, 46,* 383–394.

Harper, D. C., & Wadsworth, J. S. (1992). Improving health care communication for persons with mental retardation. *Public Health Reports, 107,* 297–302.

Hayden, M. F. (1998). Mortality among people with mental retardation living in the United States: Research review and policy application. *Mental Retardation, 36,* 345–359.

Hayden, M. F., & Heller, T. (1997). Support, problem-solving/coping ability, and personal burden of younger and older caregivers of adults with mental retardation. *Mental Retardation, 35,* 364–372.

Heller, T., & Factor, A. (1991). Permanency planning for adults with mental retardation living with family caregivers. *American Journal on Mental Retardation, 96*, 163–176.

Heller, T., Hsieh, K., & Rowitz, L. (1997). Maternal and paternal caregiving of persons with mental retardation across the lifespan. *Family Relations, 46*, 407–415.

Heller, T., Miller, A. S., & Factor, A. (1997). Adults with mental retardation as supports to their parents: Effects on parental caregiving appraisal. *Mental Retardation, 35*, 338–346.

Henderson, C. M., & Davidson, P. W. (2000). Comprehensive adult and geriatric assessment. In M. P. Janicki & E. F. Ansello (Eds.), *Community supports for older adults with lifelong disabilities* (pp. 373–386). Baltimore: Paul H. Brookes.

Holland, A. J., Karlinsky, H., & Berg, J. M. (1993). Alzheimer's disease in persons with Down syndrome: Diagnostic and management considerations. In J. M. Berg, H. Karlinsky, & A. J. Holland (Eds.), *Alzheimer's disease, Down syndrome, and their relationship* (pp. 96–114). New York: Oxford University Press.

Iglehart, A. P., & Becerra, R. M. (1996). Social work and the ethnic agency: A history of neglect. *Journal of Multicultural Social Work, 4*, 1–20.

Janicki, M. P., & Dalton, A. J. (1999). Dementia and public policy considerations. In M. P. Janicki & A. J. Dalton (Eds.), *Dementia, aging, and intellectual disabilities* (pp. 388–414). Philadelphia: Brunner-Mazel.

Janicki, M. P., & Dalton, A. J. (2000). Prevalence of dementia and impact on intellectual disability services. *Mental Retardation, 38*, 277–289.

Janicki, M. P., Henderson, C. M., Davidson, P. W., McCallion, P., Taets, J. D., Force, L. T., et al. (2002). Health characteristics and health services utilization in older adults with intellectual disabilities living in community residences. *Journal of Intellectual Disabilities Research, 46*(4), 287–298.

Janicki, M. P., McCallion, P., & Dalton, A. J. (2000). Supporting people with dementia in community settings. In M. P. Janicki & E. F. Ansello (Eds.), *Community supports for aging adults with lifelong disabilities* (pp. 387–413). Baltimore: Paul H. Brookes.

Janicki, M. P., McCallion, P., & Dalton, A. J. (in press). Dementia-related care decision-making in group homes for persons with intellectual disabilities. *Journal of Gerontological Social Work.*

Janicki, M. P., McCallion, P., Grant-Griffin, L., & Kolomer, S. R. (2000). Grandparent caregivers I: Characteristics of the grandparents and the children with disabilities they care for. *Journal of Gerontological Social Work, 33*(3), 35–56.

Kaufman, A., Adams, J., & Campbell, V. (1991). Permanency planning by older parents who care for adult children with mental retardation. *Mental Retardation, 29*, 293–300.

Kolomer, S. R. (2000). Kinship foster care and its impact on grandmother caregivers. *Journal of Gerontological Social Work, 33*(3), 85–102.

Kolomer, S. R., McCallion, P., & Janicki, M. P. (in press). African-American grandmother carers of children with disabilities: Predictors of depressive symptoms. *Journal of Gerontological Social Work.*

Krauss, M. W., Seltzer, M. M., Gordon, R., & Friedman, D. H. (1996). Binding ties: The roles of adult siblings of persons with mental retardation. *Mental Retardation, 34*, 83–93.

McCallion, P. (1993). *Social worker orientations to permanency planning with older parents caring at home for family members with developmental disabilities.* Unpublished doctoral dissertation, University at Albany, New York.

McCallion, P. (1999). Maintaining communication. In M. P. Janicki & A. J. Dalton (Eds.), *Mental retardation, aging, and dementia: A handbook* (pp. 261–277). New York: Taylor & Francis.

McCallion, P., & Grant-Griffin, L. (2000). Redesigning services to meet the needs of multi-cultural families. In M. P. Janicki & E. F. Ansello (Eds.), *Community supports for older adults with lifelong disabilities* (pp. 97–108). Baltimore: Paul H. Brookes.

McCallion, P., & Janicki, M. P. (1997). Area Agencies on Aging: Meeting the needs of persons with developmental disabilities and their aging caregivers. *Journal of Applied Gerontology, 16*, 270–284.

McCallion, P., & Janicki, M. P. (2002). *Intellectual disabilities and dementia: A CD-ROM training package.* Albany: New York State Developmental Disabilities Planning Council.

McCallion, P., Janicki, M. P., & Dalton, A. J. (2001). *Intellectual disabilities and dementia: What can we do?* Albany: New York State Developmental Disabilities Planning Council.

McCallion, P., Janicki, M. P., & Grant-Griffin, L. (1997). Exploring the impact of culture and acculturation on older families caregiving for persons with developmental disabilities. *Family Relations, 46*, 347–357.

McCallion, P., Janicki, M. P., Grant-Griffin, L., & Kolomer, S. R. (2000). Grandparent Caregivers II: Service needs and service provision issues. *Journal of Gerontological Social Work, 33*(3), 57–84.

McCallion, P., & Kolomer, S. R. (2001, May). *Caregiving grandfathers of children with developmental disabilities.* Paper presented at American Association on Mental Retardation National Conference, Denver, Colorado.

McCallion, P., & Tobin, S. (1995). Social worker orientations to permanency planning by older parents caring at home for sons and daughters with developmental disabilities. *Mental Retardation, 33*(3), 153–162.

McCallion, P., & Toseland, R. W. (1993). An empowered model for social work services to families of adolescents and adults with developmental disabilities. *Families in Society, 74*, 579–589.

McCarron, M. (1999). Some issues in caring for people with the dual disability of Down's syndrome and Alzheimer's dementia. *Journal of Learning Disabilities for Nursing, Health and Social Care, 3*(3), 123–129.

Roberto, K. A. (Ed.). (1993). *The elderly caregiver: Caring for adults with developmental disabilities.* Newbury Park, CA: Sage.

Seltzer, G., Begun, A., Magan, R., & Luchterhand, C. (1993). Social supports and expectations of family involvement after out of home placement. In E. Sutton, T. Heller, A. Factor, B. Seltzer, & G. Hawkins (Eds.), *Older adults with developmental disabilities* (pp. 123–140). Baltimore: Paul H. Brookes.

Seltzer, G., Begun, A., Seltzer, M. M., & Krauss, M. W. (1991). The impacts of siblings on adults with mental retardation and their aging mothers. *Family Relations, 40,* 310–317.

Seltzer, M. M., Greenberg, J. S., & Krauss, M. W. (1995). A comparison of coping strategies of aging mothers of adults with mental illness or mental retardation. *Psychology and Aging, 10,* 64–75.

Seltzer, M. M., Greenberg, J. S., Krauss, M. W., & Hong, J. (1997). Predictors and outcomes of the end of coresident caregiving in aging families of adults with mental retardation or mental illness. *Family Relations, 46,* 13–22.

Seltzer, M. M., & Krauss, M. W. (1994). Aging parents with coresident adult children: The impact of lifelong caregiving. In M. M. Seltzer, M. W. Krauss, & M. P. Janicki (Eds.), *Life course perspectives on adulthood and old age* (pp. 3–18). Washington, DC: American Association on Mental Retardation.

Smith, G. C., & Tobin, S. S. (1989). Permanency planning among older parents of adults with lifelong disabilities. *Journal of Gerontological Social Work, 14*(3), 35–39.

Smith, G. C., & Tobin, S. S. (1993). Case managers' perceptions of practice with older parents of adults with lifelong disabilities. In K. A. Roberto (Ed.), *The elderly caregiver: Caring for adults with developmental disabilities* (pp. 146–169). Newbury Park, CA: Sage.

Strauss, D., & Kastner, T. A. (1996). Comparative mortality of people with developmental disabilities in institutions and the community. *American Journal on Mental Retardation, 101,* 269–281.

Udell, L. (1999). Supports in small group home settings. In M. P. Janicki & A. J. Dalton (Eds.), *Dementia, aging, and intellectual disabilities* (pp. 316–329). Philadelphia: Brunner-Mazel.

University of Stirling. (2001). *The Edinburgh Principles: Guidelines of the Edinburgh Working Group on Dementia Care Practices.* Stirling, Scotland: University of Stirling, Centre for Social Research on Dementia.

Walsh, P. N., Conliffe, C., & Birkbeck, G. (1993). Permanency planning and maternal well-being: A study of caregivers of people with intellectual disability in Ireland and Northern Ireland. *Irish Journal of Psychology, 14,* 176–188.

Zitlin, A. G. (1986). Mentally retarded adults and their siblings. *American Journal of Mental Deficiency, 91,* 217–225.

Chapter 10

STRAINS AND GAINS OF GRANDMOTHERS RAISING GRANDCHILDREN IN THE HIV PANDEMIC

Cynthia Cannon Poindexter
and Nancy Capobianco Boyer

SIGNIFICANCE TO GERONTOLOGY, HEALTH CARE, AND PROFESSIONALS

Despite encouraging pharmaceutical and medical advances in the treatment of HIV disease, the HIV pandemic remains a public health, economic, social policy, and humanitarian catastrophe in the United States. Older persons constitute the preponderance of family caregivers for adults living with HIV disease (Allers, 1990; Brabant, 1994) and for the minor children of these adults (Caliandro & Hughes, 1998; Joslin, Mevi-Triano, & Berman, 1997). Most of these older caregivers are women, including grandmothers who are caring for HIV-affected and HIV-infected children (Chalfie, 1994). It has been conservatively estimated that between 13,530 and 20,625 grandmothers are custodial parents to somewhere between 27,060 and 41,250 children who were orphaned by AIDS in the United States (Joslin, 2000). Despite the growing problem, however, social work, gerontology, and the HIV field pay insufficient attention to older HIV-affected caregivers in research, practice, and educational efforts (Brabant, 1994; Gutheil & Chichin, 1991).

Gerontology has done an outstanding job of exploring the experiences of those who take care of elders. In addition, gerontologists are now attending to grandparents who are raising grandchildren because of the permanent or temporary absence of parents (e.g., Burnette, 1997; Burton, Dilworth-Anderson, & Merriwether-deVries, 1995; Dressel & Barnhill, 1994; Fuller-Thomson, Minkler, & Driver, 1997; Goldberg-Glen, Sands, Cole, & Cristofalo, 1998; Minkler, Roe, & Price, 1992). The HIV pandemic has contributed to the phenomenon of grandparents raising grandchildren, but the ramifications of this new care situation are less studied and understood. Elders who are giving care to minor children who are infected with HIV or who have lost parents to HIV should be of concern to gerontologists. These elders are often silently and invisibly burdened with HIV care and may not be prepared and supported financially, physically, socially, or emotionally to be parents to children who have been orphaned and/or are living with an infectious, life-threatening illness. Practitioners who work in geriatrics need information on how to recognize, assess, support, and study this increasing group of caregivers.

Providing custodial care to grandchildren often has negative consequences for the older caregiver's mental and physical health, such as depression (Burton, 1992), insomnia (Minkler & Roe, 1996), and increase in disabling conditions (Kelley, Yorker, & Whitley, 1997). HIV-affected grandparents not only face these circumstances, but also HIV stigma (labeled *AIDS-related stigma* by Herek and Glunt in 1988), increased social isolation, grieving for the deceased or ill adult child, stressful relationships with the grandchild's biological parent, and worry about the HIV-positive child's health and survival (Caliandro & Hughes, 1998; Emlet, 1996; Joslin & Harrison, 1998; Poindexter, 2002; Reidy, Taggart, & Asselin, 1991). Hughes and Caliandro (1996) found that the caregivers of HIV-infected children had higher levels of stress, depression, and anxiety than comparison groups. This population, although struggling with increased physical and mental health challenges, tends to be invisible and underserved by the truncated social service system (Linsk, Poindexter, & Mason, 2002). If professionals in health care, gerontology, HIV, and social work could better reach older HIV-affected caregivers and design services and research that recognized their existence and assessed their need, the health and well-being of these caregivers might improve.

Attention from practitioners and scholars is important for the sake of the caregivers as well as for the HIV-infected adults and children who rely on them. Without services and support, the health, well-being, and longevity of HIV-affected grandmothers can be negatively affected, which will leave the already bereaved HIV-infected and HIV-affected grandchildren without care and facing more familial upheaval. Not only will practitioners be neglecting the grandmothers if their needs are not attended to, but the grandchildren also will then be thrown into the overburdened child welfare system or left to fend for themselves. Health care professionals who are working with adults or children with HIV are positioned especially well to identify and serve HIV-affected older caregivers. Practitioners are encouraged to assess the level of HIV caregivers' burden, stress, and strain; determine the extent of any health and aging impairments; and evaluate their knowledge about HIV and their readiness and ability to contend with the unpredictability and difficulty of the disease in its end state (Brabant, 1994).

Caregivers typically accompany their HIV-positive family members to medical and social service appointments, even when they do not have the time and resources to attend to their own medical needs (Ogu & Wolfe, 1994). These caregivers often face daily logistical challenges, which are also barriers to accessing services. They are less likely to consider their own service needs when they are consumed with providing care, and they may not have the luxury of researching to find possible programs for help (Joslin et al., 1997; Poindexter, 1997). They may not have transportation or be able to leave the care recipient alone. These realities mean that service providers cannot wait for older HIV-affected caregivers to come to them, but may need to reach out to this population and strive to design relevant services for them.

Social workers are in a unique position to address the intersection of HIV and aging because we operate out of an ecological model, are family-centered, work with the most hidden and vulnerable, and have a strong value of social justice and equal access to care. Social workers may have opportunities through practice to raise the awareness of other helpers (such as physicians, nursing home staff and administrators, recreation providers, and outreach workers) about the intersection of HIV and aging. Gerontological social workers should be charging ahead to push the aging network, established scholarly societies, and academic educators and researchers to face HIV disease and its devastating effects on elders. Social workers in the aging network, in hospitals and clinics, and in AIDS service organizations should work hard to identify vulnerable caregivers who are supporting family members with HIV and offer them support groups, information, advocacy, counseling, and care management. Because older persons are often either unfamiliar with HIV-related services or afraid of seeking help from them, social workers in the HIV field need to reach out to this population in creative ways that are welcoming.

PRIOR RESEARCH AND KNOWLEDGE BASE

Research on HIV-affected grandparents has documented many challenges in HIV caregiving. Caring for an adult child with HIV when one has already launched children may add another level of family responsibility, stress, burden, and obligation to what might have been an empty nest (McKinlay, Skinner, Riley, & Zablotsky, 1993). Older caregivers may have physical limitations that make it difficult to perform logistical personal care tasks (Powell-Cope & Brown, 1992). They may be living with the physical and emotional pain of the care recipient (Lego, 1994) and conflicts associated with reintegration of the person with AIDS into the household (Cates, Graham, Boeglin, & Tielker, 1990). They may be overburdened with grief, anticipating the death of an adult child from AIDS, or they may be already grieving such a death while they are parenting grandchildren, and they may fear the death of one of those minor children as well (Brabant, 1994; Caliandro & Hughes, 1998; Gutheil & Chichin, 1991; Joslin & Harrison, 1998; Levine, 1995a; Michaels & Levine, 1992).

Older HIV-affected caregivers are sometimes also caring for someone other than HIV-positive loved ones, such as a frail partner, a disabled adult child, or other grandchildren or great-grandchildren for whom they have parenting responsibilities (McKinlay et al., 1993; Ogu & Wolfe, 1994; Poindexter, 1997). Although not bearing HIV stigma directly, HIV-affected grandmothers can feel associative stigma acutely (Poindexter, 2002). They may fear rejection, practice secrecy, lack trust, and report reduced social supports (Joslin, 2000; Poindexter & Linsk, 1999). The HIV diagnosis may trigger disclosure of sexual orientation or drug use, which can be difficult subjects for elders to accept or discuss and may influence their ability to accept the care recipient into the home (Allers, 1990; Gutheil & Chichin, 1991;

McKinlay et al., 1993). They may have an uncertain future if the children or grandchildren upon whom they counted for their own personal and financial care have become disabled or have died because of HIV (Levine, 1995b). Finally, they tend to deny their own needs and withdraw from social interaction as the needs of the children or adults with HIV become more pronounced; they seek help for their own needs late in the process if at all (Ogu & Wolfe, 1994; Reidy et al., 1991). Raising a minor who has HIV or who has been orphaned due to HIV brings many challenges. However, recent studies have also suggested that the stresses are accompanied by inner resources, spiritual strength, and resilience (Poindexter, 2001; Poindexter & Linsk, 1999).

CURRENT RESEARCH

This chapter reports on an exploratory qualitative study funded by the Hartford Geriatric Social Work Faculty Scholars Program (for a full discussion of methods and findings, see Boyer, 2002), which highlights the complex situations of grandparents raising grandchildren because of HIV. Six grandmothers, aged 53 to 73, who had been providing full-time custodial care for a year or longer to a school-aged grandchild, participated in open-ended interviews in Massachusetts in 2001. Half had become adoptive parents to the grandchildren and half were legal guardians. Three respondents (pseudonyms Linda, Nina, Susan) were raising an HIV-infected child; two (pseudonyms Barbara and Katie) were raising one HIV-affected child; and one (pseudonym Eileen) was raising two HIV-affected and one HIV-infected child. The HIV-positive mothers of the grandchildren of four respondents had died. Three grandmothers were of African descent and three were of European descent. They had been providing custodial care to these grandchildren for 1 to 15 years. The study relied on grounded theory, so themes, patterns, and concepts emerged from the coding of the data (Strauss & Corbin, 1990). This chapter presents challenges and benefits of HIV caregiving that were harvested from the respondents' accounts.

Caregiving Challenges

Four major challenges emerged from the grandmother's open-ended interviews: being unprepared to take on parenting again late in life;

facing one's own health and functional difficulties while raising a child; feeling burdened by the uncertain trajectory of the disease; and guarding against HIV-related discrimination.

Being Unprepared

For each of these grandmothers, the decision to take over full-time care was unexpected, precipitated by an emergency with the parent who was HIV-positive and/or using substances. Not only were they shocked by the crisis of having to take in the grandchild at a stage of life when they had moved beyond child-rearing duties, but they were also looking forward to the traditional grandmother role and focusing on themselves. Linda's comment about this unplanned situation is illustrative of the surprise and stress:

> I never dreamed I'd be doing this. I thought I would be a grandmother maybe. But not full care. I get jealous and angry with my friends who do all the fun things with their grandchildren. . . . I finally got all my kids out of the house, all grown, no more school work. I was starting to take care of me, doing what I wanted to do for the first time in my life. . . . Then all of a sudden I am back to square one again.

The caregivers were also not expecting to change from the grandmother role to the mother role. The responsibilities and relationships can be quite different when one is a noncustodial grandparent. Barbara illustrates the losses associated with the change:

> I used to spoil [my granddaughter] more and give her more, give into her more. But now I am more firmer with her. I was thinking today that maybe one day, once in a while I will just be a grandmother role. I want to switch back and forth sometime, I don't know how that will work though but we give it a try. . . . Nothing special but just to be a grandmother and she can talk to me and tell me anything like she used to.

These grandmothers were surprised at having to become a primary parent later in life, and they also described problematic or ambivalent relationships with the surviving but absent biological parents, often feeling that they were left holding the bag as caregivers and that the grandchildren were ignored by these parents. In addition, the grandmothers realized that the children will be bereft of good memories when the parent dies. Eileen explains this concern: "Parents should be involved whenever they can, even if they are strung out. . . . Because when something happens to the parent, [the children] have nothing. There is nothing there."

Caregiver Health

All participants, regardless of age, were somewhat affected by diseases or disabilities. There was a continuum of impairments, including high blood pressure managed through medication (Eileen and Barbara); sleep disorders and chronic hip pain (Katie); heart disease requiring bypass surgery (Susan); diabetes, high blood pressure, weight gain, and high cholesterol (Nina); and weight gain, depression, anxiety, panic attacks, chronic pain, high blood pressure, and fatigue (Linda). These chronic conditions, which tend to become more common in older adulthood, can affect one's ability to keep up with the demands of raising a child, especially when the child also moves in and out of acute illness, periodically needing more attention and care. Having concerns about one's own health also raises worry about one's ability to care for a special-needs child over time. Linda realized that she was not taking care of herself, and that this could affect her ability to parent her grandson Joseph, yet she is not yet able to take action: "For some reason I am not doing what I need to do. . . . Why don't I take care of myself so I can take care of him? . . . Joseph is suffering because I'm not taking care of me."

The Nature of HIV

Participants spoke at length about child-rearing challenges that could exist for any custodial grandparent, such as discipline conflicts, advising the child or teen about sex and dating, watching for drug use, and managing problems at school, as well as the strain of taking on a child when one is past the usual parenting age and stage. In addition to these challenges, however, the fact that the care was framed in HIV complicated the responsibilities and relationships. Barbara, Eileen, Nina, and Katie were raising children whose parents had died of HIV; Linda and Susan were raising HIV-infected children whose parents were completely absent. This meant that the grandmothers and grandchildren were missing and grieving their middle generation. Four caregivers were raising HIV-infected minors, which required them to be constantly on their guard about health and sexuality.

These grandmothers spoke about the difficulties of managing and making decisions about a complicated, life-threatening illness; supervising complicated medication protocols and possible side effects; discerning normal childhood illnesses from medication side effects or HIV-related infections; trying to give the grandchild as normal a life as possible; worrying about their practicing safer sex; and living with fears and uncertainty about the child's health and survival. Nina expressed the constant anxiety about having a child with HIV and never knowing what is going to go wrong physically:

> Everything happening you think it's coming from the virus. . . . "Oh my god, what is this now?" . . . You get nervous. It's just not like a normal child. If something happened to one of my kids, I said, "There's nothing wrong," but if something happens here, I stay home most of the day because you never know when you are going to get a call from the school. . . . A typical day with a sick child is not easy. And you know this is something that she is not going to get over soon. . . . You don't know what day or what hour or what minute that something is going to go—Bam!

Disclosure Decisions

Managing a complicated, infectious, fatal illness is a challenge for a custodial grandparent, but there is an added dimension with HIV. The threat of HIV-related stigma and discrimination complicates the situation, because disclosure decisions are complex and constant. Unlike with other childhood diseases, the disclosure of the HIV-positive child's diagnosis can lead to hurt feelings, rejection, or discriminatory action. All respondents spoke of being constantly aware of others who were ignorant, rude, and fearful of HIV. All had disclosed the HIV status of the adult children and minor grandchildren to immediate family members, but reported making careful decisions about who to tell outside the family, due to fear of reprisal, mistreatment, or ostracism. The grandmothers often learned through experience that they had to be careful with disclosure. One illustration of this comes from Susan, whose granddaughter was rejected by a private school after she disclosed her HIV status:

> I made a mistake, see. When I was going to send her to parochial school, . . . I talked with the nun that she did have the AIDS virus and I would like the nun to know that. Oh no, no, no, no, no, they wouldn't take her. And you couldn't do a damn thing because it is private. . . . They made such a big thing about this that I never again was honest with the thing again.

The grandmothers managed stigma through disclosing the presence of HIV to selected persons only, not admitting what disease had killed their adult child, avoiding situations where people might ask personal questions, coaching the child about how to avoid disclosure, and making sure medication was given in private. As Eileen summarized succinctly, "You really have to be careful of who you tell." Many grandmothers decided that it was not wise to tell the child's friends or their friends' parents, out of fear that they would be cut off socially. An example of coaching a child comes from Katie, who told her granddaughter when she went to school, " 'I wouldn't tell everybody that your mother died of AIDS because you never know.' I didn't want her to be hurt."

Caregiving Benefits

Although participants were surprised by having to parent again and were forthcoming about the challenges of providing that care, none of them regretted the decision to take in their grandchildren. They noted four overarching positive aspects of HIV caregiving. One was emotional reward, such as satisfaction or joy. The respondents said that loving, caring for, and taking care of their grandchildren was mutually emotionally rewarding and sustaining, that they felt good at being able to provide for the children, and that they derived joy from watching the children grow, learn, and blossom. Linda spoke with joy of living with her grandson: "He's always here with me . . . he's really a pleasure. . . . It's really uplifting, it really is." A second benefit was the relationship and companionship with the grandchildren, which helped to ameliorate the caregivers' loneliness and partially filled the void left by the deceased children. Eileen comments on the value of the relationship: "We love each other. See, so that makes a big difference." A third benefit was that parenting helped them to stay active and busy. The effort associated with unexpected parenting in later life was reframed into a positive aspect. Nina listed her grandchild's energy as a benefit to her and her husband:

> Good things—that he is here with me and my husband, having a small kid in the house gives us something to do . . . she keeps us going, keeps us on our toes. And she is a lot of fun for my husband because every time he looks she wants to follow him.

Despite being aware of HIV stigma and making careful decisions about how to manage its effects, three participants mentioned a fourth benefit: being able to support and be partners with their grandchildren in HIV education and activism. They had ventured out into the HIV world by wearing slogans on buttons or participating in the AIDS Walk and wanted to do more. Two of the HIV-negative granddaughters had done some public speaking about their mothers' illnesses: Katie's granddaughter spoke at her school, and Barbara's granddaughter read a letter at her mother's memorial service. Barbara and Nina had expressed to their grandchildren a hope that someday they would educate others about what it is like to live with the disease or to be the orphaned child of someone who died from AIDS. Barbara planned to move into more activism herself, alongside her grandchild: "The more I talk about it will help somebody else and let people know it is nothing to be ashamed about, that there is help out there in the community. . . . I told her that it is a mission for me and her both to do and go out and teach people about AIDS, to tell them about our story about AIDS."

In sum, this exploratory study (Boyer, 2002) contributes to a small but growing knowledge base by opening a window into the lives of HIV-affected custodial grandmothers. The data led to a recognition of four major areas of struggle and four mediating factors for HIV-affected custodial grandmothers. Their situations were complex and can be categorized neither as completely challenging nor completely beneficial. This study's findings support other research (see Poindexter & Linsk, 1999) that grandmothers have mixed responses to their caregiving role: parenting an HIV-infected or HIV-affected grandchild is an achievement that they do not regret, despite feeling challenged, stressed, and isolated. HIV caregiving is full of pitfalls as well as opportunities for growth, a mix of strain and gain.

FURTHER RESEARCH NEEDS

The next step is designing societal interventions to lessen the deleterious effects of HIV caregiving and to help families negotiate the emotional and medical minefields. Asking what HIV-affected grandmothers think about possible service and policy responses could assist this effort. Participatory, collaborative research is necessary to determine gaps in service systems and in public policy. There are many questions left unanswered concerning gerontological theory, grandparent caregiving in general, HIV caregiving in particular, and responses from service systems.

1. Theory: What existing gerontological theory is applicable to understanding this population? Are there models, frameworks, and interventions from other areas that can illuminate the experience of living with a life-threatening, stigmatized illness?

2. Grandparent caregiving: What affects the health and well-being of grandparents who are providing unexpected custodial care? What factors and combinations of circumstances determine whether an element of the care context is perceived as strain or gain or both? Does passage of time have a positive or negative effect on coping? Is coping related to age, individual characteristics, or family history? Do older men experience custodial grandparenting differently than women do?

3. HIV caregiving: Are the strains of raising an HIV-infected child different when the caregiver is an elder? Do HIV-affected elders experience HIV stigma more acutely than younger caregivers? What factors affect a grandmother's ability to cope successfully with HIV caregiving? Do caregivers' philosophies concerning illness, HIV stigma, and family duty have an impact on physical, mental, emotional, and spiritual coping? Does culture, ethnicity, or socioeconomic status make a difference?

4. Systems: What informal and formal supports could maximize the caregiver's maintenance of physical and mental health? Are there useful models that can be tested or adapted for bridging the gaps between the child welfare, HIV, aging, and income maintenance systems? What would make grandparent caregivers feel more comfortable approaching a social service system and asking for support?

POLICY IMPLICATIONS

At this time, there are few avenues available to address the unique needs of older caregivers and help them feel connected to each other and the community and more able to provide adequate care. HIV-affected custodial grandparents could benefit from respite services, child care, home health, support groups, benefits advocacy, counseling, education about HIV and caregiving, bereavement support, transportation, and financial assistance. However, a potent mix of ageism and HIV stigma influences access to social services for HIV-affected grandparents, who may feel out of place both in the AIDS service network, which they perceive to be tailored to younger people; and in the aging network, which they see as unreceptive to, or judgmental of, HIV concerns. Furthermore, few programs in either system have been designed for the specific needs of older HIV-affected caregivers. Consequently, persons with needs related both to aging and to HIV are often inadequately served.

The HIV and aging fields often compete with each other for scarce resources, fail to acknowledge their common ground, and neglect to communicate and coordinate (Gutheil & Chichin, 1991). The multilayered needs in HIV-affected families suggest the need for collaboration. Barriers have been created by a service system that is divided by funding source and legislative authority (i.e., AIDS service organizations, child welfare network, and aging network). Most home- and community-based services determine eligibility through the situation of the HIV-infected child or adult, and the family context is not as readily considered. Policies should address the caregiver as well as the care recipient so that practitioners and planners in The Aging Network, hospitals, and HIV service organizations can consider families as a unit. HIV and aging-service systems should develop family-centered care plans across service systems. In addition, service providers should strive to see that the needs of both older caregivers and younger care recipients are included in the overall plan.

It would be beneficial to modify reimbursement and funding mechanisms to accommodate the needs of older HIV-affected caregivers and increase the options to support caregivers for the care of others and themselves. It would also be advantageous for AIDS service organizations to expand services so that care management and support does not stop with the death of the infected person.

Existing provisions in the aging and HIV service networks could be used to support older HIV-affected caregivers. The Older Americans Act of 1965 (OAA) could be used to support older HIV-affected caregivers, even though that is not the original or primary intent of the legislation. The typical services that OAA funds, such as educational programs in senior centers, family-oriented care management, information and referral, advocacy, legal services, outreach, and nutrition and home-delivered meals, could be used to educate and support HIV-affected caregivers older than 60. In addition, the OAA was recently expanded to include the National Family Caregiver Support Program. This new program (Part E of Title III) provides services for relative caregivers of a child younger than 18, which could ease the burden for older grandparent caregivers who are raising grandchildren due to the illness or death of the parents (Older Americans Act, 2000).

Educational sessions for professionals in the aging network, funded by Title IV of OAA, could include information on older caregivers, both HIV-affected and others. State units on aging and area agencies on aging could evaluate their eligibility criteria to facilitate serving older caregivers.

The Ryan White Comprehensive AIDS Resources Emergency (CARE) Act of 1990 [CIS 90 (1990)] targets persons with HIV, but contains diverse possibilities for responding more effectively to family caregivers; however, most of these are not explicit. Title I planning councils and Title II consortia, charged with assessing and meeting community needs, are often concerned about HIV caregivers, but may not be aware of the hidden population of older caregivers. Education and advocacy are needed to challenge these bodies to incorporate outreach and support to this population. Title IV in particular is family-centered in intention and could provide care management, counseling, logistical support, respite, day care, parenting education, and perma-nency planning if the definition of family were broadened to include older caregiving relatives. Because the CARE Act is targeted to persons with HIV, the caregiver no longer has access to these services when the HIV-infected adult or child dies or leaves the home. Service providers could, if funding permits, incorporate bereavement support for older caregivers. The National AIDS Education and Training Centers are funded to teach professionals in all disciplines about the needs of persons with HIV and could include information on isolated and stressed older caregivers.

Housing Opportunities for People with AIDS (HOPWA) funds may be used for a broad range of housing, including emergency shelter, shared housing, apartments, single-room occupancy units, group homes, and housing combined with supportive services. HOPWA does not specifically target grandparent caregivers, but it has the goal of housing at-risk HIV-affected families, especially those who are homeless or at great risk of becoming homeless. HIV-affected families may live together in a HOPWA-supported housing arrangement, which can include parent and grandparent caregivers. Unfortunately, when the adult or child with HIV is absent or deceased, HIV-negative caregivers cannot receive HOPWA support. An important step in alleviating the service gaps for older HIV-affected caregivers is to be aware that they exist and to strive to provide outreach and a safe environment for them so that they are not overlooked.

Any service provider in any network could use the following strategies:

1. Provide HIV-related educational programs in senior centers and nutrition sites so that the topic is less taboo. Caregivers may in this way be encouraged to come forward and disclose to staff members or peers that they are struggling or bereaved.

2. Respectfully ask older persons if they have any HIV questions or concerns. In this way, providers can help normalize the issue and break the silence. Older caregivers may feel that they have permission to speak about caring for a family member who has HIV.

3. Offer workshops on HIV and aging to social workers, health care practitioners, and gerontologists through continuing education programs and professional conferences to raise awareness and to foster problem solving and coalition building.

4. Offer a support network or group for HIV-affected elders.

INTEGRATING KNOWLEDGE INTO THE CURRICULUM

As a discipline concerned with all levels of problems and solutions, including families, organizations, and communities, social work should in general be concerned about HIV-affected grandparent caregivers. Introductory and general courses could include articles, case studies, and discussions of the assets and needs of this population.

Gerontological texts and classes tend to view caregiving as flowing toward the elder. Many elders do become frail and require caregiving; however, that is not the only reality of aging. There is not enough recognition of elders as caregivers for younger family members, which is another common situation. In addition, courses on aging have tended to neglect HIV as a concern for older adulthood, whether the elders are infected or affected. Gerontological courses should incorporate information on grandparent caregivers in the context of HIV and other situations and highlight the commitment, resilience, and contributions of elders who are struggling without adequate support in an overwhelming pandemic.

Courses on human behavior in the social environment, which are organized around developmental stages and emphasize human diversity, should take care not to isolate aging as a one-class topic, but rather integrate information on multigenerational families and their needs and assets. Human behavior courses should include grandparent caregiving as an increasing reality in later life, as well as study this family configuration within the context of cultural competence.

Specialized courses addressing substance use and HIV should broaden the focus to include more than the individual and incorporate material on elders who are family caregivers in these contexts. Courses in individual counseling, family therapy, group work, and community organizing could acknowledge the unique struggles of HIV-affected multigenerational families, present the resilience and needs of older caregivers, and examine service models for them.

Courses and content on social work ethics can include case examples of the dilemmas faced by workers and consumers when elders are overburdened by HIV care or when truncated systems fail to meet their needs. Learners in the classroom and field can be challenged to examine their preconceived notions of aging and of HIV-affected families.

Throughout social work curricula, where systems and empowerment theories are the organizing concepts, it is helpful to use the situation of HIV-affected grandparent caregivers as an illustration of how truncated social-service systems can fail to provide safety nets for families, how stigma and secrecy can short-circuit social support and stymie personal agency, and how social service providers can inadvertently wear the same blinders that society does regarding hidden populations. Because all courses are built on values-based practice, an ethical approach to this population can be infused throughout the curriculum.

Social work interns in AIDS service organizations, in the aging-network, and in generic social service agencies could be sensitized to the hidden nature of HIV-affected older caregivers so that they could be more prepared to recognize and serve these caregivers. Integrative seminars for students in field placements could use case studies of HIV-affected grandparents.

CONCLUSIONS

The challenges of HIV caregiving could be partially ameliorated by the efforts of scholars, educators, and practitioners who could identify and address the needs of HIV-affected custodial grandparents. Because this topic is relatively new in scholarship and the studies are exploratory, the implications for research, educational efforts, and policy must also be viewed as tentative. There are both strains and gains to be found in HIV caregiving. The grandmothers in the exploratory qualitative study reported here did not feel prepared to take on child-rearing later in life, had significant health impairments of their own, were struggling mightily with the uncertainty and fear surrounding HIV disease in the family, and were constantly aware of the need for secrecy in order to protect the family from stigma. Nevertheless, they were glad that they were providing the care and reported positive benefits stemming from satisfaction, joy, companionship, relationship, staying active, and—for some of them—feeling part of an activist community.

Although HIV-affected custodial grandmothers can be remarkably strong, resourceful, and dedicated, we should not, as practitioners and policy makers, take for granted their shouldering this care without appropriate and adequate services. Policy makers should be aware of the tendency of overburdened older caregivers to neglect their own needs, because this situation could lead to physical and mental melt-down. Practitioners should advocate to include older caregivers in legislative authorization for HIV programs and older adult programs and to encourage organizations to incorporate their needs as part of a family-centered approach.

Custodial grandmothers, who each day face uncertainty, stigma, and challenges to their well-being to raise a grandchild because the HIV-positive adult parent has died or is absent, are among the most challenged and hidden of our elders. This group is little studied, so there are many unanswered questions. However, we know that they are stressed, stigmatized, and neglected, so perhaps we know enough to proceed with outreach, advocacy, and targeted services. Because they are familiar with finding, serving, and advocating for older adults, gerontological social workers could be in the forefront of these efforts.

ACKNOWLEDGMENTS

The study reported here was funded by the Gerontological Society of America, John A. Hartford Geriatric Social Work Scholars Program. The authors thank the six HIV-affected grandmothers who were willing to teach us about their struggles and blessings.

REFERENCES

Allers, C. T. (1990). AIDS and the older adult. *Gerontologist, 30,* 405–407.
Boyer, N. C. (2002). *The experiences of older caregivers of HIV-affected and infected minor children: Permanency planning, stigma, and support.* Unpublished doctoral

dissertation, Boston University, School of Social Work and Department of Sociology.

Brabant, S. (1994). An overlooked AIDS affected population: The elderly parent as caregiver. *Journal of Gerontological Social Work, 22*(1/2), 131–145.

Burnette, D. (1997). Grandmother caregivers in inner-city Latino families: A descriptive profile and informal social supports. *Journal of Multicultural Social Work, 5*(3/4), 121–137.

Burton, L. M. (1992). Black grandparents rearing children of drug-addicted parents: Stressors, outcomes and social service needs. *Gerontologist, 32,* 744–751.

Burton, L. M., Dilworth-Anderson, P., & Merriwether-deVries, C. (1995). Context and surrogate parenting among contemporary grandparents. *Marriage and Family Review, 20*(3/4), 349–366.

Caliandro, G., & Hughes, C. (1998). The experience of being a grandmother who is the primary caregiver for her HIV-positive grandchild. *Nursing Research, 47*(2), 107–113.

Cates, J. A., Graham, L. L., Boeglin, D., & Tielker, S. (1990, April). The effect of AIDS on the family system. *Families in Society: The Journal of Contemporary Human Services,* 195–201.

Chalfie, D. (1994). *Going it alone: A closer look at grandparents parenting grandchildren.* Washington, DC: American Association of Retired Persons.

CIS 90 (1990). PL101-381, Ryan White CARE Act of 1990, Washington, DC: Government Printing Office.

Dressel, P. L., & Barnhill, S. K. (1994). Reframing gerontological thought and practice: The case of grandmothers with daughters in prison. *Gerontologist, 34,* 685–690.

Emlet, C. A. (1996). Case managing older people with AIDS: Bridging systems—recognizing diversity. *Journal of Gerontological Social Work, 27*(1/2), 55–71.

Fuller-Thomson, E., Minkler, M., & Driver, D. (1997). A profile of grandparents raising grandchildren in the United States. *Gerontologist, 37,* 406–411.

Goldberg-Glen, R., Sands, R. G., Cole, R. D., & Cristofalo, C. (1998, September–October). Multigenerational patterns and internal structures in families in which grandparents raise grandchildren. *Families in Society: Journal of Contemporary Human Services,* 477–489.

Gutheil, I. A., & Chichin, E. R. (1991). AIDS, older people, and social work. *Health and Social Work, 16*(4), 237–244.

Herek, G. M., & Glunt, E. K. (1988). An epidemic of stigma: Public reactions to AIDS. *American Psychologist, 43,* 886–891.

Hughes, C. B., & Caliandro, G. (1996). Effects of social support, stress, and level of illness on caregiving of children with AIDS. *Journal of Pediatric Nursing, 11,* 347–358.

Joslin, D. (2000). Grandparents raising grandchildren orphaned and affected by HIV/AIDS. In C. Cox (Ed.), *To grandmother's house we go and stay: Perspectives on custodial grandparents* (pp. 167–183). New York: Springer.

Joslin, D., & Harrison, R. (1998). The "hidden patient": Older relatives raising children orphaned by AIDS. *Journal of the American Medical Women's Association, 53*(2), 65–71, 76.

Joslin, D., Mevi-Triano, C., & Berman, J. (1997, November). *Grandparents raising children orphaned by HIV/AIDS: Health risks and service needs.* Paper presented at the 50th Annual Scientific Meeting of the Gerontological Society of America, Cincinnati, OH.

Kelley, S. J., Yorker, B. C., & Whitley, D. (1997, September). To grandmother's house we go . . . and stay: Children raised in intergenerational families. *Journal of Gerontological Nursing,* 12–20.

Lego, S. (1994). AIDS-related anxiety and coping methods in a support group for caregivers. *Archives of Psychiatric Nursing, VIII*(3), 200–207.

Levine, C. (1995a). In whose care and custody? Orphans of the HIV epidemic. *AIDS Clinical Care, 7*(10), 83.

Levine, C. (1995b). Today's challenges, tomorrow's dilemmas. In S. Geballe, J. Gruendel, & W. Andiman (Eds.), *Forgotten children of the AIDS epidemic* (pp. 190–204). New Haven, CT: Yale University Press.

Linsk, N., Poindexter, C. C., & Mason, S. (2002). Policy implications. In D. Joslin (Ed.), *Invisible caregivers: Older adults raising children in the wake of HIV/AIDS* (pp. 248–277). New York: Columbia University Press.

McKinlay, J. B., Skinner, K., Riley, J. W., & Zablotsky, D. (1993). On the relevance of social science concepts and perspectives. In M. W. Riley, M. G. Ory, & D. Zablotsky (Eds.), *AIDS in an aging society.* New York: Springer.

Michaels, D., & Levine, C. (1992). Estimates of the number of motherless youth orphaned by AIDS in the United States. *Journal of the American Medical Association, 268,* 3456–3461.

Minkler, M., & Roe, K. M. (1996, Spring). Grandparents as surrogate parents. *Generations, 22,* 34–38.

Minkler, M., Roe, K. M., & Price, M. (1992). The physical and emotional health of grandmothers raising grandchildren in the crack cocaine epidemic. *Gerontologist, 32,* 351–358.

Ogu, C., & Wolfe, L. R. (1994). *Midlife and older women and HIV/AIDS.* Washington, DC: American Association of Retired Persons.

Older Americans Act, 42 U.S.C., Subchapter I, § 3001 (2000); Subchapter III, § 3026, part F; Subchapter VII, § 3058g; Subchapter III, Subpart 1, § 372.

Poindexter, C. (1997). *Stigma and support as experienced by HIV-affected older minority caregivers.* Unpublished doctoral dissertation, University of Illinois at Chicago.

Poindexter, C. C. (2001). "I'm still blessed": The assets and needs of HIV-affected caregivers over fifty. *Families in Society, 82,* 525–536.

Poindexter, C. C. (2002). Stigma, isolation, and support in HIV-affected elder parental surrogates. In D. Joslin (Ed.), *Invisible caregivers: Older adults raising children in the wake of HIV/AIDS* (pp. 42–63). New York: Columbia University Press.

Poindexter, C. C., & Linsk, N. (1999). "I'm just glad that I'm here": Stories of seven African-American HIV-affected grandmothers. *Journal of Gerontological Social Work, 32*(1), 63–81.

Powell-Cope, G. M., & Brown, M. A. (1992). Going public as an AIDS family caregiver. *Social Science Medicine, 34*(5), 571–580.

Reidy, M., Taggart, M. E., & Asselin, L. (1991). Psychosocial needs expressed by the natural caregivers of HIV infected children. *AIDS Care, 3,* 331–343.

Strauss, A., & Corbin, J. (1990). *Basics of qualitative research.* Newbury Park, CA: Sage.

Chapter 11

ELDER MISTREATMENT AND THE ROLE OF SOCIAL WORK

Gregory J. Paveza and Carla VandeWeerd

A CASE HISTORY

Sally is an 83-year-old woman who presented to a shelter with bruising to her forearms, chest, abdomen, and jaw that was in various stages of healing. When asked about her condition she replied that she had been living with her daughter and son-in-law and had been experiencing this form of violent treatment for more than 4 years. When asked why she had taken so long to leave, she stated that she never felt she had anywhere else to go, and that perhaps in exchange for the burden of her care, she should expect the occasional outburst. When asked what had finally changed her mind, she said it was simple: One day a social worker in an emergency room finally asked her privately about her situation, and then showed her she had options.

SIGNIFICANCE TO GERONTOLOGY

Concern about elder mistreatment developed in the late 1970s when persons working with older adults became concerned with what was then called "granny bashing." Among the American leaders in the field was Dr. Rosalie Wolf, who would become a central figure in the field of elder mistreatment for more than 25 years. She played pivotal roles in attracting many of the current senior researchers in elder mistreatment into the field, the senior author of this article included. Moreover, Dr. Wolf was crucial to bridging the gap between the research and practice communities. It was her vision of the need to address elder abuse as a matter of national policy that led to her work to establish both the National Center on Elder Abuse (NCEA) and the National Committee for the Prevention of Elder Abuse (NCPEA). Dr. Wolf remained a vital and contributing member to the field until her death in 2001.

At the same time Dr. Wolf was engaging in her efforts to focus attention on elder mistreatment, elder abuse research broke into public view with the hearings of the House Select Committee on Aging (Pepper & Oakar, 1981). The committee report was the first to call national attention to the problem in the policy-making arena. It was also one of the first to offer initial estimates of the numbers of persons affected by elder abuse and suggested that as many as 1 million individuals older than age 65 were physically abused each year. Although this report was one of the first to provide any prevalence data on elder abuse, of more importance was the critical impact of the national hearings, which raised the level of discussion and made elder abuse and neglect legitimate areas of scientific inquiry and a focus for calls for intervention.

Although elder mistreatment has been a focus of research inquiry and clinical practice for 25 years, we are still no closer to accurate incidence data, the number of new cases in a given time frame; and prevalence data, the total number of cases in a given time frame. Prevalence estimates range from as high as 9% to less than 1% of the population older than 65 (Gioglio & Blakemore, 1983; Hickey & Douglas, 1981; Homer & Gilleard, 1990; Lau & Kosberg, 1979; National Center on Elder Abuse, 1998; Pepper & Oakar, 1981; Pillemer & Finkelhor, 1988). This large disparity in prevalence and incidence estimates has resulted in suggestions by some policy makers that the whole issue of elder mistreatment is little more than a tempest in a teapot. Other policy makers see mistreatment as a grave problem and react as if every older adult is being mistreated. Neither position seems particularly useful for adequately addressing the problem. It is important to recognize that the estimates used to bolster both positions are methodologically flawed. Currently, the prevalence estimate that is considered the strongest by standards of scientific methodological rigor is the one provided by Pillemer and Finkelhor, derived from their random telephone survey of persons living in the Boston area. Their estimate puts abuse at about 2.5% of the population over the age of 65 (Pillemer & Finkelhor, 1988). In terms of incidence, the widely distributed estimate from a national incidence study suggests that the incidence of all forms of mistreatment is about 500,000 persons per year (National Center on Elder Abuse, 1998). This study however, has been criticized on a number of methodological grounds including sampling issues and the choice of sentinels (surrogates from whom data about suspected cases of abuse were collected) (Cook-Daniels, 1999; Otto & Quinn, 1999) and has left the prevailing sense that this incidence estimate remains an underestimate.

The use of the term *elder mistreatment* is rather new in the lexicon of social work. It has come to mean the group of behaviors that cause harm to older adults and includes physical and sexual abuse, neglect, and financial exploitation. The term and the behaviors associated with it are further limited by requiring that the person committing the act be in a trust or caregiving relationship to that older person. Among those who might be included in this category of trusted others are siblings, spouses, children, grandchildren, other relatives, friends, attorneys, and formal caregivers such as home health aides, homemakers, certified nursing assistants, nurses, doctors, social workers, trust officers, and others. Acts of self-neglect are excluded from our discussion according to the definition we use. Also excluded are those physically or sexually abusive acts committed by strangers, or acts of a financial nature that are either illegal or prey on older adults but are committed by strangers. This is not to say that these are unimportant behaviors for social work consideration when working with older adults. Rather it is our belief that these acts stem from a different theoretical and intervention perspective than the majority of elder mistreatment behavior. Generally, when strangers commit acts of abuse or financial exploitation, these acts need to be viewed within their criminal context and treated as such. Indeed many states have included enhanced penalties in their criminal statutes when criminal actions are targeted at vulnerable populations, including older adults. Moreover, when acts involve self-neglect, they need to be viewed from the appropriate mental health or social welfare background.

As a result of these methodological and definitional inconsistencies, the impact of elder abuse becomes difficult to define. The field lacks estimates of the proportion of older adults admitted to nursing homes as a result of elder mistreatment. No estimates exist of the numbers of older persons who may have filed for bankruptcy, or experienced some lesser financial hardship, as a result of the unscrupulous actions of family or fiduciaries. There are no estimates of the acute medical care or long-term-care costs that can be attributed to elder mistreatment. Lachs and colleagues have provided one important indication of the impact of elder mistreatment (Lachs, Williamson, O'Brien, Pillemer, & Charlson, 1998). Their research suggests that persons subject to abuse are at significantly greater risk for death than other members of their age cohort who did not experience abuse or who self-neglected.

Although exact information on the impact of elder mistreatment on elders remains sparse, the impact on caregivers of being accused of elder mistreatment or of having committed elder mistreatment has not been studied. To further complicate the treatment and prevention of elder mistreatment, no significant research exists in the scientific literature on interventions or other programs to assist the victims of elder mistreatment or those who engage in abusive, neglectful, or exploitive behaviors. And although the information we have on domestic elder mistreatment is sparse, the field has even less information on elder mistreatment in institutional settings, both acute and long-term-care. The research that does exist suggests that some of the abuse in long-term care settings is the result of the stress experienced by workers in these settings (Pillemer & Moore, 1992). To date, much of the information needed to inform practice is inadequate, largely anecdotal, or based on unevaluated clinical experience, with little or no confirmatory research. Thus, as can be seen, though a concern about elder mistreatment has existed among policy makers at both federal and state levels for more than 20 years, research has offered little help in understanding the scope of the problem.

SIGNIFICANCE TO HEALTH CARE AND HEALTH PROFESSIONALS

The lack of solid research evidence of the numbers of older adults affected, of clear identification of the risk factors associated with elder mistreatment by type, and of clearly specified intervention strategies contributes to the general lack of training in schools of social work and other health professions. Recent research suggests that the amount of time devoted to elder abuse as a topic in social work education is often less than 2 hours per year in all social work courses, including human behavior, practice theory and methods, field seminar, and research (Milonas, 2001; Paveza, VandeWeerd, & Milonas, 2001a, 2001b). This lack of attention is systemic, however, to most of the helping professions and includes not only elder mistreatment, but all areas of family violence, as was documented in the recent Institute of Medicine report on health professionals' education on family violence (Institute of Medicine [IOM], 2002). Although this report notes that there are an increasing number of educational programs available to assist in providing vital information to health-professionals, it further notes that few health professional education and training programs, including social work, have instituted such programs (IOM, 2002).

Older adults, especially mistreated older adults, are among vulnerable and oppressed populations and, as such, are among those populations with which social work as a profession should be most concerned. Moreover, it is social workers and those persons in social service positions who are most often charged with addressing the problem. It is social workers who make up the bulk of Adult Protective Service Workers, therapists, and case managers. Much of the Adult Protective Services and elder abuse legislation came about as the result of the House Select Committee hearings (IOM, 2002) and the calls by many social workers working with disabled and older adults for the states to address a growing problem. Moreover, many of these same workers endeavored to have mandatory reporting provisions written into the elder mistreatment statutes. All 50 states and the District of Columbia have some form of elder mistreatment legislation and as noted in the IOM (2002) report, only 10 states have no clear mandatory reporting provision. In all states with mandatory reporting, social workers are among the named mandated reporters.

PRIOR RESEARCH

Research in the field of elder abuse first emerged in the middle and late 1970s. To a large extent, it has followed a classic developmental pattern for many areas of the social and behavioral sciences, including child abuse and intimate partner violence. The early research was largely descriptive in nature. It used key informants for obtaining information, including social service professionals, clergy, and health care professionals. These informants were asked to identify persons with whom they had had contact who they believed had been abused. The researchers provided a definition of abuse, and the informants provided information about their contacts who met the definition. This research provided some initial demographic information, which ultimately shaped the profiles of both abusers and those at risk for abuse (Gioglio & Blakemore, 1983; Hickey & Douglas, 1981; Lau & Kosberg, 1979; Pepper & Oakar, 1981). Although these studies were critical for the early definition of the problem, they lacked scientific rigor because they used convenience samples and obtained data from third persons. Moreover, most of these early studies failed to include a nonabused group with which comparisons could be made. This research also aggregated all individual forms of elder mistreatment under one broad mistreatment heading, so the profiles provided were aggregate profiles as opposed to behavior-specific ones. Thus the ability to use these profiles to identify an older adult at risk for a specific form of elder mistreatment is limited.

These initial studies were followed by a series of small-sample explanatory studies that often produced contradictory results based on the limitations of the sample (Anetzberger, 1987; Pillemer & Wolf, 1986; Steinmetz, 1988). These studies were valuable, however, because they pushed the field to question some of the earlier conceptualizations derived from the descriptive studies. At the same time, it was with the publication of these studies that the field of elder mistreatment diverged from the other areas of family violence. If one looks at the fields of child abuse and intimate partner violence, it is apparent that after the small-sample exploratory studies, these areas initiated more rigorous, population-based studies to better determine at-risk characteristics, outcomes, and interventions for victims. Elder abuse research has lagged behind in this area. Although there have been studies attempting to address these areas (Coyne, Reichman, & Berbig, 1993; Dayton, Anetzberger, & Matthey, 1997; Lachs et al., 1998; Paveza et al., 1992; Pillemer & Finkelhor, 1988; Pillemer & Suitor, 1992; Quayhagen et al., 1997; Reis & Nahmiash, 1997), the number of studies in elder mistreatment is quite small when compared with the research output in the companion areas of child abuse and intimate partner violence at similar points in their historic development.

The lack of research development may reflect the difficulty that the field of elder mistreatment has had in developing adequate theoretical underpinnings. A number of factors have played into this lack of theoretical development, including the nature of the early research, which suggested that those who were abused were older women being abused by overwhelmed and burdened female caregivers (Gioglio & Blakemore, 1983; Hickey & Douglas, 1981; Lau & Kosberg, 1979). These data suggested that elder mistreatment theory should be similar to theory underlying work in child abuse and neglect such as that of Garbarino and Gilliam (1980), Green (1980), and Nelson (1984). However, later data in the field (Pillemer & Finkelhor, 1988; Pillemer & Wolf, 1986) began to suggest that elder mistreatment theory might need to reflect more closely the theories underlying research in intimate partner violence (Borkowski, Murch, & Walker, 1983; Dobash & Dobash, 1979; Roberts, 1984), which focused on issues of power and control. More recently, theoretical explanations have begun to attempt to use models that incorporate both issues by adopting a vulnerabilities and risk model of development (Fulmer & Paveza, 1998; Pillemer & Suitor, 1992). These models allow for a variety of factors to be considered and enhance the capability of elder mistreatment researchers to move forward with both explanatory and causal research.

The continuing discussion of whether elder mistreatment is a social and behavioral problem or largely a legal problem adds to the difficulty of developing an adequate theory. In the estimation of these authors, this debate has at time diverted energy from the need to develop useful explanatory theories. Additionally, the concern about the impact of this phenomenon on a highly vulnerable population has at times pushed the field to concentrate on interventions without proper evaluation. Furthermore, self-neglect among some older adults, a phenomenon we do not discuss in this chapter, has placed practitioners and administrators in the position of directing attention and resources to this population of older adults. The call for research then often devolves into a debate between clinical issues—such as forensic markers and intervention evaluation—and explanatory research to provide models that define risk that could then inform and guide interventions. Both of these areas of inquiry are critical to the field and both need to receive research support from government and private funders. Though theory and research have been slow to develop, this does not imply that no research is currently underway.

CURRENT RESEARCH

One of the noticeable deficiencies when looking at current research is that not one of the major foundations that support research in aging has made elder mistreatment a priority area for the investment of research funds. Though many foundations have supported some research in the field from time to time, their lack of significant commitment tends to reinforce the concept that this is not a vital research issue.

Most of the major funding for research in the field comes from the National Institute on Aging (NIA); the second most significant provider is the Department of Justice, through either the Office of Victim Assistance or the National Institute of Justice. Considering the size of the problem, the total number of projects is hard to determine. Stahl (Stahl, Prenda, & Cooper, 2001), in a recent internal report for the NIA, was able to determine 12 recently completed or currently active projects on elder mistreatment funded by the NIA. Two of the projects directly involve the authors of this chapter and are discussed in detail with the remaining 10 in Appendix A.

At the time this chapter was being written, all of the current NIA-supported research in elder mistreatment being conducted by social workers was being done by the Elder Mistreatment Research Laboratory of the School of Social Work at the University of South Florida. However, there are a limited number of social work researchers being supported by nonfederal sources.

The Elder Mistreatment Laboratory

The Elder Mistreatment Research Laboratory (EMRL) in the School of Social Work at the University of South Florida (USF) is one of the few research endeavors specifically targeting research in elder mistreatment. EMRL had its beginning in a single research project supported by the Florida Mental Health Institute of USF and the Research and Creative Scholarship Fund of USF Research Council. The initial project (Paveza & Harrison-Hughes, 1997) was an attempt to develop a typology of financial exploitation, using police records gathered from the Hillsborough County (Florida) Sheriff's Office. The internal university funding provided the platform that permitted this small research endeavor to move to the next level when it became the recipient of NIA funding to study violence and aggression in families caring for a member with Alzheimer's disease. This 3-year project was an extension and expansion of an earlier project that looked at the same issue as part of a much larger Alzheimer's disease registry project (Cohen et al., 1990; Paveza et al., 1992). The Violence in Community

Based Alzheimer's Disease Families Study was developed to obtain a larger statewide caregiving sample and to measure more specifically the risk factors believed to be associated with the physical abuse of an older adult. Additionally, this research will look at changes in conflict resolution patterns over the course of a family's life when one member of the family develops Alzheimer's disease.

Data collection for the Violence in Community Based Alzheimer's Disease Families Study project began in 1997 and continued through 2001. However, as this project moved into the later stages of data collection, the research team began some initial data analysis. The underlying rationale for this analysis was twofold, both scientific and educational. The first purpose was to permit the investigators to explore some initial hypotheses concerning risk for violence and aggression in families caring for a member with Alzheimer's disease, with the hopes that these initial peeks would assist in offering direction for subsequent analyses of the full data set. The second purpose was to provide research opportunities to the MSW students working in the lab for use in their graduate research project. Initial analysis of the data provided some interesting information that has been presented at several annual scientific meetings of the Gerontological Society of America (GSA) (Paveza, VandeWeerd, & Bruschi, 2000; Paveza, VandeWeerd, & Kirkwood, 1999; VandeWeerd, Paveza, & McGeever, 2001).

The findings from these studies have reaffirmed the link between depression and increased risk for elder abuse in terms of the choice of conflict resolution styles: Depressed individuals are more likely than less depressed individuals to resort to violent forms of conflict resolution (Paveza et al., 1999); persons with an increased sense of burden from caregiving and lower self-esteem are more likely to have impaired caregiving (Paveza et al., 2000); and conflict resolution styles are affected by alcohol use (VandeWeerd et al., 2001).

The first NIA-supported grant was essential for the establishment of EMRL as well because it permitted EMRL to expand its research endeavors through the use of fixed- and administrative-cost money funneled back into EMRL by the university. Through the use of these funds, the earlier data on financial exploitation were revisited and studied in relation to the burden of elder mistreatment borne by women. In this study, we demonstrated consistently that women bear more of the burden, that is, they are the victims of elder mistreatment more often than men are (VandeWeerd & Paveza, 1999).

The NIA funds also permitted EMRL to launch a study to look at the amount of family violence training taking place in schools of social work. That study was presented in November 2001 at the Gerontological Society of America's 54th Annual Scientific Meeting in Chicago and, as discussed elsewhere, showed that little education is being provided to social work students at either the bachelor's or master's level (Paveza et al., 2001b). The provision of fixed- and administrative-cost funds to EMRL permitted it to engage in a study, using police records, of domestic violence targeted at older adults. This study provided some interesting insights into physical violence in the home. It reaffirmed that much of the physical violence directed at older adults is perpetrated by either spouses or children, and that the reason for the violence is most often related to power and control issues rather than to obtaining money (VandeWeerd, Dorrough, & Paveza, 2000).

While these projects were underway, EMRL received funding in 1998 from the Retirement Research Foundation, through the 13th Judicial Circuit of Florida (Hillsborough County), to conduct an evaluation of the Elder Justice Center. This center was established through the administrative office of the court to provide referral services to older adults coming in contact with the courts, to help familiarize older adults with court proceedings when needed, to provide education to the public about probate issues, and to provide case management (oversight) of guardianship cases. This project is nearing its first major milestone with the preparation of a report on the case management services. Initial data have shown support for improvements in the care of wards when monitoring is done by specialists with training in elder issues (Berko, 2002).

In 1999, EMRL was also part of a consortium of institutions that received a grant from NIA to study caregiver neglect. The participants in this grant are the Division of Nursing of New York University, represented by Terry Fulmer, who is also serving as the primary principal investigator on this study; the Epsilon Group, represented by Ivo Abraham; and EMRL. The study is currently underway and is actively collecting data. Using the theory developed by Fulmer and Paveza (1998), the study will define risks and vulnerabilities for neglect in nondementing older adults and their caregivers and provides opportunities for MSW students to serve as research assistants, giving them training in the recognition of elder neglect.

In the future, EMRL hopes to seek funding to look at caregiver neglect in Alzheimer's families and to participate in studies seeking to provide better estimates of elder mistreatment, the risk factors associated with the various forms of elder mistreatment, and the sequelae to being mistreated.

FURTHER RESEARCH NEEDS

Research in elder mistreatment has been going on for 25 to 30 years, yet when one reviews the current state of knowledge in the field, it is possible to feel as though one is still without answers and clear direction. The development of the field has been haphazard, and one is taken somewhat aback and ends up asking how the field should progress from here. Indeed, the field has been so slow and haphazard in its development that in 2001, the National Institute on Aging requested the National Research Council of the National Academies of Science to convene a panel to study the current state of knowledge in the field of elder mistreatment and to make recommendations concerning the research directions for the field. The establishment of that committee offers hope for defining the future direction of elder mistreatment research. That being said, a discussion about the research needs in the field cannot be put on hold, so we will address the issue from our personal perspective.[1] The authors of this chapter believe that there are four critical areas that must be addressed by the field of elder abuse if it is to dispel the concept that this issue is principally a tempest in a teapot. First, there is the lack of recent and accurate estimates of incidence and prevalence. The principal study used for prevalence estimates is now more than 10 years old (Pillemer & Finkelhor, 1988). No methodologically rigorous prevalence studies have been attempted since. Until new estimates are forthcoming that reflect the national picture, it will be difficult to achieve the necessary buy-in of policy makers and funders to permit other areas of elder mistreatment research to move forward.

Second, more information is needed about risk and protective factors. Much of the early risk research was based on third-party information and was constructed without the use of a comparison group. There was a brief period of well-constructed retrospective studies in

---

[1] The opinions offered here are those of the authors only and do not necessarily reflect those of the Panel on the Risk and Prevalence of Elder Abuse and Neglect, of which the senior author of this chapter is a member.

the late 1980s and early 1990s (Coyne et al., 1993; Homer & Gilleard, 1990; Paveza et al., 1992; Pillemer & Suitor, 1992; Pillemer & Wolf, 1986), which looked at specific forms of elder mistreatment often in the subpopulation of dementia caregivers, but more recent research has failed to build on this tradition. Rather, recent research appears to have reverted to previous study designs using noncomparison group designs. Additionally, even some of the better-constructed recent studies fail to differentiate by form of mistreatment (Comijs, Pot, Smit, & Jonker, 1998). Thus, the risk factors reflect whatever the dominant form of mistreatment is in that sample, which means that the risk factors established by a particular study may not have equal applicability to the other forms of elder mistreatment included in the study. This makes it difficult to plan intervention and prevention programs and to develop screening mechanisms because the target behavior for the screen, prevention strategy, or intervention may not be actually associated with the particular form of abuse or neglect one is seeking to identify, prevent, or change. The lack of specificity also contributes to the lack of policy in the field.

Outcomes or sequelae of abuse and neglect is a third research area that needs greater attention. To date, only one well-constructed study has looked at the long-term impact of elder mistreatment on victims (Lachs et al., 1998). Without studies that look at health care costs, at the development of emotional problems, including post-traumatic stress disorder and depression, and at other sequelae, it becomes difficult to draw the necessary funds into the field for interventions. The prevailing attitude often appears ageist in that it suggests that elder mistreatment is a small problem with few consequences for the affected population. Cost-benefit analyses of treatment programs are clearly needed.

The final area of research that we believe is essential is evaluation of programs. Although the amount of funding provided for programs continues to be minimal, funds that are provided often go to programs that remain unevaluated, and in some cases the funding agency expressly forbids the use of funds for evaluation. Any program that is developed should include an evaluative component that will permit both service providers and funders to determine whether the goals of the program are being met, whether those goals are sustainable, and the cost to achieve the goals. For a number of years, the senior author has suggested that the difficulties facing many of the programs supported by the social work profession are directly attributable to a lack of evaluation (Paveza, 1997). Thus, when the occasional program-matic failure occurs, the program is labeled a failure because there are no solid, methodologically sound data to suggest that more people succeed than fail and that failure is the exception rather than the rule. And when a success *is* examined, the cost of obtaining that success is frequently labeled excessive because reasonable cost-benefit analysis is missing. In many instances, the lack of evaluation has resulted in the redirection of funds from social services intervention to law enforcement and criminal prosecution. Often this shift results in little benefit to the older adult who is the victim of abuse and neglect. The older adult continues to experience a reduction in quality of life, but the larger community can continue to believe that it has done something.

In addition to the evaluation research suggested here, the field of elder abuse also requires that best-practices information be more forthcoming. Programs and interventions that do have an impact are disseminated ineffectively, if they are disseminated at all. This contin-ues to leave the field without intervention strategies for practitioners to employ, and it is one of the contributing factors that keeps the field of elder mistreatment on the fringes of social work education.

POLICY IMPLICATIONS

Almost 20 years ago, Barbara Nelson (1984) wrote an important work detailing how child abuse became a matter of national policy. One of the most telling features of her discussion is her suggestion that the political climate must be right in order for national policy to be imple-mented and sustained. She notes that what helped make child abuse a national priority were the congressional hearings conducted by then-Senator Walter Mondale during an administration that was sympa-thetic to social causes. This confluence of factors resulted in both national social policy and legislation (Nelson, 1984). One can see simi-lar parallels in the development of policy around intimate partner violence, especially wife abuse. Hearings were held at a time when the climate was favorable for "law and order" issues. It is important to recognize that the intimate partner violence movement wanted the issue addressed as a criminal matter, at least when it came to the perpetrators. Thus, it became possible to formulate policy at both the national and local levels.

It is exactly the lack of confluence of politics and policy that we believe has made it difficult for elder mistreatment to develop or sustain a national policy. It has been more than 20 years since Pepper first proposed the need for national legislation to address elder mistreatment (Pepper & Oakar, 1981). At that time, the administration was largely unsympathetic to social issues and was generally opposed to new social programs. This worked against the passage of national legislation. Furthermore, the general ageism of society made it all the more difficult to develop national policy from which local policy would flow.

Adding to this difficulty today are divisions within the elder mistreatment community itself. These divisions were interestingly reflected by the senior author several years ago at an annual meeting of the American Society on Aging in a panel discussion convened to discuss whether it was time to revisit the debate on a national model statute for elder abuse. Members included on the panel were from Adult Protective Services, law enforcement, and the research and practice communities. Although members of that panel worked together, continue to work together, and hold each other in high regard, the panel had difficulty reaching consensus about whether elder mistreatment should be considered a social problem, a legal and law enforcement problem, or a health problem. This inability to reach agreement is only heightened by the lack of substantive information about prevalence, risk factors, and societal and economic costs. Thus, the debate is often clouded by what we think we know and what we actually do know, which makes the formation of policy difficult: few policy makers are prepared to establish policy on what they perceive as largely unstable ground. In sum, insufficient data impedes the development of policy. Until those data are collected, it is likely that the field of elder mistreatment in both social work and in society at large will remain underdeveloped.

INTEGRATING KNOWLEDGE INTO THE CURRICULUM

Incorporating information about elder mistreatment into the body of social work education faces significant challenges over and above those encountered in incorporating gerontological material. These issues are closely related to the difficulty of having material on family violence included not only in social work education but also in the education of physicians, dentists, nurses, lawyers, and other helping professionals. The Institute of Medicine (2002) report on training issues around family violence is exceedingly clear: Not one of the major health care professions—medicine, social work, nursing, dentistry, psychology—performs adequately in this area. This failure to provide adequate training includes not only basic preparation, but also continuing education and other forms of postprofessional-degree training as well (IOM, 2002). The report further suggests that when training does occur, it is often focused on helping professionals to avoid asking questions that require them to make a report to Adult Protective Services (IOM, 2002).

Our own study, for example, affirms not only the lack of attention paid to elder mistreatment, but also to other areas of family violence, as well in social work education (Milonas, 2001). Most training in family violence, including elder mistreatment, in social work education is consigned to elective courses. These courses are often quite specific, focusing on child abuse, intimate partner violence or elder mistreatment. Students taking these courses usually have a special interest in the topic. A few programs have a broad course in family violence that addresses all of the major topics, but again, those registering for the course are students with either a general interest in family violence or an interest in one of the subtypes (Milonas, 2001). Inclusion in the core curricula is rare, however, and as Milonas (2001) noted, often amounts to less than 2 hours per topic in the 2 years of graduate social-work education, and an equivalent amount in undergraduate social work education. Few reasons have been given for this lack of inclusion, but as the IOM (2002) report noted, a common complaint was that there is insufficient time to incorporate all of the requested materials. This argument seems somewhat specious because it assumes that the only way to incorporate new essential information is to take other essential information out. Alternatives—including shifting the types of examples used to describe situations, noting how various clinical assessment and intervention skills can be used across the life span, and expanding placement options, as well as other techniques that do not require removing essential materials but rather involve simple modifications to the way information is presented—can be utilized to infuse this content into social work education to ensure it covers a range of current problems.

There are, however, other reasons that also explain the difficulty in incorporating elder abuse materials into the core curricula, or even in building substantive electives. One reason that has been consistently noted in this chapter is the dearth of substantive material available on best practices for assessment and intervention programs. Moreover, much of the information that is available has yet to be rigorously evaluated. This means that there are few practices and programs that can be described and recommended for implementation. Similarly, theoretical formulations explaining the development of elder mistreatment also are in short supply. In sum, the lack of well-documented and disseminated information for practice and theory makes it difficult for those teaching human behavior and clinical practice courses to incorporate much information into their pedagogy.

There are some materials that are available for inclusion in human behavior classes which provide theoretical frameworks for consideration in explaining elder mistreatment, including work by Pillemer and colleagues (Pillemer & Suitor, 1992; Pillemer & Wolf, 1986), Fulmer and colleagues (Fulmer & Paveza, 1998; Fulmer & O'Malley, 1987), and others (Aitken & Griffin, 1996; Anetzberger, 1987; Biggs, Phillipson, & Kingston, 1995; Carp, 2000; Filinson & Ingman, 1989; Steinmetz, 1988). These include materials that clearly describe theories about the evolution of elder mistreatment and posit risk factors such as isolation, addiction, control, low self-esteem, feelings of burden, and history of violence as examples that social workers should be trained to recognize in clinical practice as indicators of increased abuse risk.

Information also exists that can be used by those who are teaching practice as examples of collaborative programs in assessment (Dyer et al., 1999; Dyer & Goins, 2000; Fulmer, Paveza, Abraham, & Fairchild, 2000; Vladescu, Eveleigh, Ploeg, & Patterson, 1999), in working with agencies that are not usually involved in social problems (Alfonso, 2000; Allen, 2000; Aziz, 2000), and in community initiatives to grapple with the problem (Dayton et al., 1997). Through the use of such materials as examples of programs and practice, students are encouraged to view aging and the problems of aging as just one more set of social and behavioral problems with which social workers contend.

There is still, however, the broader problem with the infusion of elder mistreatment materials in the curriculum. In order to include elder mistreatment effectively in social work education, it is necessary first to overcome the barriers to including material on general family violence in instructional content (IOM, 2002; Milonas, 2001; Paveza et al., 2001a, 2001b). This difficulty in social work is reflected in the broader society by the lack of any substantive national policy on elder mistreatment.

CONCLUSION

Elder mistreatment is a vitally important element in social work education and practice, because older adults who are the victims of elder
mistreatment are among those vulnerable populations that are at the
heart of the social work profession's ethics and values. At the same
time, the authors of this chapter have noted that critical areas in the
field of elder mistreatment remain largely underexamined. Research
in the field, including estimates of incidence and prevalence, risk
factors, and effective intervention and prevention programs, lags far
behind other areas of family violence (IOM, 2002). The lack of crucial
data has contributed to the apparent lack of information in core curricula on the identification, assessment, and intervention with the victims
of elder mistreatment (Milonas, 2001). This deficiency in the social
work curriculum leaves most practitioners inadequately prepared to
work with a population with whom they are likely to have contact
based on current demographic trends. Moreover, this lack of education
on elder mistreatment has prevented social work from taking a leadership role in elder mistreatment research and programs.

Elder abuse research currently funded by the NIA is dominated by
nurses, physicians, and psychologists; the social workers at EMRL are
the only members of the profession who are receiving NIA funding
in this area. The authors believe that it is time for social work to
change this imbalance. However, to do so will require that social work
specifically address the issue of elder mistreatment as vital to the
health and well-being of older adults. Until it does, social work will
remain, unfortunately, a second-tier player in an area where it should
be a leader.

REFERENCES

Aitken, L., & Griffin, G. (1996). *Gender issues in elder abuse.* London: Sage.
Alfonso, H. I. (2000). Mortgage fraud prevention program: Volunteer legal services
    program of the Bar Association of San Francisco. *Journal of Elder Abuse and
    Neglect, 12*(2), 75–78.
Allen, J. V. (2000). Financial abuse of elders and dependent adults: The FAST
    (financial abuse specialist team) approach. *Journal of Elder Abuse and Neglect,
    12*(2), 85–91.
Anetzberger, G. J. (1987). *The etiology of elder abuse by adult offspring.* Springfield,
    IL: Charles C Thomas.

Aziz, S. J. (2000). Los Angeles County Fiduciary Abuse Specialist Team: A model for collaboration. *Journal of Elder Abuse and Neglect, 12*(2), 79–83.

Berko, L. (2002). *Elder guardianship: An intervention in Hillsborough County.* Unpublished master's research project, University of South Florida, Tampa, School of Social Work.

Biggs, S., Phillipson, C., & Kingston, P. (1995). *Elder abuse in perspective.* Buckingham, England: Open University Press.

Borkowski, M., Murch, M., & Walker, V. (1983). *Marital violence: The community response.* London: Tavistock.

Carp, F. M. (2000). *Elder abuse in the family: An interdisciplinary model for research.* New York: Springer.

Cohen, D., Paveza, G., Levy, P. S., Ashford, J. W., Brody, J. A., Eisdorfer, C., et al. (1990). An Alzheimer's disease patient registry: The Prototype Alzheimer Collaborative Team (PACT). *Aging: Clinical and Experimental Research, 2,* 312–316.

Comijs, H. C., Pot, A. M., Smit, H. H., & Jonker, C. (1998). Elder abuse in the community: Prevalence and consequences. *Journal of the American Geriatrics Society, 46,* 885–888.

Cook-Daniels, L. (1999). Interpreting the National Elder Abuse Incidence Study. *Victimization of the Elderly and Disabled, 2,* 1, 2, 14–15.

Coyne, A. C., Reichman, W. E., & Berbig, L. J. (1993). The relationship between dementia and elder abuse. *American Journal of Psychiatry, 150,* 643–646.

Dayton, C., Anetzberger, G., & Matthey, D. (1997). A model for service coordination between mental health and adult protective services. *Journal of Mental Health and Aging, 3*(3), 295–308.

Dobash, R. E., & Dobash, R. (1979). *Violence against wives: A case against the patriarchy.* New York: The Free Press.

Dyer, C. B., Barth, J., Portal, B., Hyman, D. J., Pavlik, V. N., Murphy, K., et al. (1999). A case series of abused or neglected elders treated by an interdisciplinary geriatric team. *Journal of Elder Abuse and Neglect, 10*(3/4), 131–139.

Dyer, C. B., & Goins, A. M. (2000). The role of the interdisciplinary geriatric assessment in addressing self-neglect of the elderly. *Generations, 24*(11), 23–32.

Filinson, R., & Ingman, S. R. (Eds.). (1989). *Elder abuse: Practice and policy.* New York: Human Sciences Press.

Fulmer, T., & Paveza, G. (1998). Neglect in the elderly patient. *Nursing Clinics of North America, 33,* 457–466.

Fulmer, T. T., & O'Malley, T. A. (1987). *Inadequate care of the elderly: A health care perspective on abuse and neglect.* New York: Springer.

Fulmer, T. T., Paveza, G. J., Abraham, I., & Fairchild, S. (2000). Elder neglect assessment in the emergency department. *Journal of Emergency Nursing, 26,* 436–443.

Garbarino, J., & Gilliam, G. (1980). *Understanding abusive families.* Lexington, MA: Lexington Books.

Gioglio, G., & Blakemore, P. (1983). *Elder abuse in New Jersey: The knowledge and experience of abuse among older New Jerseyans.* Unpublished manuscript, Trenton, NJ.

Green, A. H. (1980). *Child maltreatment: A handbook for mental health and child care professionals*. New York: Jason Aronson.

Hickey, T., & Douglas, R. (1981). Neglect and abuse of older family members: Professionals' perspectives and case experiences. *Gerontologist, 21,* 171–183.

Homer, A. C., & Gilleard, C. (1990). Abuse of elderly people by their carers. *British Medical Journal, 301,* 1359–1362.

Institute of Medicine. (2002). *Confronting chronic neglect: The education and training of health professionals on family violence*. Washington, DC: National Academies Press.

Lachs, M. S., Williamson, C. S., O'Brien, S., Pillemer, K. A., & Charlson, M. E. (1998). The mortality of elder mistreatment. *Journal of the American Medical Association, 280,* 428–432.

Lau, E., & Kosberg, J. (1979, September–October). Abuse of the elderly by informal care providers. *Aging, 10–15.*

Milonas, S. T. (2001). *Violence: Are we prepared? A meta-analysis of training offered by schools of social work in family violence*. Unpublished master's research project, University of South Florida, Tampa.

National Center on Elder Abuse. (1998). *The National Elder Abuse Incidence Study* (Final Report). Washington, DC: Administration on Aging, Department of Health and Human Services.

Nelson, B. J. (1984). *Making an issue of child abuse: Political agenda setting for social problems*. Chicago: The University of Chicago Press.

Otto, J. M., & Quinn, K. (1999). An evaluation of National Elder Abuse Incidence Study by National Association of Adult Protective Services Administrators. *Victimization of the Elderly and Disabled, 2*(1), 4, 15.

Paveza, G., VandeWeerd, C., & Kirkwood, K. (1999). Correlation of depression and negative conflict resolution in community-based Alzheimer's caregivers [Abstract]. [Special Issue I]. *Gerontologist, 39,* 127.

Paveza, G. J. (Ed.). (1997). Mistreatment of older adults. *Journal of Mental Health and Aging, 3*(3), 3–5.

Paveza, G. J., Cohen, D., Eisdorfer, C., Freels, S., Semla, T., Ashford, J. W., et al. (1992). Severe family violence and Alzheimer's disease: Prevalence and risk factors. *Gerontologist, 32,* 493–497.

Paveza, G. J., & Harrison-Hughes, V. (1997). Financial exploitation of the elderly: A descriptive study of victims and abusers in an urban area [Abstract]. [Special Issue I]. *Gerontologist, 37,* 101.

Paveza, G. J., VandeWeerd, C., & Bruschi, D. (2000). Impaired caregiving: The impact of self-esteem, burden of care and coping style on depression outcomes in caregivers of community-residing Alzheimer's patients [Abstract]. [Special Issue I]. *Gerontologist, 40,* 278.

Paveza, G. J., VandeWeerd, C., & Milonas, S. T. (2001a). Elder abuse education in schools of social work: A look at current levels of training and implications for practice. *Victimization of the Elderly and Disabled, 4*(2), 1, 30–32.

Paveza, G. J., VandeWeerd, C., & Milonas, S. T. (2001b). Elder mistreatment: An analysis of training offered by accredited schools of social work [Abstract]. [Special Issue I]. *Gerontologist, 41,* 220.

Pepper, C., & Oakar, M. R. (1981). *Elder abuse: An estimation of a hidden problem.* In the Proceedings of the House Select Committee on Aging, U.S. House of Representatives. Washington, DC: U.S. Government Printing Office.

Pillemer, K., & Finkelhor, D. (1988). The prevalence of elder abuse: A random sample survey. *Gerontologist, 28,* 51–57.

Pillemer, K., & Moore, D. W. (1992). Abuse of patients in nursing homes: Findings from a survey of staff. *Gerontologist, 29,* 314–320.

Pillemer, K., & Suitor, J. J. (1992). Violence and violent feelings: What causes them among family caregivers? *Journal of Gerontology: Social Sciences, 47,* S165–S172.

Pillemer, K. A., & Wolf, R. S. (Eds.). (1986). *Elder abuse: Conflict in the family.* Dover, MA: Auburn House.

Quayhagen, M., Quayhagen, M. P., Patterson, T. L., Irwin, M., Hauger, R. L., & Grant, I. (1997). Coping with dementia: Family caregiver burnout and abuse. *Journal of Mental Health and Aging, 3,* 357–364.

Reis, M., & Nahmiash, D. (1997). Abuse of seniors: Personality, stress and other indicators. *Journal of Mental Health and Aging, 3,* 337–356.

Roberts, A. R. (Ed.). (1984). *Battered women and their families: Intervention strategies and treatment programs* (Vol. 1). New York: Springer.

Stahl, S. M., Prenda, K. M., & Cooper, H. (2001). *Research directions on elder abuse and neglect* [Report]. Bethesda, MD: National Institute on Aging of the National Institutes of Health.

Steinmetz, S. K. (1988). *Duty bound: Elder abuse and family care.* Newbury Park, CA: Sage.

VandeWeerd, C., Dorrough, E., & Paveza, G. J. (2000). Elder abuse: A look at trends in violent crimes against the elderly [Abstract]. [Special Issue I]. *Gerontologist, 40,* 170.

VandeWeerd, C., & Paveza, G. J. (1999). Physical violence in old age: A look at the burden of women [Abstract]. [Special Issue I]. *Gerontologist, 39,* 403.

VandeWeerd, C., Paveza, G. J., & McGeever, P. (2001). The correlation between alcohol use and conflict resolution style in Alzheimer's family caregivers [Abstract]. [Special Issue I]. *Gerontologist, 41,* 276.

Vladescu, D., Eveleigh, K., Ploeg, J., & Patterson, C. (1999). An evaluation of a client-centered case management program for elder abuse. *Journal of Elder Abuse and Neglect, 11*(4), 5–22.

APPENDIX A SELECTED LIST OF RESOURCES FOR TEACHERS

This bibliography is composed of books and articles, which in the opinion of the authors are readily available and offer important information that can be incorporated into the general curricula of social work. In some cases, materials that were referenced in the body of this article are excluded from this bibliography because obtaining the material is exceptionally difficult, if not impossible.

Aitken, L., & Griffin, G. (1996). *Gender issues in elder abuse.* London: Sage.

Alfonso, H. I. (2000). Mortgage fraud prevention program: Volunteer legal services program of the Bar Association of San Francisco. *Journal of Elder Abuse and Neglect, 12*(2), 75–78.

Allen, J. V. (2000). Financial abuse of elders and dependent adults: The FAST (financial abuse specialist team) approach. *Journal of Elder Abuse and Neglect, 12*(2), 85–91.

Anetzberger, G. J. (1987). *The etiology of elder abuse by adult offspring.* Springfield, IL: Charles C Thomas.

Aziz, S. J. (2000). Los Angeles County Fiduciary Abuse Specialist Team: A model for collaboration. *Journal of Elder Abuse and Neglect, 12*(2), 79–83.

Barer, B. M. (1997). The secret shame of the very old: "I've never told this to anyone else." *Journal of Mental Health and Aging, 3,* 365–375.

Biggs, S., Phillipson, C., & Kingston, P. (1995). *Elder abuse in perspective.* Buckingham, England: Open University Press.

Carp, F. M. (2000). *Elder abuse in the family: An interdisciplinary model for research.* New York: Springer.

Cook-Daniels, L. (1999). Interpreting the National Elder Abuse Incidence Study. *Victimization of the Elderly and Disabled, 2,* 1, 2, 14–15.

Coyne, A. C., Reichman, W. E., & Berbig, L. J. (1993). The relationship between dementia and elder abuse. *American Journal of Psychiatry, 150,* 643–646.

Dayton, C., Anetzberger, G., & Matthey, D. (1997). A model for service coordination between mental health and adult protective services. *Journal of Mental Health and Aging, 3*(3), 295–308.

Dyer, C. B., Barth, J., Portal, B., Hyman, D. J., Pavlik, V. N., Murphy, K., et al. (1999). A case series of abused or neglected elders treated by an interdisciplinary geriatric team. *Journal of Elder Abuse and Neglect, 10*(3/4), 131–139.

Dyer, C. B., & Goins, A. M. (2000). The role of the interdisciplinary geriatric assessment in addressing self-neglect of the elderly. *Generations, 24*(11), 23–32.

Ejaz, F. K., Bass, D. M., Anetzberger, G. J., & Nagpaul, K. (2001). Evaluating the Ohio elder abuse and domestic violence in late life screening tolls and referral protocol. *Journal of Elder Abuse and Neglect, 13*(2), 39–57.

Filinson, R., & Ingman, S. R. (Eds.). (1989). *Elder abuse: Practice and policy.* New York: Human Sciences Press.

Fulmer, T., & Paveza, G. (1998). Neglect in the elderly patient. *Nursing Clinics of North America, 33,* 457–466.

Fulmer, T. T., & O'Malley, T. A. (1987). *Inadequate care of the elderly: A health care perspective on abuse and neglect.* New York: Springer.

Goldstein, M. Z. (1996). Elder maltreatment and posttraumatic stress disorder. In P. E. Ruskin & J. A. Talbott (Eds.), *Aging and posttraumatic stress disorder* (pp. 127–135). Washington, DC: American Psychiatric Press.

Hickey, T., & Douglas, R. (1981). Neglect and abuse of older family members: Professionals' perspectives and case experiences. *Gerontologist, 21,* 171–183.

Homer, A. C., & Gilleard, C. (1990). Abuse of elderly people by their carers. *British Medical Journal, 301,* 1359–1362.

Institute of Medicine. (2002a). *Confronting chronic neglect: The education and training of health professionals on family violence.* Washington, DC: National Academies Press.

Institute of Medicine. (2002b). *Confronting chronic neglect: The education and training of health professionals on family violence—Executive summary.* Washington, DC: National Academies Press.

Lachs, M. S., Williamson, C. S., O'Brien, S., Pillemer, K. A., & Charlson, M. E. (1998). The mortality of elder mistreatment. *Journal of the American Medical Association, 280,* 428–432.

Lau, E., & Kosberg, J. (1979, September–October). Abuse of the elderly by informal care providers. *Aging,* 10–15.

National Center on Elder Abuse. (1998). *The National Elder Abuse Incidence Study* [Final Report]. Washington, DC: Department of Health and Human Services, Administration on Aging.

Otto, J. M., & Quinn, K. (1999). An evaluation of National Elder Abuse Incidence Study by National Association of Adult Protective Services Administrators. *Victimization of the Elderly and Disabled, 2*(1), 4, 15.

Paveza, G. J., Cohen, D., Eisdorfer, C., Freels, S., Semla, T., Ashford, J. W., et al. (1992). Severe family violence and Alzheimer's disease: Prevalence and risk factors. *Gerontologist, 32,* 493–497.

Paveza, G. J., VandeWeerd, C., & Milonas, S. T. (2001). Elder abuse education in schools of social work: A look at current levels of training and implications for practice. *Victimization of the Elderly and Disabled, 4*(2), 1, 30–32.

Pepper, C., & Oakar, M. R. (1981). *Elder abuse: An estimation of a hidden problem.* In the Proceedings of the House Select Committee on Aging, U.S. House of Representatives. Washington, DC: U.S. Government Printing Office.

Pillemer, K., & Finkelhor, D. (1988). The prevalence of elder abuse: A random sample survey. *Gerontologist, 28,* 51–57.

Pillemer, K., & Moore, D. W. (1992). Abuse of patients in nursing homes: Findings from a survey of staff. *Gerontologist, 29,* 314–320.

Pillemer, K., & Suitor, J. J. (1992). Violence and violent feelings: What causes them among family caregivers? *Journal of Gerontology: Social Sciences, 47,* S165–S172.

Pillemer, K. A., & Wolf, R. S. (Eds.). (1986). *Elder abuse: Conflict in the family.* Dover, MA: Auburn House.

Pritchard, J. (1996). *Working with elder abuse: A training manual for home care, residential and day care staff.* London: Jessica Kingsley.

Quinn, M. J., & Tomita, S. K. (1997). *Elder abuse and neglect* (2nd ed.). New York: Springer.

Steinmetz, S. K. (1988). *Duty bound: Elder abuse and family care.* Newbury Park, CA: Sage.

Tatara, T. (Ed.). (1999). *Understanding elder abuse in minority populations.* Philadelphia: Taylor & Francis.

U.S. Department of Health and Human Services and U.S. Department of Justice. (Eds.). (1986). *Surgeon General's Workshop on Violence and Public Health Report.* Washington, DC: Department of Health and Human Services.

Vladescu, D., Eveleigh, K., Ploeg, J., & Patterson, C. (1999). An evaluation of a client-centered case management program for elder abuse. *Journal of Elder Abuse and Neglect, 11*(4), 5–22.

Wolf, R. S., & Pillemer, K. A. (1997). The older battered woman: Wives and mothers compared. *Journal of Mental Health and Aging, 3*, 325–336.

APPENDIX B CURRENT RESEARCH

Ronald Acierno, a psychologist at the Medical University of South Carolina, is studying how a crime victim's assessment methodology may be modified for use with older adults. It is hoped that this research will provide a way for better ascertainment of participants in risk-factor and outcome studies.

Terry Fulmer, a nurse at New York University, is studying dyadic vulnerability/risk profiling for elder neglect. This study is described in detail in the discussion of research at the Elder Mistreatment Research Laboratory, but involves utilization of the Elder Assessment Inventory in emergency rooms as a way to identify older adults who may be being mistreated.

Margaret Hudson, a nurse at the University of North Carolina at Chapel Hill, is attempting to develop and field test a brief screening protocol for elder abuse to be used by health care professionals. The screening protocol includes assessment on domains of physical and emotional abuse and will be used in a variety of settings.

Jeanie Kayser-Jones, a nurse at the University of California, San Francisco, is looking specifically at eating problems in nursing homes. Her work includes the idea that there is a potential for abuse and neglect to arise when feeding tubes are employed as part of the feeding process in institutional settings.

Mark Lachs, a physician at the Cornell Medical College, is currently receiving funding on two projects. One is an attempt to determine the independent contributions of reported elder abuse and neglect to all-cause mortality, and the other is an attempt to determine the epidemiology of crimes committed against elderly persons and the health consequences of those crimes.

Charles Mouton, a physician at the University of Texas at San Antonio, is attempting to determine baseline prevalence and 3-year self-report incidence of domestic violence in a population of older women. The study is also looking at the relationship of domestic violence, incidence of gun violence, and self-reports of health status to better understand this phenomenon.

Linda Phillips, a nurse at the University of Arizona, is studying abuse of caregivers by the persons to whom they are providing care. Her research includes an intervention to reduce the frequency and intensity of the abuse.

Michael Rodriquez, a physician at the University of California, Los Angeles, is doing research on ethnic differences in elder abuse and their impact on help-seeking behavior. In addition, he is working on identifying risk factors for elder mistreatment and developing a culturally sensitive screening tool for health care settings.

Neville Strumpf, a nurse at the University of Pennsylvania, is looking at how to maintain restraint reduction in nursing homes. Her research focuses on the idea that the use of restraints can constitute either abusive or neglectful behavior of older adults when employed improperly.

Gail Williamson, a psychologist at the University of Georgia, is looking at mental health impairment in caregivers. Such impairment in the past has been linked to risk for abuse and neglect by caregivers, and this research is seeking to reaffirm whether such increased risk exists among other impacts on both the caregiver and care recipient.

Chapter 12

STANDARDIZED GERIATRIC ASSESSMENT IN SOCIAL WORK PRACTICE WITH OLDER ADULTS

Scott Miyake Geron and Faith C. Little

Within and beyond long-term care, assessment is not the catchiest of topics. For most people, there is nothing unusual about being assessed. Answering a doctor's questions, taking a standardized test in school, completing a research questionnaire, participating in a Gallup poll—all of these are types of assessments and familiar, if not regular, experiences. Nonetheless, assessment very much merits the attention of professionals working with older adults.

Geriatric assessment is one of the primary tools used by practitioners in the field of gerontology to make services for older people responsive, appropriate, and effective. There are many types of geriatric assessments now in use. Practitioners such as social workers complete comprehensive assessments in community-based settings to understand the problems, needs, resources, and strengths of an older person in order to develop a plan of care. Medical or psychiatric diagnoses are completed by specialists. The geriatric social worker often assesses the older adult on multiple levels—physical, mental, social, environmental, and emotional—and on a wide variety of capacities, resources, and attributes. Increasingly, older adults themselves are asked to assess the strengths and weaknesses of services they receive.

In the broadest sense, geriatric assessment should help inform, guide, or contribute to making professional judgments about the appropriate course of action for an older individual. Most social workers would have no problem acknowledging that the development of an appropriate, individualized care plan for a client requires an accurate and holistic assessment of a person's health status as to physiological, social, environmental, and functional needs. But not all would agree that the use of standardized assessment measures could facilitate this process. Unfortunately, an all too common experience in social work practice is that many clinical decisions are made in spite of, rather than with the help of, an assessment tool. Practitioners know better than anyone about the irrelevance of many assessment measures, even those developed with scientific rigor and adequate resources.

Most standardized geriatric assessments used by social workers and others working with older adults are designed to assemble the information needed for practice or clinical care decisions. At the same time, assessment is the often the key to access important financial, health, and social services for an older adult, by determining eligibility to begin or continue services and justifying the need for other important tests, treatments, or interventions. The multiple purposes of geriatric assessment include the following:

1. Assessments serve important clinical functions, which include helping the social worker or other health professional develop an adequate information base to understand the problems, needs, resources, and strengths in a client's situation; and assisting social workers and clients in making decisions about the care plan.

2. Assessments are often used to establish technical eligibility for the various programs and services that social workers arrange, provide, or supervise.

3. Assessments provide a useful tool for training and supervising social workers and should create a common framework for discussing cases and improving the practice of geriatric social workers.

4. When priorities must be made for the allocation of services, assessments allow the application of fair and justifiable criteria based on need for, and likely benefit of, service.

5. Assessments generate information for state officials, legislators, and the general public about the type, extent, and distribution of needs in the community, thus assisting in ongoing program planning and refinement.

6. Assessments provide the foundation for provision of timely and relevant feedback to agencies and individual social workers about their effectiveness in client meeting needs.

Of particular concern in this chapter is how standardized geriatric assessment can aid the judgments of social workers and other long-term-care practitioners in health care as well as other related fields. Many new types of assessment tools have proliferated in the past decade, but what is the payoff for clinical care? Can geriatric assessments actually help practitioners in various fields make clinical decisions?

This chapter will discuss some major purposes of geriatric assessments and will explore the significance and implications of geriatric-specific assessment to social work. This chapter is a summary of work presented elsewhere in more detailed form (e.g., see Geron, 1997b, 1998; Geron et al., 2000), but presented here with a focus on aspects of particular relevance to a social work audience. This audience includes not only those who specialize in work with older adults but, especially, more generally trained social workers who increasingly will be encountering older people and their families in the course of their everyday practice and who must be familiar with these issues and concerns. We begin by reviewing the significance of geriatric assessment to gerontology for clinical care as well as administration and policy, and we summarize the characteristics of a well-designed geriatric assessment tool. Then we provide a brief overview of established comprehensive assessment measures, which are the measures social workers in community-based long-term care use most frequently. Next, we summarize our own research in consumer-based measures of home care quality as a new way to involve consumers in the assessment process. We then briefly review one of the most important areas of assessment research: the assessment of a frail older person's capacity to manage his or her own care. We conclude the chapter with a discussion of the policy implications of geriatric assessment and describe some ways to bolster the teaching of geriatric assessment in schools of social work.

SIGNIFICANCE TO GERONTOLOGY, HEALTH CARE, AND HEALTH PROFESSIONALS

Assessment in geriatric care has important personal consequences for the older person and his or her family. For many older adults who have entered the formal service system for help, the reality of their lives—their wishes, beliefs, history, likes, and dislikes—is reduced to the data captured in measurement tools. As a consequence of these assessments, older persons often become aware of loss of or decline in functioning in areas where previously they had been independent. They may also need to face their dependency on formal support services.

Many geriatric assessments are conducted by a team of health care providers, including social workers, physicians, nurses, physical therapists, and others. Completing successful assessments with older adults requires the utmost of the health professional's ability, skills, and perceptiveness. Social workers are often required to understand clients' physical, psychological, and social functioning and make determinations, based on these assessments, of clients' eligibility and need for services. Whatever the intervention or mode of assessment, assessments of older adults in residential or community-based settings are rarely simple matters of passively obtaining descriptive information; more often than not, they are investigations requiring clinical skill and understanding. Older adults may have multiple health problems with nonspecific origins or causes, they may have functional or cognitive limitations that make it difficult to provide accurate descriptions of their symptoms, and they may not have reliable proxy informants (Geron, 1997a; Harvey & Jellinek, 1981; Kane, Kane, & Ladd, 1998; Lawton, 1991).

Is there an ideal geriatric assessment tool for use by social workers? Clearly there isn't. As described earlier, assessments typically serve multiple functions in addition to their clinical utility, many of which impose competing requirements on the design, content, and length of the instrument. Additionally, every measurement tool must accommodate clients whose problems range from simple to complex, as well as assessors with different levels of experience and ability. Notwithstanding these challenges, assessment tools can be designed that enhance clinical decision-making and facilitate professional judgment. In our experience, geriatric assessments that successfully facilitate both clinical decision-making and serve policy objectives include the following characteristics:

1. *They are comprehensive in scope.* To serve useful clinical functions, assessments should be comprehensive enough to help social workers and other health professionals develop an adequate information base

to understand the problems, needs, resources, and strengths of a client's situation, and to guide the practitioners and the client in making decisions about a care plan. This means assessments should cover multiple dimensions or domains, including, at a minimum, demographic information, health status, functional performance, cognitive functioning, mental health status, social and informal supports, environmental assessment, and financial status. Not all components are measurements in a formal sense. Some items address necessary descriptive information such as income sources, household composition, marital status, and so on.

2. *They are functional in design.* Properly designed, an assessment tool can inform clinical judgments in many ways, some of them quite simple. For example, the design of the assessment should support clinical decision-making. The order of the domains and of questions within domains should be consistent with the normal flow of a clinical interview. Assessment forms should acknowledge the practitioner's expertise by providing space to record his or her perceptions, observations, judgements, and notes. In forms where such space is not provided, the practitioner's judgments and observations should be identified as such and should be separate from statements made by consumers, family members, or others participating in the assessment. The assessment tool should provide clear skip patterns so the assessor knows which questions to ask or avoid, based on answers the client provides to questions; and it should facilitate branching to allow the assessor to explore areas in depth if warranted. Newer computerized assessments have great potential to include help programs and diagnostic questions to help focus the assessor.

Assessments can also inhibit or enhance clinical decision-making in more complex ways. For example, the assessment should not include simplistic scoring schemes that tie the hands of practitioners and force them to "game" the scoring to promote or prevent placement or treatment decisions. To give another example, many assessments include a review of the client's medication use, with forms that simply leave a few lines to record this information (dosage, amount and frequency, route administration, etc.) without specifying how the information is to be obtained or from whom. A better approach would be to include language on the assessment tool that directs the assessor to ask clients to *show* them all of their medications. Skilled practitioners who work with older adults know that the bottles provide more accurate information and often contain important evidence about potential illnesses.

Computerized assessments can include red flags, if certain medications or doses of medication are used, that direct the practitioners to seek an additional assessment or prompt the assessors to ask additional questions.

The functionality of an instrument for clinical purposes also refers to its adaptability across users, from the most advanced to the most inexperienced. The best instruments are designed for the latter but are useable even by the most senior and experienced assessor. Again, computers offer great potential for modifying an instrument so that it is appropriate to the user's experience level.

3. *They are uniform across users.* It is desirable that a common assessment protocol be used at least within a particular agency and preferably throughout a statewide program. Developing a uniform, well-designed assessment instrument facilitates intervention and clinical decision-making in a number of ways. Uniformity provides a safety check to ensure that all important elements of an assessment are consistently collected. Uniformity also minimizes subjectivity and establishes a common language that permits communication across disciplines and agencies, creating a common framework for discussing cases and improving the social worker's clinical practice. The use of standardized assessment measures makes it possible to develop meaningful and substantial data bases about client functioning over time, which can support clinical practice as well as management, evaluation, and research.

Uniformity also means that the assessment instrument should incorporate standardized questions and response options whenever possible. In assessments, the way in which a question is asked influences the answer; similarly, the response options provided also constrain the answers made by consumers or others. This is true for simple demographic questions (e.g., marital status, ethnicity), for more difficult items such as functional capacity (e.g., dressing, eating), and for subjective questions about the consumer's health or well-being. Although the way a question is asked can and should be addressed in training, the assessment instrument should include the actual phrasing of questions and a list of response options to the greatest extent possible.

4. *They incorporate established measures.* Whenever possible, the assessment instrument should include standardized scales and measures that have proven validity and reliability, are widely used, and have been shown to be appropriate for older adults. Numerous standard-

ized measures have been developed to assess many of the important domains included in comprehensive assessments (e.g., mental status questionnaires, depression, physical functioning). If a social worker needs a specific or comprehensive assessment measure, the best strategy is to use a well-tested, established tool if one is available, but the social worker should supplement that instrument with program-, agency-, or project-specific items or measures as needed. This means careful planning up front when embarking on an assessment project to determine what existing tools would be appropriate.

5. *They balance psychometric precision with practicality.* Assessment is a form of measurement, and measurement precision is an important characteristic of any successful instrument. The precision of any assessment tool can be judged by how well it minimizes the chances of making a mistake, either by falsely suggesting something is the case when it is not (false positive) or falsely suggesting something is not the case when it is (false negative). The precision of a measure is determined by its validity and reliability. The accuracy or validity of an assessment is established by showing that the assessment measures what it purports to measure. The reliability of an assessment refers to the extent to which the measure produces consistent results with repeated applications (unless real change has occurred). Reliability is in part a training issue. Even when an assessment incorporates measures that are commonly recognized as valid and reliable, consistent administration of measures should be reinforced through training and periodic reliability testing of interviewers.

Assessments of older adults also should have practical utility. Assessments should be as short as possible, mindful of both the burden placed on clients and their families by the assessment process and the cost and timeliness of data collection. They should be easy to administer and parsimonious in design, requiring only as much information as needed to inform clinical decision-making and to satisfy the other purposes of the measure. These legitimate concerns can be at odds with the research objective of maximizing measurement precision. Generally, research has shown that the more items a measure has in a particular domain the more reliable and valid it is (Stewart, 1990). In the context of community-based assessment of older adults, however, it is necessary to balance the desire for psychometric precision with concerns about cost, respondent burden, and ease of administration. Fatigued clients are more likely to provide inaccurate information; adding to the length of an assessment without achieving gains in accurate information relevant to clinical decision-making is not justifiable.

6. *They support objective and multiple sources of information.* As much as possible, assessments should rely on items that can be observed by the practitioner. To the extent possible, the consumer's demonstration of functional performance should be encouraged. It is important to distinguish between activities the client is able to perform and activities he or she actually does perform, with the latter providing a less accurate assessment of functional capacity (Geron, 2002). For example, some consumers do not cook or clean but are able to do so. Similarly, the assessment should avoid the trap of having the practitioner (or a proxy informant) make ratings of the client's feelings or mental states. Subjective feelings and evaluations (e.g., how the client feels about his or her health) can legitimately come only from the client. The assessment tool can support these tasks by including direct questions to the client (surprisingly, many do not), by specifying the type of information that should come from the client, and by indicating how it should be collected. The objectivity of the assessment also can be improved by incorporating, with the client's approval, multiple sources of information whenever possible, including health providers, family members and neighbors, and other professionals who may be aware of the consumer's condition. The information obtained is used to help validate the assessor's opinion or to reconcile differing views among the client, the client's family, care providers, and others.

7. *They are easy to read and administer.* Consumers may wish to read the assessment, and practitioners may find it helpful to show the instrument to some consumers while completing one or more sections. The language in the assessment should be clear and simple. Questions or probes should be written in nontechnical language, and technical terms, even common ones like "marital status" and "activities of daily living" should be avoided or accompanied with simple definitions. Simple language facilitates understanding by clients and makes it easier to develop culturally accurate translations for non-native speakers. Orientation and detailed instructions for the use of the instrument should be provided.

For all items in the assessment, the sources of information should be clearly identified. In many assessments it is impossible to determine who completed the assessment and from whom or where the information originated. The assessment should clearly indicate when the client is not the primary source of information, and there should be decision rules for use of caregivers or others as proxy informants. The time dimensions for all questions within the assessment should be clear. This means that the assessment form should specify whether a consumer has been asked about his or her functioning in the past day, week, month, or 6 months. When a proxy informant answers for, or in addition to, a consumer, this person should be identified.

Though social workers and other health professionals are justifiably concerned about the length of any assessment, the importance of the brevity of administration time is not the same as minimizing the number of pages of the assessment form. In general, the clarity of the layout of an instrument is more important than its length. A jumbled measure with small characters that are difficult to read is more likely to result in missed or inaccurate information.

8. *They are culturally sensitive.* Though the diversity of the United States is increasingly acknowledged, efforts to design culturally equivalent assessment tools have lagged behind. Health care services research has demonstrated that ethnicity and socioeconomic status are related to rates of disability, morbidity, mortality, and health care utilization (Burstin, Lipsitz, & Brennan, 1992; Fox & Stein, 1991; Yee, 1992). Like other health and social service professionals, assessors too often feel uncomfortable, avoid issues related to minority culture, and do not understand how cultural differences may impede health care access and utilization. The best assessment protocols acknowledge cultural diversity and consider the implications for the instrument when used with non-English-speaking and minority clients. These assessments include training for social workers, nurses and case managers and others that addresses (a) how the assessor's values, beliefs, and attitudes may impede the ability of minority elders to respond to assessment questions; (b) an appreciation of cultural diversity among elders and how cultural, linguistic, and other modes of expression vary among minority elders; and (c) how these differences may affect minority elders' answers to assessment questions, shape their acceptance of the conclusions in the assessment and subsequent care plan options, and ultimately influence their ability to obtain services (Boyle & Springer, 2001; Sodowsky, Taffe, Gutkin, & Wise, 1994; Sue & Sue, 1999).

PRIOR RESEARCH AND KNOWLEDGE BASE

In the past decade, the number of standardized geriatric assessment measures has evolved and multiplied, and there is a wide variety of research-validated assessment instruments now in use (e.g., see American Psychiatric Association, 2000). In this section, we will focus primarily on the type of assessments conducted by "generalist" practitioners, most often social workers. These assessments typically involve comprehensive multidimensional social and health assessments of older adults in community-based settings, do not require specialist medical or psychiatric training, and usually take place in face-to-face interviews in the client's home (but they may also occur in the hospital, nursing home, or physician's office). Increasingly, these types of assessments are conducted over the telephone or by using software that allows the interviewer to input client responses directly into a computer.

In a review of this length, it is impossible to describe all of the recent developments in sufficient depth to do them justice, much less help readers seeking recommendations about specific measures. Fortunately, a number of comprehensive reviews are available. We recommend M. Powell Lawton and Jeanne A. Teresi's (1994) edited volume, *Annual Review of Gerontology and Geriatrics: Focus on Assessment Techniques*. In addition, Scott Miyake Geron's (1997b) review of geriatric assessment in the journal *Generations* contains specific articles by leading gerontologists on different types of geriatric assessment. Charles Emlet and colleagues (Emlet, Crabtree, Condon, & Treml, 1996) have written *In Home Assessment of Older Adults: An Interdisciplinary Approach*, which is a practical resource for those approaching the field of in-home care from a variety of disciplines and levels of education. Each of these reviews provides a summary of the research on many instruments, includes extensive citations on each, and reviews the psychometric properties of the measures.

Comprehensive multidimensional geriatric assessments endeavor to obtain a complete picture of the health and social situation of an older person. Comprehensiveness is one of their principal advantages—it is what makes them attractive for home- and community-based assessments of older adults in which clients' strengths and weaknesses need to be considered across a range of health and social dimensions. Another desirable feature of multidimensional assessment instruments is that they provide assessors with a uniform recording format to make comparisons across domains and to arrive at a rating of the clients' overall functioning or well-being (George, 1994). Multidimensional assessments that are adaptable to different users and clients have been developed, and many address clinical purposes as well as general research or evaluation concerns, although not all do so equally well. For a majority of the most established measures, reliability and validity statistics are available and are generally impressive.

Although the benefits of using a standardized, comprehensive instrument are considerable, their appeal to practitioners is still problematic. The length of multidimensional assessments is a drawback to many users. Although it is arguable whether the collection of equivalent relevant information could be accomplished more quickly without the aid of a standardized form, respondent fatigue is a legitimate concern in using multidimensional assessments. Most of the measures presented in this review can be completed in about an hour or less, or have versions that can be completed in that time, but practitioners know that their sessions with clients often last much longer than the time it takes to complete the instrument. More important, many practitioners working with older adults in home- and community-based settings find that multidimensional assessment instruments were not designed to help them make decisions about a client's eligibility and need for specific services or interventions, or to help them coordinate and plan services and care. Some of the major comprehensive assessments now in use include the following:

The Older Americans Resources and Services (OARS) Multidimensional Functional Assessment Questionnaire (MFAQ)

Developed by researchers at Duke University (Duke University Center for the Study of Aging and Human Development, 1978; Pfeiffer, 1975), the OARS is one of the most widely used multidimensional assessment instruments. The OARS measures functional status of older adults on five dimensions, contains 70 questions answered by the respondent, 10 about the respondent answered by an informant, and 14 about the respondent answered by the interviewer. The OARS MFAQ was designed to be administered as an interview in about 45 minutes. Many of the assessments developed by states incorporate elements of the OARS.

Comprehensive Assessment and Referral Evaluation (CARE)

Another measure that deserves mention is the CARE instrument, originally developed for a study of clinical judgments in Britain and the

United States (Gurland, Golden, Teresi, & Challop, 1984; Gurland et al., 1977). The CARE measure was designed to identify problems in older adults that are of concern to the health professionals (Gurland & Wilder, 1984). The most frequently used version is the CORE-CARE, a 314-item measure comprised of separate scales for 22 domains (Golden, Teresi, & Gurland, 1984). The CORE-CARE takes an average of 90 minutes to complete. Another version, labeled SHORT-CARE, uses 6 scales from CORE-CARE plus additional items for diagnostic purposes and takes about 30 minutes to complete.

Multilevel Assessment Instrument (MAI)

The MAI was developed by Dr. Lawton and his colleagues (Lawton, Moss, Fulcomer, & Kleban, 1982) at the Philadelphia Geriatric Center and is based on the developers' conceptual understanding of well-being of older people (Lawton, 1972). The MAI measures function on seven dimensions: physical health, cognition, activities of daily living, time use, social interaction, personal adjustment, and perceptions of the environment. The full-length MAI includes 135 items and requires an average of 50 minutes for administration. Mid-length and short-length versions are available; reliability and validity data for the shorter forms of the test are quite similar to the full version.

Medical Outcomes Study (MOS)

The MOS measures (Stewart & Ware, 1992) are a set of health scales that assess functional capacity and perceptions of health for adults with chronic conditions, including the elderly. The measures grew out of the MOS, a large observational study of variations in physician practice styles and patient outcomes in different systems of care. The full MOS measures address 12 dimensions of functioning and well-being and contain 149 items. Shorter versions include the 36-item MOS Short Form (SF-36), one of the most widely used measures of health and quality of life, and more recently the SF-12 and the MOS 6-item General Health Form (Jenkinson et al., 1997; Stewart & Ware, 1992; Tarlov et al., 1989; Ware & Sherbourne, 1992).

Anyone who is considering using a comprehensive multidimensional assessment instrument should review closely these and some of the other established instruments. These are the measures that have been thoroughly tested, are the most widely used, and have achieved, in most cases, impressive reliability and validity. However, there are important differences between them that only a more careful review will identify. For example, the domains assessed differ widely, reflecting differences in the conceptualization and approach used. Even within dimensions with the same title (e.g., mental health), the scope and type of assessment may vary widely. For example, the CARE measure focuses on diagnostic categories, while the MOS views quality of life through the rubric of health.

CURRENT RESEARCH: THE CONSUMER PERSPECTIVE

One of the most important developments in social work during the past decade has been the movement to empower consumers in all areas of practice (Becerra & Zambrana, 1985; Gutierrez, 1990). In geriatric social work, particularly in the area of long-term care, this trend manifests itself in the growing recognition of the importance of obtaining the consumer's perspective in assessing and monitoring services and providers (Applebaum, Straker, & Geron, 2000; Geron, 1998; Strasser, Aharony, & Greenberger, 1993). The assessment of consumer satisfaction with services is one of the most direct methods of giving voice to consumers' concerns about the quality of services they receive.

In this section, we discuss the development of the Home Care Satisfaction Measure (HCSM), a multi-item measure to assess satisfaction with home care services that was developed by Scott Geron and other colleagues at Boston University and the New England Research Institutes (Geron et al., 2000). Although considerable attention has been given to the development of client satisfaction measures in acute care (Cleary & McNeil, 1988; Cryns, Nichols, Katz, & Calkins, 1989; Davies & Ware, 1988; Ware, Snyder, & Wright, 1976) and mental health (Larsen, Attkisson, Hargreaves, & Nguyen, 1979; Lebow, 1983; Love, Caid, & Davis, 1979), existing measures of older consumers' satisfaction with home and community-based long-term-care services have suffered from several shortcomings.

First, many of the satisfaction instruments used in home care were adapted from measures developed to assess client satisfaction with medical care services, even though care provided in the home or nursing home is different in many respects from acute care or office-based health or mental health care (Kane, Illston, Eustis, & Kane, 1991). Compared to the circumscribed episode of a physician visit or acute medical episode, long-term home care centers on a consumer's daily living situation and is frequently of long duration. Moreover, though long-term home care does sometimes require the use of sophisticated technologies, much of the service is low tech, often provided by personnel with limited training and without professionally derived standards of practice.

Second, most measures in home care have been developed for a particular research or programmatic purpose (Linn, 1985; Linn, Linn, Stein, & Stein, 1989; Lucas, Morris, & Alexander, 1988; Pablo, 1975; Rinke & Wilson, 1988; Woerner & Phillips, 1989). Ad hoc measures, though contributing to our understanding of home care client satisfaction, do not allow for comparison across studies. Single-item global rating satisfaction measures have also been used frequently; unfortunately, these have not been found adequate to capture the complexity of services like health, mental health care (Andrews & Withey, 1976; Stewart & Ware, 1992) or long-term care.

Third, most available measures are based on researcher or provider perspectives of satisfaction, not the perceptions of older recipients of services. Equally important, even when consumer involvement has been utilized (Woerner & Phillips, 1989), the perspectives of minorities have been absent. The involvement of consumers is now widely recognized as necessary to ensure that the measure fully represents the dimensions of quality that are considered important to service recipients (Geron, 2000; Miller-Hohl, 1992; Riley, Fortinsky, & Coburn, 1992; Rinke & Wilson, 1988). Because satisfaction may have different meanings to different consumers (Geron, 1995; Gutek, 1978), the need to explore the meanings that consumers attach to terms such as "satisfaction," "satisfied," or "like" is a critical first step in developing a home-care satisfaction instrument.

Finally, none of the existing measures that were developed to evaluate consumer satisfaction with services received by frail older adults in their homes have been rigorously tested for reliability and validity. Adequate psychometric testing is a prerequisite to evaluating program or treatment effects accurately; establishing norms for satisfaction ratings across services, client populations, and ethnic groups; investigating correlates of satisfaction; or evaluating causal models of satisfaction.

The HCSM was designed to overcome shortcomings identified in the existing literature. Funded by a 3-year R01 grant from the National

Institute on Aging, the HCSM is based on consumer-defined notions of home care satisfaction, including the perspectives of ethnic minorities (Geron et al., 2000). After an initial review of the literature and prior pilot study information, separate focus groups were held with African American, Hispanic, and non-Hispanic White elders (Jewish, Italian American, and Irish American) to probe differences in the meaning of satisfaction across racial and ethnic groups. Group membership ranged from four to eight consumers.

"Grounded theory" methods were used to identify satisfaction dimensions that guided the development of the instrument (Charmaz, 1990; Orona, 1990). Focus group sessions were audiotaped and transcribed and were analyzed separately by the principal investigator and research associate into content and theme categories. As each theme was explored, discussed, and refined, the quotes of the study participants were used to define and explicate the meaning of the theme. Ultimately, eight dimensions of home care satisfaction were identified, although not all dimensions applied to all five services: competency, humaneness, dependability, service adequacy, continuity of care, choice, accessibility, and advocacy. Two independent raters repeated the analysis of the transcripts and identified seven of the eight dimensions.

The instrument was field-tested with 238 cognitively intact, community-dwelling adults (approximately equal numbers of African American, Hispanic, and White elders) 60 years of age or older who had received one or more of the selected in-home services for at least 6 months. The field-test version of the instrument included a section about each of five long-term home care services: Homemaker, Home Health Aide, Home-Delivered Meals, Grocery Service, and Care Management. Each service section contained 30–40 items that addressed specific dimensions of care received. To assess test-retest reliability, one half of the participants were randomly selected to participate in a second administration of the survey instrument within 5–9 days of the first.

Two methods were used to evaluate the initial pool of items, identify the dimensions of satisfaction, and select the final items for the measure. First, for each service, correlations were computed among all items in the pool. Each matrix was used to test convergent validity (large correlations among items hypothesized to measure the same dimension) and divergent validity (small correlations among items measuring different dimensions). Several items that were not related to their intended dimensions or that appeared to tap several dimensions were eliminated from the pool, as were others that were confusing to respondents. The remaining items were then subjected to a factor analysis using oblique (Promax) rotation estimated by maximum likelihood. Separate factor analyses were performed for each service. Oblique rotation was used because the dimensions of satisfaction were presumed to be correlated with one another. Items were selected to measure each service dimension based on the magnitude of the factor loadings and the unidimensionality of the items. The selected items were also designed to balance the number of positive and negative items for each dimension.

The final version of the HCSM consists of 60 items measuring dimensions of satisfaction with five major home health services. The HCSM provides an overall home-care satisfaction score and subscale scores for five common services, all scored on a scale of 0 to 100. The subscales of the HCSM for Homemaker Service (HCSM-HM13), Home Health Aide Service (HCSM-HHA13), and Case Management Service (HCSM-CM13) each contain 13 items. The subscale of the HCSM for Home-Delivered Meal Service (HCSM-MS11) contains 11 items, and the subscale for Grocery Service (HCSM-GS10) contains 10 items. Each of the subscales (except those in the Grocery Service module) contains a balance of positively and negatively worded items. All items use the same 5-point Likert-type response option: *Yes, definitely; Yes, I think so; Maybe yes, Maybe no; No, I don't think so; and No, definitely not.*

The HCSM provides a standardized assessment of home care satisfaction that is relatively brief, is easy to administer, and meets standard psychometric criteria for validity and reliability. Each subscale of the HCSM can be completed in 3–5 minutes. The HCSM can be supplemented by open-ended questions or items of particular interest to a particular service program. The measure is currently available in English, Spanish, and Russian, and can be administered in a face-to-face or telephone interview with a trained assessor. Based on the development sample, the HCSM service score test-retest reliabilities were all large, ranging from .68 (in the smallest service group) to .88, and the HCSM service and dimension scores possessed an acceptable to high degree of internal consistency. Substantial concurrent validity was achieved for HCSM subscale scores. In regression analyses with each HCSM subscale, home care satisfaction was not found to be related to age, gender, disability, or race, but was associated with a measure of social desirability.

The HCSM is designed to be used by agencies and organizations that arrange or provide community-based home care services to frail older adults who are residing in the community, as well as by researchers and practitioners studying consumer evaluations of home care services (either interprogram or sample-to-sample). With recent support from the Retirement Research Foundation, training materials and guidelines have been developed. The HCSM was recently adopted for use by the U.S. Administration on Aging as a key performance outcome measure. To date, more than 13,000 administrations of the HCSM have been completed, and the measure has been used or is being used in more than 20 states and programs. Currently, benchmarks are being developed that will permit agencies to compare their performance to national home care satisfaction standards. We are continuing to conduct research on the HCSM and to work with users to use the results productively to improve the quality of home care services provided.

FURTHER RESEARCH NEEDS

Geriatric assessment is constantly evolving to improve the utility and precision of existing measures, and there is now a dizzying array of established and well-tested tools available. New areas of geriatric assessment also continue to be addressed. One critically important area is the assessment of cultural competency, which Peter Maramaldi discusses in the next chapter. Another emerging area of research is the assessment of a frail elder's capacity for self-care. In this section, we highlight this important area in assessment research, which should be of paramount interest to social work practitioners who work with older adults in community-based settings.

The development of consumer-directed care is one of the major new developments in long-term care. Consumer-directed care is a reaction to decades of professionally driven services, where the views of consumers were rarely addressed or considered (Geron, 2000). Developed in large part from the independent living movement (ILM) and other rights advocates for those who are disabled in the United States (Batavia, DeJong, & McKnew, 1991), *consumer-directed care* refers to the development of services in which older adults who are frail assume control over the services provided to them. In the most extreme forms, consumers are allowed to hire, train, supervise, and pay their own workers and, if necessary, to fire them.

Several recent studies have shown that consumers prefer consumer-directed care over more traditional agency-provided services and have obtained better outcomes (Doty, Benjamin, Matthias, & Franke, 1999; Doty, Kasper, & Litvak, 1996). Our own research has shown that when elderly consumers who are frail are more satisfied with the home care services they receive from agencies, they also have a stronger sense of personal control (Geron, 2000).

In terms of assessment, determining the cognitive capacity of consumers to exercise full autonomy and choice will be one of the biggest challenges to consumer-directed long-term-care programs. The desire of payers and family members for assurance that service users are cognitively intact and capable of using information to make decisions is understandable. Programs must distinguish between two basic types of users—those who are cognitively impaired and unable to directly manage their own care, and those who are capable of controlling or directing their personal assistance. There are numerous well-established assessments of cognitive capacity (e.g., see Geron, 1997b; Lawton & Teresi, 1994); however, the majority of the most widely used cognitive assessments are relatively brief "screens" used to identify persons with dementia or severe cognitive impairments. The notion that consumers should have to "pass" or exceed a cutoff score on some kind of competency assessment of this kind is appealing, but unrealistic.

The judgment, knowledge, and skills required to manage one's care are complex and multifaceted, and it is likely that most consumers—even those with moderate to severe cognitive impairments—will be able to express their preferences or be able to manage at least some aspects of the long-term care they receive. For this reason, more complex assessments of capacity are needed that will identify specific areas where the consumer has trouble managing his or her care. The focus of these new cognitive assessments should be to highlight the areas in which consumers may need assistance, rather than whether they are competent to manage at all.

POLICY IMPLICATIONS

The aging of our society, and concomitant increases in the need for services and care by older adults, is one of the major challenges of the twenty-first century. The aging of the baby boom generation will drive the potential demand for health and long-term-care services over the next half century (Stone, 2000). In the coming decades, geriatric assessment will play a critical role in identifying the service and treatment needs of older adults.

A number of factors have contributed to the increased importance of assessment in long-term-care policy. The emergence of community-based long-term-care demonstration projects under Medicaid waivers in the 1970s and 1980s stimulated the growth of formalized comprehensive assessment to determine the needs of clients for services and to provide a uniform basis to make decisions about the appropriate type and intensity of services. The design and conduct of assessment have emerged as core elements of long-term-care programs. More recently, the changing policy and financing context in which long-term care is provided—efforts to reduce federal and state spending in general, and the growth of managed care in health and long-term care—have transformed the rationale and methods of assessment. Formalized and mandated client assessments are now conducted in part because health care insurers are demanding them for reimbursement. Agencies and programs use assessments to help justify what they do as they compete with insurance companies and managed care corporations for scarce public and private dollars. These same trends have also increased pressure on agencies to replace face-to-face assessments with telephone interviews, and to replace comprehensive assessments with short screens to identify those who require more complete assessments.

One of the most common types of assessments used to make policy decisions is the assessment of functional impairment. Basic functional abilities usually include getting out of bed, taking baths or showers, using the toilet, dressing, preparing meals, and eating. These types of functional tasks allow people to socialize, work, or engage in a myriad of other productive and social activities. The capacity to perform these fundamental self-care activities, though mundane and ordinary to most of us, has been confirmed in numerous studies to have broad implications for functioning, reflecting a person's ability to live independently in the community (Kane et al., 1998; Stone, 2000). Disability or functional impairment refers to a person's inability to perform these and other basic tasks without assistance, whether the reason is due to aging, illness, accident, or conditions at birth (Kovar & Lawton, 1994). The use of functional impairment as an eligibility criterion for long-term-care services is widespread (Justice, 1993; Kane et al., 1998).

Impairment eligibility standards vary from state to state, but are usually defined as needing assistance in two or three activities of daily living (ADL). Most states have created their own ADL measures, although these usually rely on other previously established measures.

The growth of consumer-directed care also poses policy challenges (Geron, 2000). Allowing adult users of long-term-care services a greater voice in managing and controlling the services they need will require changes in laws, politics, and public opinion (Kapp, 1997, 1999; Sabatino, 1996; Sabatino & Litvak, 1992). Establishing consumer rights to make these judgments has proved controversial and difficult, as the efforts to address the legal and statutory barriers to establishing models of consumer-directed care have shown (Flanagan, 1994; Flanagan & Green, 1997) and as the concerns of state administrators have demonstrated (Lagoyda, Nadash, Rosenberg, & Yatsco, 1999).

INTEGRATING KNOWLEDGE INTO THE CURRICULUM

The social work curriculum can offer students a variety of ways in which to gain the knowledge and skills needed to administer geriatric assessment measures successfully. Social work education about geriatric assessment should begin with foundation courses and then build on this knowledge to train social work students in the specific assessment challenges encountered when working with older adults. In addition, students' field placements offer an excellent way to gain valuable firsthand experience engaging with older adults in a variety of situations, including the geriatric assessment. Infusion of geriatric assessment content into the academic curriculum and the field placement is discussed below.

Integrating General Information on Aging into Foundation Course Content

Social work practice with older adults requires a fundamental understanding of the aging process, including the multitude of biological, physiological, psychological, and political and economic aspects of aging (Lowy, 1985). Students thus will need specific information on various theories of development across the life span, family, community, and social welfare systems, as well as on the physical aspects of aging (Ivry, 1992). The foundation courses in Human Behavior and the Social Environment (HBSE) are the best place to introduce this content to 1st-year students. Specific content on older individuals can be provided on development in later life, on families in later life, and on the role of the community in the older adult's well-being. Recent treatments of this material offer a competence-centered view of the adult in later life, which stresses the strengths and potentialities of each individual, rather than presenting old age as a medical "problem" (Maluccio, Pine, & Warsh, 1996).

Other foundation courses can also incorporate information related to conducting assessments with older adults. Most social-welfare policy courses at the foundation level currently offer basic material on social policies and entitlements that apply to older people, for example, Medicare, Social Security, and the programs of the Older Americans Act. However, the policy framework that influences programs and services for older people is often presented as an add-on to those regarding children and families and not as a central piece of the policy puzzle. A separate module is needed on policies and programs for older adults, which employs a historical view of aging policy and analyzes in depth the current political climate toward aging programs and services. Foundation courses in ethics can also address important information related to geriatric assessment. Ethics courses provide students with the tools to reason ethically about practice and policy decisions, including those required in geriatric assessment. It is crucial that they be familiar with the concepts of confidentiality and the rights of clients to participate in an informed way in the assessment process. Ethics training is also essential to reinforce the ethical and clinical obligation of social work to intercede when using poorly designed or faulty assessments. Though common sense tells us that assessment results should never entirely supersede or replace the role of clinical or professional social work judgment—or the right of consumers to question the results—too often this does happen (e.g., a false positive on a test result), sometimes with catastrophic results for a client.

Integrating Geriatric Assessment into Specialized Clinical Courses

At the advanced level, graduate schools of social worker have a responsibility to devote more attention to the topic of standardized assessment. There are some specific content areas and practical skills needed in interviewing and assessing older adults that should be included in any advanced practice course on assessment. Good interviewing skills form the basis of any client encounter, and there are basic techniques that all social work students must learn in order to become good practitioners with any age group (Geron, 1997b; Ivry, 1992). Among the most basic skills is the ability to read the questions exactly as written and in the order indicated, as the slightest wording change could bias the study or confuse the client. The ability to probe for completeness, clarity, and correctness in responses is also needed. Practitioners need to use a neutral tone of voice in asking the questions, avoiding any behavior, spoken or unspoken, conscious or unconscious, that could affect the way a client answers the questions. In order to avoid bias, the practitioner should *never* express his or her own opinions, suggest answers, or use leading probes.

The teaching of geriatric assessment to social work students should also consider specific practice issues involved in working with older adults (Gwyther, 1988; Kropf, 1996). One of the special challenges of working with older adults is the need to be aware of any specific physical difficulties or impairments in the older interviewee. For example, the social work practitioner who is conducting a geriatric assessment should speak clearly and slowly (but not shout) to an older client, and it is often a good idea to sit directly in front of the person so he or she can see the assessor's lips and other facial cues. Older adults also may tire more quickly, especially in a long assessment. The practitioner should watch for signs of fatigue or lack of concentration (e.g., frequently asking for the question to be repeated, increasing difficulty understanding the answer choices) and should be prepared to postpone the remainder of the assessment to another time. The interviewer also must be watchful for cues that might signify the respondent has a cognitive impairment that might affect his or her responses. Some cognitive deficits are subtle and not readily apparent, and the assessor may go through several questions before realizing the client is not capable of answering the questions appropriately.

Field Placement: Practice in Geriatric Assessment Skills

The student's field placement is, of course, the ideal point at which to begin to practice the skills of geriatric assessment learned in coursework. It is essential that students who want to specialize in the field of aging be exposed to the full continuum of long-term care for elders, from home- and community-based programs and services to those provided by rehabilitation and nursing facilities. Students need experience in assessment at all of these levels of care, and a field practicum that exposes students to the full continuum of care for elders would also provide them with needed exposure to the wide variety of assessment tools used in different settings. Clearly this type of wide exposure is difficult in traditional placements that involve a particular practice setting. However, whenever possible, the field practicum should arrange for students to spend some time in other agencies or other services.

CONCLUSION

This chapter has highlighted the importance of geriatric assessment, the characteristics of a useful assessment measure for practice, and some of the existing and emerging areas of assessment research. Through its mission, values and practice, the social work profession is ideally suited to play an important role in making these assessments. Social workers already provide an array of clinical, social, case management, and advocacy services to individuals, families, and communities, and their expertise and training make social workers highly effective members of interdisciplinary service-delivery teams. Historically, social work is unique among health and mental health professions because its practitioners are trained to consider holistically the entire range of physical, mental, social and environmental needs of clients. This comprehensive view of human needs is essential in the assessment of older adults and their families. After conducting the geriatric assessment, social workers often serve as a critical link between the informal (i.e., elders, families, and friends) and formal care systems (i.e., hospitals, nursing homes, and home health services). The relevance of a broader "social health care model" versus the narrower "medical care model" indicates that social work should and will be centrally involved in making geriatric assessments that are designed to improve and promote the quality of life for older Americans.

REFERENCES

American Psychiatric Association. (2000). *Handbook of psychiatric measures.* Washington, DC: Author.

Andrews, F., & Withey, S. (1976). *Social indicators of well-being.* New York: Plenum Press.

Applebaum, R. A., Straker, J. K., & Geron, S. M. (2000). *Assessing satisfaction in health and long-term care: Practical approaches to hearing the voices of consumers.* New York: Springer.

Batavia, A. I., DeJong, G., & McKnew, L. B. (1991). Toward a national personal assistance program: The independent living model of long-term care for persons with disabilities. *Journal of Health Politics, Policy, and Law, 16,* 523–542.

Becerra, R. M., & Zambrana, R. E. (1985). Methodological approaches to research on Hispanics. *Social Work Research and Abstracts, 21*(2), 42–49.

Boyle, D. P., & Springer, A. (2001). Toward a cultural competence measure for social work with special populations. *Journal of Ethnic and Cultural Diversity in Social Work, 9*(3/4), 53–71.

Burstin, H. R., Lipsitz, S. R., & Brennan, T. A. (1992). Socioeconomic status and risk for substandard medical care. *Journal of the American Medical Association, 268,* 2383–2387.

Charmaz, K. (1990). Discovering chronic illness: Using grounded theory. *Social Science and Medicine, 30,* 1161–1172.

Cleary, P. D., & McNeil, B. J. (1988). Patient satisfaction as an indicator of quality care. *Inquiry, 25,* 1161–1172.

Cryns, A. G., Nichols, R. C., Katz, L. A., & Calkins, E. (1989). The hierarchical structures of geriatric patient satisfaction: An older patient satisfaction scale designed for HMOs. *Medical Care, 27,* 802–816.

Davies, A. R., & Ware, J. E. (1988). Involving consumers in quality of care assessment. *Health Affairs, 13*(Spring), 33–48.

Doty, P., Benjamin, A. E., Matthias, R. E., & Franke, T. M. (1999). *In-home supportive services for the elderly and disabled: A comparison of client-directed and professional management models of service delivery. Non-technical summary report.* Washington, DC: U.S. Department of Health and Human Services, Office of the Assistant Secretary for Planning and Evaluation.

Doty, P., Kasper, J., & Litvak, S. (1996). Consumer-directed models of personal care: Lessons from Medicaid. *Milbank Quarterly, 74,* 377–409.

Duke University Center for the Study of Aging and Human Development. (1978). *Multidimensional functional assessment: The OARS methodology* (2nd ed.). Durham, NC: Duke University.

Emlet, C. A., Crabtree, J. L., Condon, V., & Treml, L. (1996). *In-home assessment of older adults: An Interdisciplinary approach.* Gaithersburg, MD: Aspen.

Flanagan, S. (1994). *Consumer-directed attendant services: How states address tax, legal, and quality assurance issues.* Cambridge, MA: SysteMetrics.

Flanagan, S. A., & Green, P. S. (1997). *Consumer-directed personal assistance services: Key operational issues for state CD-PAS programs using intermediary service organizations.* Washington, DC: SysteMetrics.

Fox, S., & Stein, J. (1991). The effect of physician-patient communication on mammography utilization by different ethnic groups. *Medical Care, 29,* 1065–1082.

George, L. K. (1994). Multidimensional assessment instruments: Present status and future prospects. In M. P. Lawton & J. A. Teresi (Vol. Eds.), *Annual review of gerontology and geriatrics: Vol. 14. Focus on assessment techniques* (pp. 353–375). New York: Springer.

Geron, S. M. (1995, March). *Utilizing elder focus groups to develop client satisfaction measures for home-based services.* Paper presented at the 41st Annual Meeting of the American Society on Aging, Atlanta, GA.

Geron, S. M. (1997a). Multidimensional assessment measures. *Generations, 21*(1), 52–54.

Geron, S. M. (Ed.). (1997b). Using assessment to improve practice: New developments and measures. *Generations, 21*(1).

Geron, S. M. (1998). Assessing the satisfaction of older adults with long-term care services: Measurement and design challenges for social work. *Research on Social Work Practice, 8*, 103–119.

Geron, S. M. (2000). The quality of consumer-directed care. *Generations, 24*(3), 66–73.

Geron, S. M. (2002). Functional abilities. In D. J. Ekerdt, R. A. Applebaum, K. C. Holden, S. G. Post, K. Rockwood, R. Schulz, R. L. Sprott, & P. Uhlenberg (Eds.), *Encyclopedia of aging* (Vol. II, pp. 517–519). New York: Macmillan Reference USA.

Geron, S. M., Smith, K., Tennstedt, S., Jette, A., Chassler, D., & Kasten, L. (2000). The Home Care Satisfaction Measure (HCSM): A client-centered approach to assessing the satisfaction of frail older adults with home care services. *Journal of Gerontology: Social Sciences, 55B*, S259–S270.

Golden, R. R., Teresi, J. A., & Gurland, B. J. (1984). Development of indicator scales for the Comprehensive Assessment and Referral Evaluation (CARE) Interview Schedule. *Journals of Gerontology, 39*, 138–146.

Gurland, B., Golden, R., Teresi, J., & Challop, J. (1984). The SHORT-CARE: An efficient instrument of the assessment of depression, dementia, and disability. *Journal of Gerontology, 39*, 166–169.

Gurland, B. J., Kuriansky, J., Sharpe, L., Simon, R., Stiller, P., & Birkett, P. (1977). The Comprehensive Assessment and Referral Evaluation (CARE): Rationale, development, and reliability. *International Journal of Aging and Human Development, 8*, 9–42.

Gurland, B. J., & Wilder, D. E. (1984). The CARE interview revisited: Development of an efficient, systematic clinical assessment. *Journal of Gerontology, 39*, 129–137.

Gutek, B. A. (1978). Strategies for studying client satisfaction. *Journal of Social Issues, 34*(4), 44–56.

Gutierrez, L. M. (1990). Working with women of color: An empowerment perspective. *Social Work, 35*, 149–153.

Gwyther, L. O. (1988). Assessment: Content, purpose, outcomes. *Generations, 12*, 11–15.

Harvey, R., & Jellinek, H. (1981). Functional performance assessment: A program approach. *Archives of Physical Medicine and Rehabilitation, 62*, 456–461.

Ivry, J. (1992). Teaching geriatric assessment. *Journal of Gerontological Social Work, 18*(3/4), 3–22.

Jenkinson, C., Layte, R., Jenkinson, D., Lawrence, K., Petersen, S., Paice, C., et al. (1997). A shorter form health survey: Can the SF-12 replicate results from the SF-36 in longitudinal studies? *Journal of Public Health Medicine, 19*(2), 179–186.

Justice, D. (1993). *Case management standards in state community based long-term care programs for older persons with disabilities.* Washington, DC: National Association of State Units on Aging.

Kane, R., Illston, L., Eustis, N., & Kane, R. (1991). *Quality of home care: Concept and measurement.* Minneapolis: University of Minnesota.

Kane, R. A., Kane, R. L., & Ladd, R. (1998). *The heart of long-term care.* Oxford, England: Oxford University Press.

Kapp, M. (1997). Who is responsible for this? Assigning rights and consequences in elder care. *Journal of Aging and Social Policy, 9*(2), 51–65.

Kapp, M. B. (1999). From medical patients to health care consumers: Decisional capacity and choices to purchase coverage and services. *Aging and Mental Health, 3*(4), 294–300.

Kovar, M. G., & Lawton, P. M. (1994). Functional disability: Activities and instrumental activities of daily living. In P. M. Lawton & J. A. Teresi (Eds.), *Annual review of geriatrics and gerontology: Vol. 14. Focus on assessment techniques* (pp. 57–75). New York: Springer.

Kropf, N. (1996). Infusing content on older people with developmental disabilities into the curriculum. *Journal of Social Work Education, 32*, 215–226.

Lagoyda, R., Nadash, P., Rosenberg, L., & Yatsco, T. (1999). *Survey of state administrators: Consumer-directed home and community-based services.* Washington, DC: National Institute on Consumer-Directed Long-Term Services, The National Council on the Aging, and National Institute for Disability and Rehabilitation Research.

Larsen, D. L., Attkisson, C. C., Hargreaves, W. A., & Nguyen, T. D. (1979). Assessment of client-patient satisfaction: Development of a general scale. *Evaluation and Program Planning, 2,* 197–207.

Lawton, M. P. (1972). Assessing the competence of older people. In D. Kent, R. Kastenbaum, & S. Sherwood (Eds.), *Research, planning and action for the elderly* (pp. 122–143). New York: Behavioral Publications.

Lawton, M. P. (1991). A multidimensional view of quality of life in frail elders. In J. E. Biren et al. (Eds.), *The concept and measurement of quality of life* (pp. 4–27). New York: Academic Press.

Lawton, M. P., Moss, M., Fulcomer, M., & Kleban, M. H. (1982). A research and service oriented multilevel assessment instrument. *Journal of Gerontology, 37,* 91–99.

Lawton, M. P., & Teresi, J. A. (Eds.). (1994). *Annual review of gerontology and geriatrics: Vol. 14. Focus on assessment techniques.* New York: Springer.

Lebow, J. L. (1983). Similarities and differences between mental health and health care evaluation studies assessing consumer satisfaction. *Evaluation and Program Planning, 6,* 237–243.

Linn, M. W. (1985). Nursing home care as an alternative to psychiatric hospitalization. *Archives of General Psychiatry, 42,* 544–551.

Linn, M. W., Linn, B. S., Stein, S., & Stein, E. M. (1989). Effect of nursing home staff training on quality of patient survival. *International Journal of Aging and Human Development, 28*(4), 305–315.

Love, R. E., Caid, C. D., & Davis, A. (1979). The user satisfaction survey: Consumer evaluation of an inner city community mental health center. *Evaluation and the Health Professions, 1,* 42–54.

Lowy, L. (1985). *Social work with the aging* (2nd ed.). New York: Longman.

Lucas, M. D., Morris, C. M., & Alexander, J. W. (1988). Exercise in self-care agency and client satisfaction with nursing care. *Nursing Administration Quarterly, 12*(3), 23–30.

Maluccio, A., Pine, B., & Warsh, R. (1996). Incorporating content on family reunification into the social work curriculum. *Journal of Social Work Education, 32,* 363–374.

Miller-Hohl, D. A. (1992). Patient satisfaction and quality care. *Caring, 11*(1), 34–37.

Orona, C. (1990). Temporality and identity loss due to Alzheimer's disease. *Social Science and Medicine, 30*(11), 1247–1256.

Pablo, R. Y. (1975, March). Assessing patient satisfaction in long-term care institutions. *Hospital Administration in Canada,* 22–32.

Pfeiffer, E. (Ed.). (1975). *Multidimensional functional assessment: The OARS methodology* (1st ed.). Durham, NC: Duke University Center for the Study of Aging and Human Development.

Riley, P. A., Fortinsky, R. H., & Coburn, A. F. (1992). Developing consumer-centered quality assurance strategies for home care: A case management model. *Journal of Case Management, 1*(2), 39–48.

Rinke, L., & Wilson, A. (1988). Client-oriented project objectives. *Caring, 7*(1), 25–29.

Sabatino, C. P. (1996). Competency: Refining our legal fictions. In M. Smyer, K. W. Schaie, & M. B. Kapp (Eds.), *Older adults' decision-making and the law* (pp. 1–47). New York: Springer.

Sabatino, C. P., & Litvak, S. (1992). Consumer-directed homecare: What makes it possible? *Generations, 16*(3), 53–58.

Sodowsky, G. R., Taffe, R. C., Gutkin, T. B., & Wise, S. L. (1994). Development of the Multicultural Counseling Inventory: A self-report measure of multicultural competencies. *Journal of Counseling Psychology, 41,* 137–148.

Stewart, A. L. (1990). Psychometric considerations in functional status instruments. In M. Lipkin (Ed.), *Functional status measurement in primary care.* New York: Springer-Verlag.

Stewart, A. L., & Ware, J. E. (1992). *Measuring functioning and well-being: The medical outcomes study approach.* Durham, NC: Duke University Press.

Stone, R. I. (2000). *Long-term care for the elderly with disabilities: Current policy, emerging trends, and the implications for the twenty-first century.* New York: Milbank Memorial Fund.

Strasser, S., Aharony, L., & Greenberger, D. (1993). The patient satisfaction process: Moving toward a comprehensive model. *Medical Care Review, 50,* 219–248.

Sue, D. W., & Sue, D. (1999). *Counseling the culturally different: Theory and practice* (2nd ed.). New York: Wiley.

Tarlov, A. R., Ware, J. E., Jr., Greenfield, S., Nelson, E. C., Perrin, E., & Zubkoff, M. (1989). The medical outcomes study: An application of methods for monitoring the results of medical care. *Journal of the American Medical Association, 262,* 925–930.

Ware, J. E., & Sherbourne, C. D. (1992). The MOS 36-Item short-form health survey (SF-36). I. Conceptual framework and item selection. *Medical Care, 30,* 473–481.

Ware, J. E., Snyder, M. K., & Wright, W. R. (1976). *Development and validation of scales to measure patient satisfaction with health care services. Volume I of a final report, Part B: Results of scales constructed from the patient satisfaction questionnaire and other health care perceptions* (NTIS Publication No. PB288-330). Springfield, MA: National Technical Information Service.

Woerner, L., & Phillips, J. (1989). Client perspectives on quality care. *Caring, 8*(6), 47–51.

Yee, D. L. (1992). Health care access and advocacy for immigrant and other underserved elders. *Journal of Health Care for the Poor and Underserved, 2,* 448–464.

Chapter 13

CULTURAL CONSIDERATIONS IN HEALTH CARE AND QUALITY OF LIFE

Peter Maramaldi and Marci Guevara

Health-related quality of life (HRQL) is a construct that often overlaps with terms such as *quality of life* or *functional health*. Although these terms are considered to be conceptually different, they are not mutually exclusive or discrete. Quality of life in health care has been conceptualized as the patient's subjective account of the attributes of daily life and is affected by the ability to adapt when discrepancies exist between one's expected and actual well-being (Padilla, Ferrell, Grant, & Rhiner, 1990). Schipper, Clinch, and Olweny (1996) integrated quality of life and functional health to conceptualize HRQL as the individual's perception of the functional effect of an illness or treatment. Two common overriding themes in the HRQL literature are (a) the patient's comparison of historical life circumstance with a current state of affairs, and (b) the patient's perceptions of his or her own situation (King et al., 1997). Each of these themes illustrates the centrality of perceptions. Patients' subjective perceptions of their health and well-being are as important as physical symptoms in determining their HRQL.

Perceptions of HRQL are driven by individual personality, worldview, and culture. Culture affects HRQL by influencing perceptions of disease, pain, depression, stress, and general health conditions (Fayers, Hand, Bjordal, & Groenvold, 1997; Gonzalez-Calvo, Gonzalez, & Lorig, 1997; Guarnaccia, 1996; King et al., 1997; Kleinman, 1988). The relevance of culture is further evidenced by its epidemiological association with general health (L. F. Berkman, 1980; Cassel, 1976; Cassel, Patrick, & Jenkins, 1960; Marmont, 1981, 1994; Susser, 1987; Syme, 1992). Because culture is a dynamic construct, constantly evolving at both the individual and group levels (Vega, 1992), it remains difficult to define operationally, a challenge to measure, and a frequent source of acrimony among practitioners, researchers, and policy makers. Although the concept of "culture" is used liberally in the social sciences, there is no universally accepted definition that we are aware of.

CONCEPTUALIZATION OF CULTURE

After finding more than 100 definitions of *culture* in the communication literature, Gudykunst and Kim (1992) framed it as a system of knowledge shared by a large group of people in what frequently—but not always—corresponds to geographic borders. During the early development of anthropology as an academic discipline, Linton (1945) offered a framework to look at a specific group or society, and conceptualized culture as the transmission of learned behaviors in relative terms. Barnouw (1985) conceptualized culture as "a way of life of a group of people, the complex of shared concepts and patterns of learned behavior that are handed down from one generation to the next through the means of language and imitation" (p. 5). He emphasized integration, cohesion, and tradition, which weigh heavily on health care because cultures pass on a language and folklore that is associated with illness, health, and healing. Shweder (1991) categorizes the post-Nietzschean influence on the conceptualization of culture in three areas: (a) culture as conditioned response—humans believe what they are told, and thus march lockstep to the cadence of their society; (b) culture as defensive mechanism—culture is a protective system that allows people to meet their needs; and (c) culture as a symbolic system—wherein humans are masters of "rhetoric" and use it through life to represent imaginative creations. Each of these conceptual exemplars is relevant to patients' perceptions of their health conditions and needs.

As members of particular cultures, individuals define health as they are conditioned to do through a socialization process in their society. The measurement of functioning in activities of daily living (ADLs), for example, would be culturally defined differently in some developing countries than in most industrialized countries. In some cultures, eating with one's hands is considered natural, sanitary, and the cultural norm. Children are taught by their parents to eat this way, often using fresh-baked flat breads to scoop food from the plate into their mouths. In other cultures, where touching food with one's hands is considered unnatural, unsanitary, and rude, the use of sophisticated utensils such as knifes, forks, spoons, or chopsticks is the norm. It clearly would be nonsensical to force someone to use utensils during an evaluation if they were socialized in a culture where the hand is used instead of utensils. So too must professionals consider whether their own culturally determined perceptions of health and well-being are in concert with their patients'. By framing health and functioning within the context of specific cultural constructs or models, professionals can better understand how patients view health and what patients—as consumers—desire in order to maintain a self-perceived sense of equilibrium within their environment. In the absence of universally accepted definitions of cultural groups, race and ethnicity will be used in this chapter as proxies to demonstrate the relatively overt cultural diversity within older populations, and the potential impact of culture on HRQL.

SIGNIFICANCE TO GERONTOLOGY

According to the 2000 United States Census, there are nearly 35 million Americans aged 65 and older (12.4% of the total population), of whom 16.4% or 5.7 million self-identified as members of minority groups (Administration on Aging [AOA], 2001c; U.S. Bureau of the Census, 2000a). The largest aging minority group is currently African Americans, comprising 8% of those 65 years and older. Hispanics (of any race) comprise 5%, Asians and Pacific Islanders comprise 2.4%, American Indians and Alaska Natives comprise 0.4%, and 0.9% were categorized as being of another race or of two or more races (U.S. Bureau of the Census, 2000a).

By the year 2050, the general U.S. population older than 65 is expected to more than double to become approximately 82 million, representing 20.3% of the total population (U.S. Bureau of the Census, 2000b). The percentage of minority Americans who will be age 65 and older by the year 2050 is expected to more than double, growing to 35.8% of the older population, numbering around 29 million. The Hispanic population is projected to be the fastest-growing minority group and is expected to comprise 16.4% of those 65 and older. African Americans are expected to comprise 12.2%, Asians and Pacific Islanders 6.5%, and American Indians and Alaska Natives 0.6% (U.S. Bureau of the Census, 2000b). And within each minority group the percentage of those who are 65 years and older is growing. By the year 2050, it is projected that 15.4% of all persons in all minority populations combined will be 65 or older, compared to 24.7% of all Whites in the same age group. Specifically, 18.7% of all African Americans will be 65 and older, 13.7% of Hispanics, 15% of Asians and Pacific Islanders, and 16.4% of American Indians and Alaska Natives (U.S. Bureau of the Census, 2000b).

Another point to consider regarding the "cultural" diversity of the older U.S. population is that current data on racial and ethnic minorities may underrepresent the true diversity of the aging segment of the populations. Older people in the United States may themselves be immigrants, or at least closer to the immigrant generations of their families of origin into this country. As a result, they are more likely to be influenced by their families' cultures of origin than more acculturated generations that have a longer pedigree in the United States.

SIGNIFICANCE TO HEALTH-RELATED QUALITY OF LIFE

As the older population grows, so will the number of people with health problems. In 1997, more than half (54.5%) of the older population reported having at least one chronic health condition (AOA, 2001b). The most common health conditions afflicting older people are hearing impairments, arthritis, heart disease, hypertension, and cataracts (National Academy on an Aging Society [NAAS], 1999). Some older individuals are limited in their daily activities because of these chronic conditions, including 34% of persons aged 65–74 and 45% of those aged 75 and older (NAAS, 1999). The proportions of older populations requiring assistance as a result of limitations in activities include 8.1% of persons aged 65–69, 10.5% of persons aged

70–74, 16.9% of persons aged 75–79, and 34.9% of persons aged 80 and older (AOA, 2001b). The occurrence of health conditions varies by race and ethnicity. For example, African American persons are more likely than Hispanic or White persons to report having diabetes, stroke, and hypertension (Federal Interagency Forum on Aging-Related Statistics, 2000).

With the passage of the Patients Outcome Research Act of 1989, the United States Congress proposed a patient-centered outcomes research program that went beyond the traditional assessment focus on biological measures of health to look at HRQL issues of functional status, well-being, and patient satisfaction (Schipper et al., 1996; Ware, 1995). Although not specifically mandated by this legislation, it became apparent that health care plans should be culturally tailored to be appropriate for patients and their families. Assessments should account for the heavy influence of culture on perceptions of health and well-being. As a result, the HRQL literature of the 1990s acknowledges the need for greater understanding of culture and how it affects perceptions of health in the emerging consumer-driven health outcomes research.

The change toward consumer-centered health care evaluation constitutes something of a paradigm shift (Kuhn, 1970) away from exclusively positivist epistemologies in health outcomes research. Positivist paradigms typically assume that phenomena such as patient outcomes can be understood by reducing them to a set of objective biological measures (Baker, 1991), such as mortality, morbidity, and tangible socioeconomic variables that can be readily operationalized and measured within and between groups or national samples (Feinstein, 1993). It is widely accepted that physiologic interventions intended to optimize survival must include patients' perceptions of treatment and treatment outcomes (Schipper et al., 1996). Patients' idiosyncratic values, beliefs, and judgments ultimately determine whether a change in health status or treatment is positive or negative (Spilker, 1996). Values, beliefs, rules, and judgments are grounded in culture (Barnouw, 1985; Cole, 1996; Geertz, 1965; Gudykunst & Kim, 1992; Hofstede, 1991; Linton, 1945; Martin, 1994; McLaughlin & Braun, 1998; Triandis, 1980). Therefore, quality of life is shaped and largely established by culture (Campos & Johnson, 1990; Guarnaccia, 1996).

Nominal categorization of cultures by racial or ethnic groups is no longer an adequate means of capturing the differences among groups in health care. For example, a Finnish immigrant and a Greek immigrant are most likely categorized as White. In reality, Scandinavian and Mediterranean cultures vary dramatically, and this variance is likely to affect patients' perceptions of health and well-being. Likewise, African Americans and African immigrants are typically grouped under the same nominal category of African American or Black. If the African immigrant comes from a developing country, he or she would have few cultural commonalities with the third- or fourth-generation African American. The last example illustrates an important point. Health care professionals have generally failed to embrace the concept of culturally determined perceptions of health and well-being and the subsequent variation among patients from different cultures such as patients from developing countries (McLaughlin & Braun, 1998). This is especially true in outcomes research.

By virtue of their training, the vast majority of health care professionals approach patients with positivist, quantitative epistemologies that are focused on the probability of desired outcomes in health care. The desired outcome is usually symptom management, delayed decline, and maintenance or gains in quality of life. In attempting to understand the older patients' HRQL and responses to illness, health care professionals give significant weight to physical and specific psychiatric symptoms. Psychiatric taxonomies are perhaps the most developed in the area of behavioral sciences due in large part to the development of reliable diagnostic tools such as the *Diagnostic and Statistical Manual of Mental Disorders* (*DSM-IV-TR*) (American Psychiatric Association, 2000) and the *ICD-10-CM* (World Health Organization, 1992). However, culturally based perceptions of health and well-being are often not measured, even though they bear significant weight in understanding the patients' needs. Within any given culture, individuals' personalities and dynamic worldviews make it difficult to develop a reliable culture taxonomy without grossly overgeneralizing or stereotyping. Although a patient's medical or psychiatric indicators are highly delineated and measurable, the same patient may have cultural features that are not accounted for in measurement. The problem is that cultural taxonomies are not as clearly defined and delineated as psychiatric taxonomies, but the absence of clear cultural parameters threatens the reliability of psychiatric taxonomies among varied cultural groups.

Kleinman (1988) gives the example of symptoms using a strict psychiatric taxonomy with added cultural interpretation. In psychiatric interviews with Native Americans following the death of a spouse, there may be reliable findings of hallucinations as the patients report hearing the voice of the deceased spouse as his or her spirit moves on to the afterworld. Hearing the voice is "normal" in the context of the patient's culture. To the contrary, *not* hearing the voice of the deceased loved one would be a greater indicator of abnormality, and thus of concern. The professional must not only focus on the physical or psychiatric indicators, but also listen to the cultural context of the patient's experience.

Individual levels of acculturation further complicate the development of cultural taxonomies. Acculturation refers to the modification of values, norms, attitudes, and behaviors when, as members of a minority group, individuals are exposed to the mainstream cultural norms (Marin, Sabogol, Marin, Otero-Sabogal, & Perez-Stable, 1987). Acculturation also refers to both an individual and a group phenomenon (Dana, 1996). It is considered a long-term fluid process in which members of a group move along at least two cultural continua. Acculturation is not a zero-sum gain away from, or toward, the poles of the culture of origin or that of the host country, but rather a simultaneous engagement of each of the cultures in the current environment. As part of the acculturation process, one's worldview changes and aspects of the original and new culture are learned and modified (Marin & Gamba, 1996). This change process is stressful (Dana, 1996). Adaptation to change can simultaneously include both old and new attitudes and beliefs about health and health care (Talavera, Elder, & Velasquez, 1997).

SIGNIFICANCE TO HEALTH PROFESSIONALS

A change in focus from finite attributes that are readily operationalized to a loosely defined and evolving phenomenon like culture (King et al., 1997) presents health care providers with new challenges to frame health care not only from the providers' perspectives, but in the context of the patients' perceptions of well-being. This means that providers must ask about a patient's culture in the same way they would ask about physical symptoms. Asking about, and understanding, culture is the first step in developing culturally tailored health messages and interventions that are efficacious. An example of a culturally tailored program is the Seattle–King County Senior Services Area Agency on Aging. This program provides funding for a dietician who works to meet the nutritional needs of elder clients with culturally appropriate meals. Clients are from many cultures, including Chinese, Japanese, Cambodian, Laotian, Filipino, Hispanic, African American, American Indian, and Samoan. By offering culturally appropriate meals to the clients through the work of the dietician, the program is able to preserve and adapt cultural traditions in order to improve the health and lives of Seattle–King County seniors (AOA, 2001a).

Framing health disparities among cultures as social justice issues illustrates the centrality of this discussion to social work. By virtue of training and ethical standards of practice, social work professionals are uniquely prepared—and also mandated—to ensure that patients' cultural values are considered in the development of patient-specific chronic care plans. As nonmedical experts on clinical teams, social work practitioners play a significant role in the assessment and understanding of patients' culturally based perceptions of health and quality of life. In addition to understanding the interaction among physiological, social, cognitive, and biological factors (B. Berkman, 1996), social workers can help the other team members understand the impact of both the providers' and the patients' cultures on the development and evaluation of chronic care services that will provide patients with the highest possible quality of life.

Social work providers are ideally suited to use Hofstede's (1984) approach to cultural relativism as a means of ensuring the patients' and caregivers' right to self-determination. Hofstede posits that cultural relativism calls for the suspension of judgment—based in one's own viewpoint—when dealing with groups that are different from one's own. Social workers must be aware of how cultural differences manifest themselves in many different ways that can be categorized, using Hofstede's model, as symbols, heroes, rituals, and values. *Symbols* are words, gestures, pictures, or objects that carry particular meaning that can only be recognized by people who share the same culture. However, symbols are the most superficial manifestations of culture. They are easily copied by other cultures, and they change or evolve with relative ease. *Heroes* serve as models, possess characteristics that are prized within a culture, and can be alive or dead, real or imagined. *Rituals*, though technically superfluous, are considered socially essential collective activities. *Values*—which are at the core of culture—are the most difficult manifestation to observe. Values are among the first things that children learn and are generally beyond the conscious awareness of the person as an adult. Values can be understood as broad tendencies for preferences, such as dirty versus clean, natural versus unnatural, or abnormal versus normal (Hofstede, 1984).

Social workers can be trained to use models such as this to understand the meaning of health conditions to patients and their family members. By working to observe and understand the symbols, heroes, and rituals of a patient's culture, social workers can gain insights into underlying core cultural values. For example, social workers can be trained to learn that the symbols of medical professionals (lab coats, stethoscopes, charts, and so forth) may be incongruent with the symbols a patient observed in health care heroes of her own culture (such as providers within state-run medical systems, shamans, or folk healers). So, too, may the rituals (such as rounds, waiting and examination rooms, and chart notations) be incongruent with more familiar rituals (such as healing ceremonies, herbal remedies, acupuncture or manipulation, or folk interventions). By understanding a patient's reactions to the symbols, heroes, rituals, and values of the health care system, professionals can gain insights into how the patient is experiencing illness, assessment, and health intervention. Professionals can use this frame to ask patients how their perceptions of the current health care culture differ from the ones they are more familiar with, such as those in their native country or region. This will open the door to discussions and greater understanding about value conflicts regarding medical assessment and intervention. By understanding the value conflict, professionals can better understand patient perceptions and needs. Both parties can better communicate their intent and work together to develop a culturally tailored response to illness, disease, or a chronic condition.

Social workers are superbly positioned by training and ethical practice standards to bring their nonmedical expertise into the medical treatment team to facilitate communication about culturally based subjective perceptions of illness and treatment among patients, caregivers, and professionals. Social work's contribution to the team can make better use of patients' cultures, which can yield more efficacious resource expenditures and optimal patient satisfaction. Patients will perceive an acceptable degree of HRQL only when health care is tailored to be in synchrony with the patients' and caregivers' cultural values.

PRIOR RESEARCH AND KNOWLEDGE BASE

Using race and ethnicity as proxies for culture, we will present prior research and knowledge in the area of breast cancer disease management as an exemplar of cultural considerations in HRQL. (The problems associated with using race and ethnicity as proxies for culture will be discussed later in this chapter in "Policy Implications.") Although White women are more likely to develop breast cancer than women in racial and ethnic minority groups (Greenlee, Hill-Harmon, Murray, & Thun, 2001), women in minority groups have higher breast cancer mortality rates than do White women (Dignam, 2000; Greenlee, Murray, Bolden, & Wingo, 2000; Landis, Murray, Bolden, & Wingo, 1999; Yood et al., 1999). Could these outcomes disparities be related to culturally driven screening disparities? The next question must then be, Whose culture is driving the screening behavior—the patient's, the professional's, or perhaps a combination of both?

In the past, it was too easy for providers to put the onus for low screening rates within a cultural group on "noncompliant" patients. However, it is increasingly evident that health care professionals play a major role in patient compliance in disease management. For example, African American women have higher breast cancer mortality rates than White women in the general population. An intervention study was implemented to maximize screening effectiveness and minimize the delay from screening to diagnosis in order to eliminate the prognostic disparities between African American woman and White women. When both groups received comparable treatment and the diagnosis was made at a similar disease stage, their prognosis was the same (Dignam, 2000). Findings like this underscore the importance of the American Cancer Society's call for improved screening initiatives with members of minority groups, diverse ethnic groups, and older women (Woolam, 2000).

Numerous cancer-screening studies have focused on populations of Latina women, providing strong evidence of a culturally driven resistance to participation in screening protocols, which may lead to increased risk for later detection and poorer prognosis (Bentley, Delfino, Taylor, Howe, & Anton-Culver, 1998; Chang et al., 1996; Chavez & Hubbell, 1997; Fox, Pitkin, Paul, Carson, & Naihua, 1998; Fox & Roetzheim, 1994; Frazier, Jiles, & Mayberry, 1996; Giachello, 1996; Hubbell, Chavez, Mishra, & Valdez, 1996; Hubbell, Mishra, Chavez, & Valdez, 1997; Lobell, Bay, Rhoads, & Keske, 1998; Mandelblatt et al., 1999; Napoles-Springer, Perez-Stable, & Washington, 1996; Pearlman, Rakowski, Ehrich, & Clark, 1996; Salazar, 1996; Sanders-Phillips, 1996; Zambrana, Breen, Fox, & Gutierrez-Mohomed, 1999). However, socioeconomic conditions can act as mediating variables, further complicating the clear identification of specific links between culture and screening behavior. Breen and Figueroa (1996) used Surveillance Epidemiology and End Results (SEER) data to determine that women living in socioeconomically disadvantaged census tracts had a 51% greater chance of being diagnosed with invasive breast cancer than those who lived elsewhere. Gray and Puente (1996) found that in addition to being culturally different from majority groups in this country, Latino populations tend to experience social and economic disadvantages that include high poverty levels, low levels of education, high unemployment, and limited access to health care due in large part to an absence of health insurance as well as language and culture barriers (Gray & Puente, 1996).

In addition, within-group differences among racial and ethnic groups have also drawn the attention of investigators who are seeking better understanding of disparities in screening and outcomes. This is an important distinction when grouping women from different countries and cultures under the rubric *Latina*. An excellent example of the possible pitfalls of using broad nominal classifications to determine patterns of health care use is found in data from the 1992 National Health Interviews Survey. In comparing four Latina groups—Mexican American, Mexican, Puerto Rican, and Cuban women—each group was different in its receipt of screening for breast or cervical cancer, with Mexican women least likely to be screened for either (Zambrana et al., 1999).

CURRENT RESEARCH

The first author's current research exploring cultural differences between the health beliefs of Latina and White women around breast cancer screening and treatment is presented as an exemplar of the significance of better understanding the influence of patients' cultures in preventive health care. In a retrospective study of women of low income who were participating in free breast and cervical cancer screening programs in California, Maramaldi (2001) found that although significantly more Latina women reported having trust in doctors than did White women, Latina women were more likely to delay getting follow-up to abnormal breast exams than were White women. This incongruity between trust and delay in follow-up procedures can be viewed through a culturally sensitive lens, albeit an interpretive one. With time, the Latina women's reported trust in doctors' recommendations may have been outweighed by culturally determined fatalistic beliefs. Chavez and Hubbell (1997) explain that fatalism puts control outside the self and frequently into the hands of God. In these cases of breast cancer disease management, initial trust in the doctor could come from being placed in the hands of an authority figure. However, the intensity of a patient's contact with medical professionals diminishes after the initial period of clinical contact. The trust in professional recommendations may give way to culturally driven values and health beliefs such as, for example, fatalism—the belief that the breast cancer is in the hands of God, so why bother going through the discomfort and expense of screening and treatment. A discussion of the rich literature on fatalism is beyond the scope of this chapter; however, we caution that professionals should not overgeneralize or stereotype Latino populations regarding fatalistic beliefs. Within-group differences must always be considered, as is the case with any group characteristic.

This self-reported trust in doctors could also be interpreted in another way, as an exemplar of what Marin and Gamba (1996) describe as Latinos' tendency to avoid perceived confrontation through acquiescent responses. A respondent from a Latino culture might be inclined to tell a professional what she thinks the professional wants to hear, in this case, that she trusts doctors. It seems likely that an acquiescent response would take the form of affirmative, compliant, and nonconfrontational comments about suggested interventions and satisfaction with services. An acquiescent response, in this case saying that she trusts the doctor, does not guarantee behavioral compliance with health care recommendations. If providers are aware that certain cultural groups are prone to give acquiescent or deferential responses, additional time and resources are needed during the clinical contact to be certain that patients understand the realities and importance of the prescribed treatment. Again, caution must be taken to avoid assumptions and stereotyping by neglecting individual and within-group differences. In psychosocial oncology, additional research is needed to understand how culture affects patient delays in seeking screening, diagnosis, treatment, and follow-up care.

FURTHER RESEARCH NEEDS

In order to develop more effective practice models in promoting and maintaining the health and well-being of older adults, social work must deepen its understanding of the interaction between culture and health. Traditional research methodologies—informed by positivist epistemologies—must be augmented to increase understanding of patients' health beliefs that are grounded in culture. The impact of the professional's health beliefs also must be considered in the context of diagnosis, treatment, and disease management. Better understanding of culturally based health beliefs—of both patient and professional—offers opportunities to eliminate disparities among groups, to improve patients' self-perceptions of their own HRQL, and to make professional clinical contacts more efficacious. In order to use cultural theory as a conceptual base in health research, mixed methodologies should be using open-ended questions and patient narratives to fill in the conceptual gaps left by questions with forced-choice response sets. For example, a survey might ask a woman if she is afraid to tell her husband she had a suspicious screening test. A *yes* response serves data analysis well, but does not answer the question *why*. Follow-up survey questions with several forced choices for *why* may be helpful, but only if the forced choices were developed through qualitative methodologies such as focus groups or narratives. As a specific example, Hubbell and colleagues (1996) found that Latina women frequently held beliefs that breast cancer was God's punishment for previous immoral behavior, and therefore feared their husbands' reactions to the assumption that a breast cancer diagnosis was related to past wrongdoings. Findings like this would not have been captured through forced-choice response sets. Researchers had to take the time to let the women tell their stories.

Culturally sensitive health services will likely benefit older patients and their caregivers by increasing their involvement in assessment and treatment, by decreasing resistance to medical protocols, and by heightening providers' awareness of patient and caregiver perceptions of health, illness, and treatment. Greater understanding of cultural nuances in chronically ill populations will improve professionals' understanding of patients' perceptions, better inform tailored health messages, and ultimately lead to more efficacious treatment interventions.

POLICY IMPLICATIONS

Competent health care policy and research requires an awareness and sensitivity to group differences in physiologic manifestation of disease as well as culturally based attitudes toward events such as illness, disability, stress, depression, and other health-related events. However, the lack of consensus about the meaning of race, ethnicity, and culture make this a complicated and politically charged task.

A recent article is a good example of the confusion about race, ethnicity, and cultural in academic medicine and other disciplines. Chin and Humikowoski (2002) warn against the pitfalls of racial profiling in clinical settings and suggest that an effective safeguard is to train medical providers in cultural competence. However, they go on to suggest that ethnicity can be used as an initial proxy for cultural and other patient attributes. Herein lies the source of much of the confusion about culture: It is often grouped with race and ethnicity in conceptual discussions. In fact, researchers and policy makers use data, such as the U.S. Census data we cited at the beginning of this chapter, as a proxy for cultural groups.

Although scholarship around race and ethnicity is the product of our own societal and political evolution, ethnicity is a relatively new concept. White Americans thought of themselves in racial contexts for centuries, but the concept of ethnicity did not appear in the social science literature of the nineteenth and early twentieth centuries (Marable, 2000). Indeed, ethnicity is an elaborate psychological construct interwoven into other equally complex constructs such as culture, identity, and minority status (Phinney, 1996). Public health professionals have yet to reach agreement about the meaning or significance of racial and ethnic categories. Recent changes in the categorization of race and ethnicity in the 2000 U.S. Census force the issue and underscore the importance of developing a better understanding of race and ethnicity (Krieger, 2000). Census 2000 adhered to the 1997 Office of Management and Budget (OMB) Directive 15, which mandates the revision of race and ethnicity standards by all federal programs no later than January 1, 2003. Under these guidelines, race and ethnicity are reported separately (Sondik, Lucas, Madans, & Smith, 2000). Between the four Hispanic options and multiple race options that were included, there were 126 possible permutations of race in Census 2000. Although 97% of Americans chose the single-race category during the actual census count, the U.S. Bureau of the Census expects the mixed-race count to increase steadily (Editor, 2001). Under the revised OMB guidelines, it will be possible for individuals to self-identify differently in future counts than they did during Census 2000, especially when *multirace* is included as a choice. This raises the question of how a person can change race between counts. Furthermore, how will this affect public health surveillance of the needs of older patients and caregivers? Sondik and colleagues (2000) identify factors that influence self-identified race to include the way respondents understand the choices offered under the OMB guidelines, the influence of biological or genetic, cultural, and societal constructs that may change over time, and the political influence of special interests to encourage multiracial people to choose one group over another.

Additional clinical challenges arise in the investigation of mediating variables through which race and ethnicity have impact, such as acculturation, socioeconomic indicators that may affect access to care, and attitudinal indicators that may influence levels of participation in health interventions (Meyerowitz, Richardson, Hudson, & Leedham, 1998). The revised OMB standards fail to provide the type of detailed information about ethnicity, acculturation, and economic position necessary to understand the relationship between race and ethnicity, culture, and health status and outcomes, yet they represent an important first step toward more accurate categorizations of race and ethnicity (Friedman, Cohen, Averbach, & Norton, 2000). Professionals working with older people and their families can transcend the limitation of racial and ethnic categories by using an anthropology lens to frame patients' cultures as a means of understanding culturally based perceptions of health and well-being.

INTEGRATING KNOWLEDGE INTO THE CURRICULUM

The Educational Policy and Accreditation Standards of the Council on Social Work Education (CSWE) require foundation content in eight curriculum areas: values and ethics, diversity, populations at risk, human behavior in the social environment, social welfare policy, social work practice, research, and field education. Viewed through an anthropological lens in the context of HRQL, culture has significant implications in each of these curriculum areas, especially—but not exclusively—for students who are training for work in health or mental health practice, research, or policy arenas.

Unfortunately, the competing demands in core areas of practice, research, and policy strain social work curricula, making it difficult to infuse anthropological epistemologies on cultural groups. Part of the curriculum problem rests in what Meenaghan (2001) calls the "artificial structuring of curriculum in graduate schools of social work" (p. 50), wherein relevant social-science material is packaged in the human-behavior classes that emphasize the individual unit of analysis in the context of human development. The cross-fertilization of knowledge with other disciplines such as anthropology would better prepare future generations of social workers to understand the ubiquity of culture in all areas of professional practice.

HRQL lends itself to social work pedagogy as a means of exploring alternative values and cultures through something that clients and students have in common: their own individual perceptions of health and well-being that are based in their cultural values. Health and well-being is a value-based state that every student can relate to on a personal level, which makes it a nonthreatening starting point from which to explore cultural differences. As an example, consider the core social-work ethical value of patients' rights to self-determination. It does not allow for the imposition of a dominant culture's values upon an individual or group that does not ascribe to those values. In the context of health care, self-determination emphasizes the importance of understanding and attending to older patients' culturally based, subjective perceptions of health and well-being, within parameters that will not place someone in danger.

Consider further the health disparities among cultural groups as social justice issues. The identification of divergent cultural perceptions of health and well-being lends itself to effective teaching examples in the CSWE curriculum areas of diversity and populations at risk. If one cultural group has different health outcomes than the dominant cultural group, the nondominant group is at risk—as was discussed with Latina women having poorer breast cancer outcomes than White women. The documentation of health disparities through rigorous public health surveillance in areas such as cancer offers rich opportunities to demonstrate the practical use of research methodologies to link the micro patient needs to macro policy decisions toward the promotion of social justice through equality in health care.

Rich anthropological literature on culture will add substance to the social work curriculum. In practice and field education, anthropological models can be used to understand the patients' subjective perceptions of health and illness in their cultural context. This approach transcends the limitations associated with blanket group classifications under rubrics that are currently used such as race, ethnicity, gender, and sexual orientation. A viable approach to infusing culture into the curriculum is a cultural relativism model such as Hofstede's (1984), which will help social work students understand their clients and frame policy issues beyond nominal group classifications. Hofstede's model is an exemplar of a rigorous, empirically developed framework by which social work students can learn to view culture in greater depth and add it to their assessment skills in clinical practice. The infusion of a culture model into all areas of the curriculum will also add substance to policy discussions and the development of research designs.

Anthropological frameworks also provide clinical social-work students with the increased self-awareness that is needed to avoid countertransference: judging the response of one's clients and family members to health and well-being by one's own culturally based health beliefs and underlying values. Framing diversity in the context of health and illness provides a nonthreatening yet personally relevant venue to apply theoretical ideas about cultural relativism. By conceptualizing health and well-being in the context of culture, individual cases become rich ground on which to explore the cultural evolution and acculturation of families by following their perceptions of health and well-being through several generations.

CONCLUSION

Anthropologist Clifford Geertz (1973) used a metaphor to contend that the webs spun by man himself are, in fact, the culture upon which he remains suspended. He argued that culture should be explored for meaning through interpretation rather than for laws through scientific analysis. Obeyesekere (1990) warns, however, that when we use the metaphor of the cultural web, we must take care to "focus on the spider" at work, for when the observer's voice is heard more clearly than the people being studied, the significance of the cultural web is lost. By understanding the patients' cultural perspective of their HRQL, professionals empower older people and their caregivers by responding to their needs, optimizing their satisfaction within the limitations of their condition and personal resources, and increasing the impact and effectiveness of precious medical resources. If the professional's desired clinical outcome is increased HRQL for all patients, the one-size-fits-all approach must be abandoned. The dominant culture of medical professionals in any given setting or region cannot be forced on all patients. Professionals must take time to ask, listen, and attempt to understand patients' health conditions in the context of the patients' cultures.

REFERENCES

Administration on Aging. (2001a, February 12). *Cultural competency—Fact sheet.* [On-line]. Available: http://www.aoa.gov/may2001/factsheets/Cultural-Competency.html (Retrieved May 11, 2002).

Administration on Aging. (2001b, December 21). *A profile of older Americans 2001: Health, health care, and disability.* [On-line]. Available: http://www.aoa.dhhs. gov/aoa/stats/profile/2001/12.html (Retrieved May 11, 2002).

Administration on Aging. (2001c, December 21). *A profile of older Americans 2001: Racial and ethnic composition.* [On-line]. Available: http://www.aoa.dhhs.gov/ aoa/stats/profile/2001/5.html (Retrieved May 11, 2002).

American Psychiatric Association. (2000). *Diagnostic and statistical manual of mental disorders* (4th ed., text revision). Washington, DC: Author.

Baker, W. J. (1991). Positivism versus people: What should psychology be about? In C. W. Tolman (Ed.), *Positivism in psychology: Historical and contemporary problems* (pp. 9–16). New York: Springer-Verlag.

Barnouw, V. (1985). *Culture and personality.* Belmont, CA: Wadsworth.

Bentley, J. R., Delfino, R. J., Taylor, T. H., Howe, S., & Anton-Culver, H. (1998). Differences in breast cancer stage at diagnosis between non-Hispanic White and Hispanic populations, San Diego County 1988–1993. *Breast Cancer Research and Treatment, 50,* 1–9.

Berkman, B. (1996). The emerging health care world: Implications for social work practice and education. *Social Work, 41,* 541–551.

Berkman, L. F. (1980). Physical health and the social environment: A social epidemiological perspective. In A. Kleinman (Ed.), *The relevance of social science for medicine* (pp. 51–75). Dordrecht, Netherlands: Reidel.

Breen, N., & Figueroa, J. B. (1996). Stage of breast and cervical cancer diagnosis in disadvantaged neighborhoods: A prevention policy perspective. *American Journal of Preventive Medicine, 12,* 319–326.

Campos, S. S., & Johnson, T. M. (1990). Cultural considerations. In B. Spilker (Ed.), *Quality of life assessments in clinical trials* (pp. 163–170). New York: Raven Press.

Cassel, J. C. (1976). The contribution of the social environment to host resistance. *American Journal of Epidemiology, 104,* 107–123.

Cassel, J. C., Patrick, R. C., & Jenkins, C. D. (1960). Epidemiologic analysis of the health implications of culture change: A conceptual model. *Annals of the New York Academy of Sciences, 84,* 938–949.

Chang, S. W., Kerlikowske, K., Napoles-Springer, A., Posner, S. F., Sickles, E. A., & Perez-Stable, E. J. (1996). Racial differences in timeliness of follow-up after abnormal screening mammography. *Cancer, 78,* 1395–1402.

Chavez, L. R., & Hubbell, F. A. (1997). The influence of fatalism on self-reported use of Papanicolaou smears. *American Journal of Preventive Medicine, 13*, 418–424.

Chin, M. H., & Humikowski, C. A. (2002). When is risk stratification by race or ethnicity justified in medical care? *Journal of the Association of American Medical Colleges, 77*, 202–208.

Cole, M. (1996). *Cultural psychology: A once and future discipline.* Cambridge, MA: Belknap Press of Harvard University Press.

Dana, R. H. (1996). Assessment of acculturation in Hispanic populations. *Hispanic Journal of Behavioral Sciences, 18*, 317–328.

Dignam, J. J. (2000). Differences in breast cancer prognosis among African-American and Caucasian women. *CA—A Cancer Journal for Clinicians, 50*(1), 50–64.

Editor, C. (2001). Primary colours. *The Economist, 358*(8213), 27–28.

Fayers, P. M., Hand, D. J., Bjordal, K., & Groenvold, M. (1997). Causal indicators in quality of life research. *Quality of Life Research, 6*, 393–406.

Federal Interagency Forum on Aging-Related Statistics. (2000). *Older Americans 2000: Key indicators of well-being.* [On-line]. Available: http://www.agingstats. gov/chartbook2000/healthstatus.html (Retrieved May 11, 2002).

Feinstein, J. S. (1993). The relationship between socioeconomic status and health: A review of the literature. *Milbank Quarterly, 71*, 279–322.

Fox, S. A., Pitkin, K., Paul, C., Carson, S., & Naihua, D. (1998). Breast cancer screening adherence: Does church attendance matter? *Health Education and Behavior, 25*, 742–758.

Fox, S. A., & Roetzheim, R. G. (1994). Screening mammography and older Hispanic women. *Cancer, 74*, 2028–2033.

Frazier, E. L., Jiles, R. B., & Mayberry, R. (1996). Use of screening mammography and clinical breast examinations among Black, Hispanic, and White women. *Preventive Medicine, 25*, 118–125.

Friedman, D. J., Cohen, B. B., Averbach, A. R., & Norton, J. M. (2000). Race/ethnicity and OMB Directive 15: Implications for state public health practice. *American Journal of Public Health, 90*, 1714–1719.

Geertz, C. (1965). The impact of the concept of culture on the concept of man. In J. R. Platt (Ed.), *New views of the nature of man* (pp. 93–118). Chicago: University of Chicago Press.

Geertz, C. (1973). *The interpretation of cultures: Selected essays.* New York: Basic Books.

Giachello, A. L. (1996). Health outcomes research on Hispanics/Latinos. *Journal of Medical Systems, 20*(5), 235–254.

Gonzalez-Calvo, J., Gonzalez, V. M., & Lorig, K. (1997). Cultural diversity issues in the development of valid and reliable measures of health status. *Arthritis Care and Research, 10*, 448–456.

Gray, J., & Puente, S. (1996). Introduction to special issue. *Journal of Medical Systems, 20*(5), 229–233.

Greenlee, R. T., Hill-Harmon, M. B., Murray, T., & Thun, M. (2001). Cancer statistics, 2001. *CA—A Cancer Journal for Clinicians, 51*(1), 15–36.

Greenlee, R. T., Murray, T., Bolden, S., & Wingo, P. A. (2000). Cancer statistics, 2000. *CA—A Cancer Journal for Clinicians, 50*(1), 7–33.

Guarnaccia, P. J. (1996). Anthropological perspective: The importance of culture in the assessment of quality of life. In B. Spilker (Ed.), *Quality of life and pharmacoeconomics in clinical trials* (pp. 523–528). Philadelphia: Lippincott-Ravin.

Gudykunst, W. B., & Kim, Y. Y. (1992). *Communicating with strangers: An approach to intercultural communication.* New York: McGraw-Hill.

Hofstede, G. (1984). *Culture's consequences: International differences in work-related values.* Beverly Hills, CA: Sage.

Hofstede, G. (1991). *Cultures and organizations: Software of the mind.* London: McGraw-Hill.

Hubbell, F. A., Chavez, L. R., Mishra, S. I., & Valdez, R. B. (1996). Differing beliefs about breast cancer among Latinas and Anglo women. *Western Journal of Medicine, 164,* 405–409.

Hubbell, F. A., Mishra, S. I., Chavez, L. R., & Valdez, R. B. (1997). The influence of knowledge and attitudes about breast cancer on mammography use among Latinas and Anglo women. *Journal of General Internal Medicine, 12,* 505–508.

King, C. R., Haberman, M., Berry, D. L., Bush, N., Butler, L., Dow, K. H., et al. (1997). Quality of life and the cancer experience: The state-of-the-knowledge. *Oncology Nursing Forum, 24*(1), 27–42.

Kleinman, A. (1988). *Rethinking psychiatry: From cultural category to personal experience.* New York: Free Press.

Krieger, N. (2000). Counting accountably: Implications of the new approaches to classifying race/ethnicity in the 2000 census. *American Journal of Public Health, 90,* 1687–1689.

Kuhn, T. S. (1970). *The structure of scientific revolutions* (2nd ed.). Chicago: University of Chicago Press.

Landis, S. H., Murray, T., Bolden, S., & Wingo, P. A. (1999). Cancer statistics, 1999. *CA—A Cancer Journal for Clinicians, 49*(1), 8–31.

Linton, R. (1945). *The cultural background of personality.* New York: Appleton-Century.

Lobell, M., Bay, R. C., Rhoads, K. V. L., & Keske, B. (1998). Barriers to cancer screening in Mexican American women. *Mayo Clinic Proceedings, 73*(4), 301–308.

Mandelblatt, J. S., Gold, K., O'Malley, A. S., Taylor, K., Cagney, K., Hopkins, J. S., et al. (1999). Breast and cervix cancer screening among multiethnic women: Role of age, health, and source of care. *Preventive Medicine, 28,* 418–425.

Marable, M. (2000). We need new and critical study of race and ethnicity. *Chronicle of Higher Education, 46*(25), B4–B7.

Maramaldi, P. (2001). *Diagnostic delays following abnormal mammography: A comparison of Latina and White women.* Unpublished doctoral dissertation, Columbia University, New York.

Marin, G., & Gamba, R. J. (1996). A new measurement of acculturation for Hispanics: The Bidimensional Acculturation Scale for Hispanics (BAS). *Hispanic Journal of Behavioral Sciences, 18,* 297–316.

Marin, G., Sabogol, F., Marin, B. V., Otero-Sabogal, R., & Perez-Stable, E. J. (1987). Development of a short acculturation scale for Hispanics. *Hispanic Journal of Behavioral Sciences, 9,* 183–205.

Marmont, M. (1981). Culture and illness: Epidemiologic evidence. In P. G. Mellett (Ed.), *Foundations of psychosomatics* (pp. 323–340). Chichester, England: Wiley.

Marmont, M. (1994). Social differentials in health within and between populations. *Daedalus, 123,* 197–216.

Martin, J. N. (1994). Intercultural communication: A unifying concept for international education. In G. Althen (Ed.), *Learning across cultures* (pp. 9–29). Washington, DC: NAFSA: Association of International Educators.

McLaughlin, L. A., & Braun, K. L. (1998). Asian and Pacific Islander cultural values: Considerations for health care decision making. *Health and Social Work, 23*(2), 116–126.

Meenaghan, T. M. (2001). Exploring possible relations among social sciences, social work, and health interventions. In G. Rosenberg & A. Weissman (Eds.), *Behavioral and social sciences in 21st century health care* (pp. 43–50). Binghamton, NY: Haworth Press.

Meyerowitz, B. E., Richardson, J., Hudson, S., & Leedham, B. (1998). Ethnicity and cancer outcomes: Behavioral and psychosocial considerations. *Psychological Bulletin, 123*(1), 47–70.

Napoles-Springer, A., Perez-Stable, E. J., & Washington, E. (1996). Risk factors for invasive cervical cancer in Latino women. *Journal of Medical Systems, 20*(5), 277–293.

National Academy on an Aging Society. (1999). *Chronic conditions: A challenge for the 21st century.* Washington, DC: Gerontological Society of America.

Obeyesekere, G. (1990). *The work of culture: Symbolic transformation in psychoanalysis and anthropology.* Chicago: University of Chicago Press.

Padilla, G. V., Ferrell, B. R., Grant, M. M., & Rhiner, M. (1990). Defining the content domain of quality of life for cancer patients with pain. *Cancer Nursing, 13*(2), 108–115.

Pearlman, D. N., Rakowski, W., Ehrich, B., & Clark, M. A. (1996). Breast cancer screening practices among Black, Hispanic, and White women: Reassessing differences. *American Journal of Preventive Medicine, 12,* 327–337.

Phinney, J. S. (1996). When we talk about American ethnic groups, what do we mean? *American Psychologist, 51,* 918–927.

Salazar, K. (1996). Hispanic women's beliefs about breast cancer and mammography. *Cancer Nursing, 19,* 437–446.

Sanders-Phillips, K. (1996). Correlates of health promotion behaviors in low-income Black women and Latinas. *American Journal of Preventive Medicine, 12,* 450–458.

Schipper, H., Clinch, J. J., & Olweny, C. L. M. (1996). Quality of life studies: Definitions and conceptual issues. In B. Spilker (Ed.), *Quality of life and pharmacoeconomics in clinical trials.* Philadelphia: Lippincott-Raven.

Shweder, R. A. (1991). *Thinking through cultures: Expeditions in cultural psychology.* Cambridge, MA: Harvard University Press.

Sondik, E. J., Lucas, J. W., Madans, J. H., & Smith, S. S. (2000). Race/ethnicity and the 2000 census: Implications for public health. *American Journal of Public Health, 90,* 1709–1713.

Spilker, B. (1996). Introduction. In B. Spilker (Ed.), *Quality of life and pharmacoeconomics in clinical trials* (pp. 1–10). Philadelphia: Lippincott-Raven.

Susser, M. (1987). Social science and public health. In M. Susser (Ed.), *Epidemiology, health, and society* (pp. 177–185). Oxford, England: Oxford University Press.

Syme, S. L. (1992). Social determinants of disease. In R. B. Wallace (Ed.), *Maxcy-Rosenau-Last: Public health and preventive medicine.* Norwalk, CT: Appleton & Lange.

Talavera, G. A., Elder, J. P., & Velasquez, R. J. (1997). Latino health beliefs and locus of control: Implications for primary care and public health practitioners. *American Journal of Preventive Medicine, 13,* 408–410.

Triandis, H. C. (1980). Introduction. In J. W. Berry (Ed.), *Handbook of cross-cultural psychology* (Vol. 1, pp. 1–14). Boston: Allyn and Bacon.

U.S. Bureau of the Census. (2000a). *Census 2000 summary file 1* (Publication No. SF 1). Washington, DC: U.S. Department of Commerce.

U.S. Bureau of the Census. (2000b). *Projections of the total resident population by 5-year age groups, race, and Hispanic origin with special age categories: Middle series, 2050 to 2070* (Publication No. NP-T4-G). Washington, DC: U.S. Department of Commerce.

Vega, W. A. (1992). Theoretical and pragmatic implications of cultural diversity for community research. *American Journal of Community Psychology, 20,* 375–391.

Ware, J. E. (1995). The status of health assessment 1994. *Annual Review of Public Health, 16,* 327–354.

Woolam, G. L. (2000). Cancer statistics, 2000: A benchmark for a new century. *CA—A Cancer Journal for Clinicians, 50*(1), 6.

World Health Organization. (1992). *The tenth revision of the international classification of diseases and related health problems.* Geneva, Switzerland: Author.

Yood, M. U., Johnson, C. C., Blount, A., Abrams, J., Wolman, E., McCarthy, B. D., et al. (1999). Race and differences in breast cancer survival in a managed care population. *Journal of the National Cancer Institute, 91,* 1487–1491.

Zambrana, R. E., Breen, N., Fox, S. A., & Gutierrez-Mohomed, M. L. (1999). Use of cancer screening practices by Hispanic women: Analyses by subgroup. *Preventive Medicine, 29,* 466–477.

Chapter 14

CENTRALITY OF SOCIAL TIES TO THE HEALTH AND WELL-BEING OF OLDER ADULTS

James Lubben and Melanie Gironda

Supportive social ties enhance physical and mental health among older adults. Conversely, social isolation, loneliness, and stressful social ties contribute to higher risk of disability, poor recovery from illness, and early death. As health researchers and policy makers move from a fixation on disease and medical-care service utilization to a serious examination of how to increase active life expectancy and improve quality of life among older adults, social ties will be shown to be even more vital. Given the growing consensus of their importance, the use of consistent tools to assess social ties is even more crucial to the appropriate practice of geriatrics and study of gerontology.

SIGNIFICANCE OF SOCIAL TIES

A national committee on future directions for behavioral and social sciences research at the National Institutes of Health (National Research Council [NRC], 2001) recently issued a report that identified a domain of research questions whose resolution could lead to major

319

improvements in the health of the U.S. population. One of the top 10 priority areas for research investment to integrate the behavioral, social, and biomedical sciences at the National Institutes of Health was that of personal ties. The NRC report noted a growing body of epidemiological findings that link social relationships with mental and physical health outcomes, including mortality. Furthermore, disruption of personal ties, loneliness, and conflictual interactions are stress-producing whereas supportive social ties are vital sources of emotional strength.

Partly because of the high complexity of social relationship phenomena, there is a lack of agreement on definitions and preferred measures for social ties (Berkman, 1985; Berkman & Glass, 2000; Ell, 1984; Heitzman & Kaplan, 1988; House, Landis, & Umberson, 1988; Levin, 2000; Lin, Ye, & Ensel, 1999; Lubben & Gironda, 1996; Vaux, 1988; Wenger, 1996). For example, this construct has been labeled as social bonds, social supports, social networks, social integration, social ties, meaningful social contacts, confidants, human companionships, reciprocity, guidance, information given, emotional support, and organizational involvement. (Caplan, 1974; Cobb, 1976; Ell, 1984; Henderson, 1977; Lowenthal & Haven, 1968; Lubben, 1988; Miller & Ingham, 1976). In one meta-analysis, Heitzmann and Kaplan (1988) identified 23 different techniques for measuring social support.

One of the most surprising observations from a review of the research is that the connection between social ties and health remains quite consistent despite the lack of clarity in defining social support networks coupled with an inconsistency in measuring health. Furthermore, the diversity of these studies adds extra significance to the convergence of their findings. Indeed, public heath experts posit that the association between social support networks and health is now as strong as the epidemiological evidence linking smoking and health at the time the Surgeon General issued his famous warning about the dangers of smoking (House et al., 1988).

More specifically, inadequate social support networks have been associated with both an increase in morbidity and an increase in mortality (Berkman, 1984, 1986; Berkman & Syme, 1979; Blazer, 1982; Bosworth & Schaie, 1997; Ceria et al., 2001; Ell, 1984; House et al., 1988; Kaplan, Seeman, Cohen, Knudsen, & Guralnik, 1987; Rook, 1994; Torres, McIntosh, & Kubena, 1992; Zuckerman, Kasl, & Ostfeld, 1984). Social scientists also report that social isolation is associated with increased symptoms of psychological distress or loneliness (Lin et al., 1999; Mor-Barak, 1997; Thoits, 1995; Turner & Marino, 1994; Wenger,

1996; Williams, Ware, & Donald, 1981). Other scholars report an association between limited social ties and poor overall health and well-being (Chappell, 1991; Chappell & Badger, 1989; Cutrona & Russell, 1986; Krause, Herzog, & Baker, 1992; Lubben, Weiler, & Chi, 1989; Rook, 1994; Stuck et al., 1999). Others document a connection between social support networks and adherence to desired health practices (Potts, Hurwicz, & Goldstein, 1992). A recent study even suggested that people with more social ties are less susceptible to the common cold (Cohen, Doyle, Skoner, Rabin, & Gwaltney, 1997).

Although much of the literature recounts the blessings of strong social support networks, there is also some that addresses negative aspects of personal ties. If relations between family members, friends, or neighbors become strained, some personal ties may actually increase stress rather than reduce stress. There are also pivotal times when family members and friends may be too eager to offer help to an older adult and such support may prove detrimental. In a study of intergenerational support, Silverstein, Chen, and Heller (1996) found that a threshold of support existed where support from children was beneficial up to a certain point, but too much support produced an increase in dependence and a reduction in well-being. Other researchers have found that some older adults may desire the perceived availability of family and peer contacts but not necessarily the actual contact (Mullins, Sheppard, & Anderson, 1991).

A number of theories have been proposed to explain the link between social ties and health. One theory suggests that strong social ties may serve to stimulate the immune system to ward off illnesses more effectively. Similarly, a buffering-effect theory suggests that strong social ties may reduce the susceptibility of an individual to stress-related illnesses (Cassel, 1976; Cobb, 1976; Krause et al., 1992; Krause & Jay, 1991; Mor-Barak & Miller, 1991; Thoits, 1982). A third theory suggests that social networks provide essential support that is needed during times of illness, thereby contributing to better adaptation and quicker recovery time. Finally, a fourth theory posits that social ties are instrumental in adherence to good health practices and the cessation of bad ones (Kelsey, Earp, & Kirkley, 1997; Potts et al., 1992).

Primary and Secondary Social Groups

Personal or social ties as a construct consist of various features of social connections between an individual and the members of various primary and secondary social groups with whom the individual is involved. Primary social groups, such as family, friends, and neighbors, are the mainstay of social and personal ties in old age. Family is often considered the most central primary group to which an individual belongs. However, intimate friends can be as vital as family ties, especially when family relations are strained or deficient for other reasons. Alternative family arrangements and the formation of nonmarried couples impart new complexity to the character of primary social groups in later life. An older adult may have membership in an array of secondary social groups such as clubs and organizations, including religious ones. Further, for those older adults who are still employed, the workplace is an important forum for social relationships.

The study of social participation of older adults has been a common theme in the social gerontological literature for several decades. Some early theories of the sociology of aging even proposed that social disengagement with advanced age was a normal, perhaps desired, part of human development. Gerontological research has generally refuted such notions, suggesting that social disengagement is neither normal nor desirable. Instead, new models of aging embrace a goal of broad integration of older adults in society as advocated in a World Health Organization (WHO) document presented at the Second World Assembly on Aging in Madrid (WHO, Ageing and the Life Course Section, 2002). Although older adults may reallocate their time from secondary group participation to more primary group participation, secondary groups remain important to health and well-being. Such organized social environments provide keen opportunities for social activity and participation that impact on the nurturing and replenishment of an older adult's social support network.

Social Networks, Social Supports, and Loneliness

The literature often distinguishes between social networks and social supports. Generally, *social networks* refer to the structural aspects of social ties, including size, density, source of ties, member homogeneity, boundedness, frequency of contacts, geographic proximity, durability, intensity, reciprocity, and multiplexity (Berkman & Glass, 2000; Ell, 1984; Vaux, 1988). Social networks have also been defined as the web of social relationships that surround a person and the objective characteristics of those social ties (Ell, 1984). Social networks describe the more objective traits of social ties.

The term *social support* is used to describe the more subjective traits of social ties, focusing on the quality and nature of interactions among members of a social network. A diversified and well-stocked reservoir of members in an older adult's social networks increases the likelihood that the appropriate social support would be available for life's various emergencies. Social support is generally drawn from a small subset of one's total social network. Berkman (1984) has defined social support as the "emotional, instrumental and financial assistance that is obtained from one's social network" (p. 414).

Loneliness is distinguished as a construct that is distinct from social networks and from supports. Indeed, one may feel lonely in the midst of a crowd. For example, Weiss (1973) states that "loneliness is not simply a desire for company, any company; rather it yields only to very specific forms of relationships" (p. 13). Perlman (1987) claims that loneliness is a discrepancy between one's desired and one's achieved levels of social contacts. Loneliness is identified as a subjective experience, whereas isolation is defined as an objective condition that involves a lack of integration into social networks (Rook, 1984).

There is likely to be some overlap between social support, social networks, and loneliness to the extent that they are all aspects of a person's total social milieu. Because social networks are the source from which social support is drawn, the two are not totally separable from one another. Similarly, because loneliness may result from deficiencies in one's social ties, loneliness is likely to be correlated with measures of either social networks or social supports. A psychometric analysis of three commonly used measures of social ties concluded that social networks, social supports, and loneliness are so sufficiently different as constructs that there is a need for discrete measures for each (Lubben & Gironda, 2000).

Using a concept they call the "loneliness threshold," Johnson and Mullins (1989, p. 113) define different levels and types of social contact needed to prevent the development of loneliness. Therefore, support programs need to be designed individually to encourage and maintain independence and a sense of control and competency over the situation and not to encourage dependence and loss of control. A one-size-fits-all approach to the problem of isolation or loneliness will not work. The amount of social contact needed by older people may vary, depending on social, physical, and economic circumstances as well as personality patterns. For example, Long and Martin (2000) found that for the oldest-old subpopulation of older adults, affectionate relationships with children were of prime importance as a buffer to loneliness. For other groups, intimate friends might be equally salient.

As noted, not all isolates are alike, and different interventions need to be developed to address distinctive types and profiles of isolates. For example, respite programs might be an appropriate strategy for older adults whose social contacts have become impaired due to caregiving responsibilities, whereas self-help groups might work best for those whose isolation is attributed to bereavement. Among some of the successful interventions in place today are respite programs, counseling, senior peer-support groups, and other self-help programs. Other programs in earlier stages of development include (a) telephone or computer communication services, (b) intergenerational mutual support programs, and (c) skill-building programs to improve social integration among older isolated adults.

Distinctive Features of Social Support Networks

The functional nature of social support is distinguished by the presence of the perceived availability of specific dimensions of support (Sherbourne & Stewart, 1991). Emotional support can consist of caring, affection, love, sympathy, understanding, esteem, and empathy. Instrumental assistance consists of more tangible support such as information, financial aid, or help with medical needs, household maintenance, or other daily living tasks, among other things. Typically, usual sources of support include spouse, children siblings, extended family, friends, and neighbors.

The perceived quality of social support is sometimes more important than the actual support provided. The perception that help was available when needed is more important than the actual help provided. Although the perception of the quality of most supportive relationships is positive—providing a sense of security and bolstering people's coping strategies—some relationships can have a negative outcome if they reinforce negative health behaviors or communicate negative feedback (Antonucci, 2001; Wallsten, Tweed, Blazer, & George, 1999).

Social support can come from a variety of sources, including family, friends, and neighbors. It appears that family, friends, and neighbors may serve different functions in older people's lives (Antonucci, 1990; Chappell, 1991). Having family support, for example, is often crucial in forestalling institutionalization (Felton & Berry, 1992; Hooyman & Kiyak, 1988). Spouses and children, particularly daughters, are often credited as primary caretakers who provide in-home personal assistance to frail older persons, enabling them to remain within the community (Stone, Cafferata, & Sangl, 1987). Immediate family members are usually the major source of help during illness and disability. Without such timely and dependable social support, the likelihood of using extensive formal services and the risk for institutionalization is higher.

Although family members often provide for most of the critical needs of an older person, a growing body of literature also testifies to the importance of having strong friendships in old age. Many scholars have noted how important friendships are to the psychological well-being of elderly adults (Antonucci, 1990; Crohan & Antonucci, 1989; Francis, 1991; Hooyman & Kiyak, 1988; Larson, Mannell, & Zuzanek, 1986; Peters & Kaiser, 1985). Furthermore, in comparing the effects of satisfaction between family and friends, Crohan and Antonucci (1989) suggest that friendships are less likely to have negative effects on the well-being of mature adults; family relationships, on the other hand, can trigger negative effects when demands are too high. Carstensen (1992) followed a group of women and men for 34 years and found that even though interaction intensity with friends varied over the years, feelings of emotional satisfaction and closeness towards friends remained relatively stable.

When it comes to the need for immediate assistance, neighbors and proximal friends may prove to be an especially important source of support (Hooyman & Kiyak, 1988). Litwak (1985) suggests that for some tasks, such as responding quickly during illness or emergencies, friends and neighbors may be more accessible and readily available than family members who either live farther away or who are away at work much of the day. Adams (1986) also notes that neighbors and nearby friends help when it is convenient to them and for predictable tasks, such as providing transportation, and thus relieve the family of some burdens in their care of elderly adults.

As individuals advance in age, they become more neighborhood-bound, and neighbors have been shown to be important links to community services (Regnier, 1980). Also, natural helping networks in neighborhoods often provide supportive and monitoring functions to community-dwelling older persons, especially those living alone, and even delay institutionalization (Ehrlich, 1979; Pyroos, Hade-Kaplan, & Fleisher, 1984). The importance of friendship and neighborhood-based helping networks is likely to increase as the proportion of older persons with adult children decreases (Gironda, Lubben, & Atchison, 1999).

Distinguishing Between Social Isolation and Loneliness

Social isolation is a term used to characterize those older adults who have extremely limited social support networks. In a clinical trial of social health risks among a large community-dwelling elderly population, 66% of the study sample were considered at low risk for social isolation, 16% were rated at moderate risk, and 8% were rated as isolated (R. L. Rubinstein, Lubben, & Mintzer, 1994). In this study, social workers were asked to identify the primary cause of the older adult's isolation. Relatively few of those deemed socially isolated were characterized as lifelong isolates. The most common responses included spousal caretaker strain, depression, and recent health conditions.

Such differences in isolation etiology have practice implications. The needs of a widow who withdraws from social contact in bereavement are likely to be quite different from those of a wife whose overwhelming caretaking responsibilities have forced her to withdraw from interaction with friends. Depression as a factor associated with isolation offers yet a different set of circumstances that are likely to influence the choice of intervention approaches (Dorfman et al., 1995).

Wenger (1996) proposed a number of determinants for social isolation and for loneliness. They included age, gender, widowhood, singleness, living alone, childlessness, retirement migration, poor health, and low morale. Older adults are especially likely to face the loss of a key family member or friend from their network, making them more vulnerable to isolation and loneliness. The challenge for social workers and gerontologists is to find ways to substitute for these losses and foster the development of new ties or strengthen those among remaining members of the older adult's social network.

Whereas social isolation is identified as a somewhat objective condition that can be observed, loneliness is conceptualized as more of a subjective experience that can be identified largely through self-report. One distinguishing aspect of loneliness is that it is oftentimes unmitigated by social activity (Weiss, 1973). Loneliness can occur even when an older adult is in the midst of people and activities. It is not simply that a person needs people around, but that specific types of social relationships need to be present.

Two types of loneliness are identified in the literature: *emotional isolation*, which is the lack of truly intimate ties; and *social loneliness*, which is the lack of a network of involvement with family, peers, friends, and neighbors (Weiss, 1973). It is in the social loneliness domain that social isolation presents as a critical issue for older adults who have lost access to significant parts of their social network. In particular, certain subpopulations of elders are at risk for social isolation, including people who are among the oldest old, who are in poorer health, not married, and with lower levels of income and education (Kaufman & Adams, 1987).

SIGNIFICANCE TO GERONTOLOGY, HEALTH CARE, AND HEALTH PROFESSIONALS

Although there is extensive evidence that social ties are extremely important to the health and well-being of older adults, this knowledge is only beginning to affect health care practice. In health care settings, minimal attention is paid to an older adult's social health status, compared with the attention to other attributes that an older person presents when seeking care. More specifically, the health care system shows much more regard for the physical and mental health dimensions of patients, but only minor attention to the social health dimensions of patients.

In an era that stresses community-based delivery of care, members of an older person's social support network may be more responsible for the successful execution of treatment plans than are members of the health care team. Social ties are often the 24-hour in-home care managers who are monitoring compliance with treatment regimes and early detection of new problems that require timely and modified interventions. Increased sensitivity to the importance of social support networks for well-being in old age might help flag those elders who are in need of a more comprehensive assessment by a social worker or other practitioner.

This marginal concern for social health is demonstrated in many facets of the health care encounter but is especially apparent in the assessment protocols used to detect an older adult's needs. Assessment is the heart and soul of geriatric practice (Solomon, 2000). Very few components of geriatric assessment instruments deal with social health matters, suggesting that they are not currently perceived to be at the heart and soul of geriatric practice.

Therefore, indicators of an older adult's social health should be as much a part of the geriatric assessment protocols as are mental and physical health markers. An abbreviated social-support-network scale can readily be incorporated into a geriatric assessment battery, allowing clinicians to gather social health information in a systematic manner in a relatively short period of time. From there, they can readily share the knowledge with other team members in quantifiable, measurable terms. Also, the systematic use of such a scale facilitates a more accurate description of aspects of social network and social support that may require tailored intervention. Additionally, global scales that quantify an older person's social environment might also be useful for monitoring systematic changes over time. Expanded use of social-support-network measurement tools in geriatric practice will enhance community care and appropriate referral to such programs as respite care, peer support, or counseling.

The use of such assessment tools may also increase the attention that the older person pays to his or her own social health. Older persons might be encouraged by the nature of inquiry in these scales to evaluate or identify (on their own) areas of weakness in social network or areas of strength or potential resources. Short-assessment tools can be used as health promotion screeners to identify cases of social isolation or loneliness that might otherwise go undetected. A good measure of one's social support network will prove useful as an initial indicator of risk for isolation and loneliness.

CURRENT RESEARCH

Although the upsurge of research on social support networks has spawned a profusion of measurement techniques, a limited number of well-documented scales exists. Further, there tends to be inadequate reporting of the psychometric properties of social support measures used in the various studies. O'Reilly (1988) laments the inadequate clarity of definition and the general lack of attention and reporting of reliability and validity analyses of most social-support-network assessment instruments. A common criticism of many of these studies is the use of instruments with unknown or unreported psychometric properties (Winemiller, Mitchell, Sutliff, & Cline, 1993). Given the growing consensus of the importance of social support networks to health and well-being, consistent tools used to conduct social assessments are becoming even more crucial to the appropriate practice of geriatrics and study of gerontology (Glass, Mendes de Leon, Seeman, & Berkman, 1997; Levin, 2000; Steiner et al., 1996). Rather than attempting to design a singular social-support-network scale that fits the demands of all settings, a feat only remotely attainable, it seems more practical to design measurement instruments for specific populations along with clear intentions on how the instrument should be used (Mitchell & Trickett, 1980).

From applied research and clinical perspectives, pressure is growing to develop short and efficient scales. Some elderly populations are unable to complete long questionnaires. Time constraints in most clinical practice settings also necessitate efficient and effective screening tools, and shorter scales require less time and energy for the administrator and the respondent. Parsimonious and effective screening tools will be more acceptable to elders and to health care providers. However, basic researchers often desire somewhat longer research instruments. Having a larger number of items and better clarity of concepts generally contributes to a scale's reliability. These longer instruments also facilitate the appraisal and analyses of subtle differences in social support networks. The need for compromise is essential if scale developers are to meet the needs of research and of patient care.

The Lubben Social Network Scale (LSNS)

The present analyses provide a case example of the careful modification of a validated measurement scale, the LSNS, to address the conflicting goals of brevity and completeness. For a relatively brief measure of kin and non-kin social ties, the LSNS-R is presented; to address the needs of clinicians and applied researchers for a very abbreviated version, the LSNS-6; and for basic social and health science researchers, an expanded version (the LSNS-18).

The LSNS has been used in a wide array of studies since it was first reported a decade ago (Ceria et al., 2001; Chou & Chi, 1999; Dorfman et al., 1995; Hurwicz & Berkanovic, 1993; Lubben, 1988;

Lubben et al., 1989; Lubben & Gironda, 1996; Luggen & Rini, 1995; Martire, Schulz, Mittelmark, & Newsom, 1999; Mor-Barak, 1997; Mor-Barak & Miller, 1991; Mor-Borak, Miller, & Syme, 1991; Okwumabua, Baker, Wong, & Pilgrim, 1997; Potts et al., 1992; L. Z. Rubenstein et al., 1994; R. L. Rubenstein et al., 1994). It has been used in research and in practice settings, and it has been translated into several languages (including Chinese, Korean, Japanese, and Spanish) for use in cross-cultural and cross-national comparative studies. Recently, Lubben, Gironda, and Lee (2002) published the revision of the original LSNS (the LSNS-R), a 12-item measure of social ties that offers enhanced administrative and psychometric properties of the original LSNS. Appendix A presents this revision.

The LSNS-6: An Abbreviated Version of LSNS-R

Although the original LSNS and the LSNS-R are relatively short instruments, there have been numerous requests to identify an even shorter scale especially for screening purposes. Also, some researchers have selectively extracted a subset of LSNS items (e.g., Martire et al., 1999). Out of concern for a possible proliferation of inconsistent shortened versions, as has happened with some other commonly used scales, a standard six-item abbreviated version of the LSNS is proposed. Clinicians and researchers have already adopted this abbreviated scale in practice and applied research settings (Lubben & Gironda, 2000). The LSNS-6 (Appendix B) can be used as a screener for social isolation in health-screening clinics, to identify cases deemed worthy of more extensive assessment and possible clinical interventions. The LSNS-6 might also be appropriate for research studies that are unable to accommodate one of the longer versions.

The items for the LSNS-6 were selected deliberately. Perceived emotional supports, perceived tangible supports, and actual network size have all been suggested as particularly salient to social networks (Heitzmann & Kaplan, 1988). Thus, three items that tap into these dimensions of social support networks were chosen for family networks and a similar set for nonkin networks.

The LSNS-18: An Expanded Version of LSNS-R

As previously described, social supports come from a variety of sources, including family, friends, and neighbors. Because family, friends, and neighbors may serve different functions in older people's lives, there was a desire to modify the LSNS so that it could better specify and distinguish the nature of family, friendship, and neighborhood-based social networks. Although the original LSNS and the newly revised version (LSNS-R) distinguish between kin and non-kin, neither of these scales distinguished between friends and neighbors. The LSNS-R has six items that deal with family and another six that deal with friends (including those who live in the neighborhood). The LSNS-18 (Appendix C) increased quantification of key structural and functional elements of family, friendship, and neighborhood-based social support networks. Furthermore, the LSNS-18 can be disaggregated into three subscales (family, friends, and neighbors) to better examine the distinctive roles of each type of social support network, making it useful in basic social and health science research. In the LSNS-18, the family items are the same as in the LSNS-R. However, the six items for friendships are split into one set that deals with neighbors (some of whom may be friends) and one set that deals with friends (excluding those who live in the respondent's neighborhood).

Psychometrics of Different Versions of LSNS

In a survey of older White non-Hispanic Americans in Los Angeles County, California, a sample of individuals aged 65 and older was interviewed between June and November 1993. The sample included ·130 women (65%) and 71 men (35%) with a mean age of 75.3 years. Additional details on the sample are reported elsewhere (Moon, Lubben, & Villa, 1998; Pourat, Lubben, Wallace, & Moon, 1999; Pourat, Lubben, Yu, & Wallace, 2000). These data are used for the following analyses.

Table 14.1 presents the summary results of the internal consistency tests. The Cronbach alpha scores for the LSNS-R ($\alpha = .78$) and the LSNS-6 ($\alpha = .78$) are presented here for comparison with the LSNS-18. They are all well within the acceptable parameters suggested by Streiner and Norman (1995) for health measurement scales. The LSNS-18 ($\alpha = .82$) presents the highest level of internal consistency of the three scales. Reliability tests were also conducted for the LSNS-18 subscales of family networks, friendship networks, and neighborhood networks. Not surprising, these more homogeneous subscales demonstrate high internal consistency: family subscale ($\alpha = .82$), friends subscale ($\alpha = .87$), and neighbors subscale ($\alpha = .80$).

TABLE 14.1   LSNS-6 Factor Matrix

Item	Family Factor	Nonkin Factor
Family: Size	.80	.03
Family: Feel close to call for help	.84	.16
Family: Discuss private matters	.84	.13
Friend/neighbor: Size	.18	.81
Friend/neighbor: Feel close to call for help	.06	.85
Friend/neighbor: Discuss private matters	.07	.77

The factor structure for the LSNS-6 is quite clean as reported in Table 14.1. The three items dealing with family all load heavily on that factor, and the three friendship items also load heavily on a friend factor. There are no discernible cross loadings.

The factor structure for the LSNS-18 was not as easily determined. Using Kaiser's rule of including all factors with eigenvalues greater than 1 produced a four-factor solution for the LSNS-18. The first factor corresponded with friendship network items, the second factor with family network items, the third with neighborhood-based confidant relationships, and the fourth with other facets of neighborhood-based networks. This four-factor solution offers good interpretability, given that the first two factors clearly contain only friendship or family items whereas the third and fourth factors only contain neighbor items. However, a scree plot suggested that a three-factor solution might be workable, and that was supported by the fourth factor barely meeting Kaiser's rule (eigenvalue = 1.3). Furthermore, there was considerable cross loading of items on the two neighbor factors, suggesting that a forced three-factor might be preferred. A distinct advantage of a three-factor solution is that it would be more easily interpreted, and so another principal component analysis was performed forcing a three-factor solution.

The results from the forced three-factor solution are shown in Table 14.2. There is very little loss of explanatory power. The three factors account for 56.5% of the total variation, whereas the previously described four-factor solution explained 63.5%. All item factor loadings for each factor are higher than 0.60, and there are no cross loadings to other factors. This time, all family, friendship, and neighborhood-based items load cleanly onto the three factors, which lends support

TABLE 14.2   LSNS-18 Factor Matrix (3 Factor Solution)

Code	Item	Friends Factor	Family Factor	Neighbors Factor
L12F	Friends: Subject has confidant	.81932	.09966	.12192
L9F	Friends: Discuss private matters	.81082	.14232	.12176
L8F	Friends: Frequency of contact	.77825	.02225	.05377
L11F	Friends: Subject is confidant	.75259	.12078	.18084
L7F	Friends: Size	.74820	.23379	−.02720
L10F	Friends: Feel close to call for help	.73821	.12775	.10129
L4	Family: Feel close to call all for help	.10720	.78354	.05675
L3	Family: Discuss private matters	.13444	.75522	.09387
L6	Family: Subject has confidant	.12349	.72561	−.09826
L1	Family: Size	.00456	.69741	.07216
L5	Family: Subject is confidant	.19466	.68931	−.05017
L2	Family: Frequency of contact	.12175	.67157	−.14488
L9N	Neighbors: Discuss private matters	.05331	−.09103	.74986
L11N	Neighbors: Subject is confidant	.05381	.09595	.74367
L12N	Neighbors: Subject has confidant	.09520	−.06750	.73892
L10N	Neighbors: Feel close to call for help	.16291	.11301	.72315
L7N	Neighbors: Size	.01572	−.00878	.66497
L8N	Neighbors: Frequency of contact	.11012	−.08216	.61167
Eigenvalues		3.18	2.15	
4.83				

for our initial prospectus of a three-latent-factor structure tapping into family, friendship, and neighborhood-based social networks.

Item-total scale correlational analyses (Table 14.3) reveal coefficients ranging from 0.34 to 0.67, indicating that items are sufficiently homogeneous, without excessive redundancy. Similarly, item-subscale total correlations with subscale scores range from 0.67 to 0.78 for the family subscale, 0.74 to 0.84 for the friend subscale, and 0.65 to 0.78 for the neighbor subscale. All correlation coefficients fall within the acceptable range to indicate internal reliability as suggested by Streiner and Norman (1995).

TABLE 14.3   LSNS-18: Item-Total Scale and Subscale Correlations

Code	Item	LSNS-18	Family	Friend	Neighbor
L1	Family: Size	.39	.67		
L2	Family: Frequency of contact	.40	.73		
L3	Family: Discuss private matters	.54	.75		
L4	Family: Feel close to call for help	.51	.79		
L5	Family: Subject is confidant	.54	.77		
L6	Family: Subject has confidant	.48	.78		
L7F	Friends: Size	.60		.77	
L8F	Friends: Frequency of contact	.56		.76	
L9F	Friends: Discuss private matters	.67		.82	
L10F	Friends: Feel close to call for help	.58		.74	
L11F	Friends: Subject is confidant	.66		.79	
L12F	Friends: Subject has confidant	.67		.84	
L7N	Neighbor: Size	.34			.65
L8N	Neighbor: Frequency of contact	.38			.66
L9N	Neighbor: Discuss private matter	.34			.71
L10N	Neighbor: Feel close to call for help	.51			.67
L11N	Neighbor: Subject is confidant	.47			.76
L12N	Neighbor: Subject has confidant	.44			.78

The various versions of the LSNS presented in this chapter are theory driven and are responsive to pragmatic administrative considerations. Each of the three scales—the LSNS-R, LSNS-18, and LSNS-6—are tailored for particular settings in which there has been an expressed desire for refined social support network measures. The

LSNS-R is a general measure of social ties that capture characteristics of *kin* and *non-kin* networks. The LSNS-18 also measures *kinship* ties but in addition distinguishes *friendship* ties from those that are *neighborhood-based*. The LSNS-6 is useful where brevity is key to obtaining the information needed.

All three scales presented in this chapter will benefit from more validation and testing. In particular, each needs further validation among a diverse set of older populations. Also, test-retest reliability is especially needed, given that it could not be conducted in the present analyses because of the cross-sectional nature of the data. The three new versions of the LSNS also need to be compared with other social support network scales. Lubben and Gironda (1996) previously compared the LSNS with the RAND Medical Outcomes Study (Sherbourne & Stewart, 1991) and with the UCLA Loneliness Scale (Russell, Peplau, & Cutrona, 1980). Similar analyses using the newer versions of the LSNS might prove helpful in better evaluating the relative strengths of the three modified versions described in this chapter. It also would be beneficial to clarify whether taxonomies of social support networks, such as the one developed by Wenger (1996), could be constructed from inquiry used in the LSNS-18. If it were possible to construct the Wenger typology or others from the LSNS-18, then it would be possible to evaluate the relative strengths of the various classification schemas with one another using data collected by the LSNS-18.

FURTHER RESEARCH NEEDS

Although there has been much progress in understanding the importance of social ties, more work needs to be done. Further clarification of the types of social isolation and the determinants or risk factors of each is necessary. It is desirable to develop the strategies to help identify high-risk populations and to ascertain whether the social isolation is malleable and under what circumstances. Once this level of knowledge has been reached, it would seem appropriate to consider designing clinical trials to study the relative benefits of different interventions and their ability to alter the factors most salient to social isolation.

Central to all of this future research will be measurement development. Scale development and validation are cumulative and ongoing processes. Social integration scales must be tested on a variety of levels, using both psychometric and practical standards to assess their actual clinical usefulness. Future analysis of the scales should include an assessment of their sensitivity to various differences within and between groups, for example, cultural and sociodemographic differences or levels of health and functional status that might affect response patterns. Improved measures of social support networks are essential to better understanding the reported link between social integration and health. Such knowledge will enhance future gerontological research and geriatric care.

POLICY IMPLICATIONS

James House (2001) recently said, "Social isolation kills." Such a strong statement carries with it obvious policy ramifications. But as House also notes, the social epidemiological evidence has repeatedly shown that social isolation is dangerous to one's health, yet researchers still do not have a clear understanding of why or how social isolation contributes to mortality or serious morbidity. Accordingly, the ramifications of a new appreciation for social ties are only beginning to be revealed. Perhaps the firmest validation of the importance of social ties is in the form of the National Research Council's (2001) call for research to clarify the mechanisms by which social isolation and health are linked.

Even if the exact mechanisms by which social isolation influences health are not known, an examination of relevant public policies can commence. For example, Balfour and Kaplan (2002) recently documented how neighborhood characteristics contributed to the loss of physical functioning of older adults. Such findings can be incorporated into urban planning policies. Building safe neighborhoods in which older adults can access public transportation and feel safe enough to venture outside to visit with neighbors and friends would contribute to maintaining social ties throughout the life course.

The socially isolated are especially vulnerable to natural disasters, and so disaster preparation policies and programs need to be reviewed to anticipate the special needs of isolated older adults. For example, the heat waves of 1995 in Chicago resulted in at least 700 heat-related deaths. Socially isolated older adults were likely victims (Semenza et al., 1996). Although the Chicago heat wave of 1999 claimed fewer lives, once again social isolation and advanced age were significant risk factors (Naughton et al., 2002). Prevention and outreach programs should be developed that could reduce the prevalence of such extreme isolation that contributes to excess vulnerability in times of natural disaster.

Adult protective-service policy and programs need to take special notice of older adults who lack adequate protective social ties, because isolated older adults are also vulnerable to misfortune of the human variety. Older persons without adequate protective social ties are often the victims of scams and other misdeeds to steal their resources. In an era of increasing identity theft, there have been reported cases of older adults losing large sums of money and in some instances having their houses sold out from under them. These are merely a few examples of why a wide array of policies at all levels need to be reconsidered from the perspective of adequate social integration of older adults.

INTEGRATING KNOWLEDGE INTO THE CURRICULUM

If health care professionals are expected to incorporate sensitivity to social ties into their assessment and treatment protocols, then professional education must also be changed to incorporate this subject matter into the curriculum. In social work, consideration of various facets of an individual's social milieu should be infused throughout curriculum. Social functioning is at the core of social work practice knowledge. Unfortunately, core social-integration content often gets lost as social work curriculum is designed around specific populations or problem areas. Depending on the specific content area of the course, there are several approaches to introduce the study of social integration of older adults into course work.

Policy courses consider a wide array of topics and issues that impact the nature of social ties with and among older populations. For example, a review of the impact of current community and housing policies might suggest how they might be modified to foster social interaction further and thus facilitate the nurturing of social ties. Such courses could also consider how existing family policies enhance or impede familial social ties among older adults. An area for new policy development is how best to facilitate stronger social ties among nonrelated individuals. The California State Assembly, for example, recently considered legislation that would formalize the rights and responsibilities of domestic partners. Another suggested classroom exercise would be to set up a mock public hearing in which a student would testify on the need for policy reform.

Research methods courses could ask students to evaluate various assessment tools and decide which measure would work best for their particular population or area of interest. Assessment tools dealing with social support networks could be evaluated from a research and a clinical practice perspective in the social work research courses. Levin (2000) provides a particularly thorough review of measures currently used for the assessment of social functioning.

In terms of a fieldwork practice exercise, students could identify specific social integration measures used at their field placement settings. Furthermore, students could examine intake, assessment, and treatment planning procedures to evaluate how well social integration is addressed in practice protocols. They also should be encouraged to suggest how they would redesign the forms to better consider social ties of older clientele in their practice settings. A needs-assessment exercise considering social integration could be constructed, which might include developing a grant proposal that addressed the unmet needs of particular subpopulations of older adults of increased social integration.

For courses specifically designed to teach social work practice methods, social integration should already be infused into the curriculum. Much of what social workers do involves social networks and social supports. However, such information may be poorly defined and collected in haphazard fashion. An exercise that would facilitate more careful scrutiny of social ties would be to have students conduct a self-appraisal using the LSNS-18 or other standardized assessment tool. The student could compare the relative strength of various dimensions (family, friends, neighbors) and identify areas they would like to work on to round out their networks. Further, they might examine how external factors may impact on their own social ties and project how their social integration profile might change over time. Similarly, the students might construct a retrospective social integration profile on one of their older adult clients.

CONCLUSION

This chapter has reviewed the growing body of evidence regarding social ties. As House (2001) laments, researchers know that social isolation kills but researchers still don't know why and how. At the present, there are increasing opportunities to generate new knowledge in this important research area. For example, Seeman, Singer, Ryff, Love, and Levy-Storms (2002) recently described a plausible biological pathway through which social integration may influence health. In the not too distant future, it may be possible to consider clinical trials to evaluate the relative merits of alternative strategies for promoting social relationships that are maximally health-promotive or, at the very least, that offer protection against the deleterious consequences of extreme social isolation.

An essential building block for such research is good measurement. Given the complexity of the construct of social integration, as well as the breadth of research settings, it is unreasonable at this time to design a single social-support-network scale. It seems far more practical to design measurement instruments for specific populations, with clear indications of how they should be used (Mitchell & Trickett, 1980). Use of such well-targeted social-support-network assessment instruments will yield more valid research results than measurement tools that are less well targeted. In this spirit, the chapter presented three different versions of the LSNS that are tailored for specific circumstances but sufficiently linked to allow for subsequent meta-analyses.

Though future research will explicate more definitive pathways, work can start on building communities and adopting practice models that acknowledge the centrality of social ties to enhancing the health and well-being of older adults. The social cost of ignoring the importance of social ties often goes unnoticed until a major tragedy occurs. Such costs can be avoided by increased sensitivity among policy makers and community planners. Much as community planners are designing community and home environments to be more barrier-free, they also need to commence designing environments that break down barriers to making and maintaining strong social ties.

Finally, all health care workers must respond to the growing body of knowledge regarding the centrality of social ties to the health and well-being of older adults. Geriatricians need to adopt practice protocols to regularly monitor the social integration of older adult clientele. Treatment plans need to consider social interventions that could improve the quality of life, as well as reduce the risk of mortality, among older adults. Much as community health nurses are being urged to screen home-health clients as well as assisted-living residents for social isolation (Tremethick, 2001), social workers and other health care professionals should similarly adopt such practice protocols.

REFERENCES

Adams, R. G. (1986). Secondary friendship networks and psychological well-being among elderly women. *Activities, Adaptation and Aging, 8*, 59–72.

Antonucci, T. C. (1990). Social supports and social relationships. In R. Binstock & L. George (Eds.), *Handbook of aging and the social sciences* (3rd. ed., pp. 205–226). San Diego, CA: Academic Press.

Antonnuci, T. C. (2001). Social relations: An examination of social networks, social support, and sense of control. In J. E. Birren & K. Warner Schaie (Eds.), *Handbook of the psychology of aging* (pp. 427–453). Orlando, FL: Academic Press.

Balfour, J. L., & Kaplan, G. A. (2002). Neighborhood environment and loss of physical function in older adults: Evidence from the Alameda County Study. *American Journal of Epidemiology, 155*, 507–515.

Berkman, L. F. (1984). Assessing the physical health effects of social networks and social support. *Annual Review of Public Health, 5*, 413–432.

Berkman, L. F. (1985). The relationship of social networks and social supports to morbidity and mortality. In S. Cohen & S. L. Syme (Eds.), *Social support and health* (pp. 241–262). Orlando, FL: Academic Press.

Berkman, L. F. (1986). Social networks, support, and health: Taking the next step forward. *American Journal of Epidemiology, 123*, 559–562.

Berkman, L. F., & Glass, T. (2000). Social integration, social networks, social supports and health. In L. F. Berkman & I. Kawachi (Eds.), *Social epidemiology* (pp. 137–173). New York: Oxford Press.

Berkman, L. F., & Syme, S. L. (1979). Social networks, host resistance, and mortality: A nine year follow-up study of Alameda County residents. *American Journal of Epidemiology, 109*, 186–204.

Blazer, D. G. (1982). Social support and mortality in an elderly community population. *American Journal of Epidemiology, 116*, 684–694.

Bosworth, H. B., & Schaie, K. W. (1997). The relationship of social environment, social networks and health outcomes in the Seattle Longitudinal Study: Two analytical approaches. *Journal of Gerontology: Psychological Sciences, 52B*, P197–P205.

Caplan, G. (1974). *Support systems and community mental health: Lectures on concept development.* New York: Behavioral.

Carstensen, L. (1992). Social and emotional patterns in adulthood: Support for socioemotional selectivity theory. *Psychology and Aging, 7*, 331–338.

Cassel, J. (1976). The contribution of the social environment to host resistance. *American Journal of Epidemiology, 104*, 107–123.

Ceria, C. D., Masaki, K. H., Rodriguez, B. L., Chen, R., Yano, K., & Curb, J. D. (2001). The relationship of psychosocial factors to total mortality among older Japanese-American men: The Honolulu Heart Program. *Journal of the American Geriatrics Society, 49*, 725–731.

Chappell, N. L. (1991). The role of family and friends in quality of life. In J. E. Birren, J. E. Lubben, J. C. Rowe, & D. E. Deutchman (Eds.), *The concept and measurement of quality of life in the frail elderly* (pp. 171–190). New York: Academic Press.

Chappell, N. L., & Badger, M. (1989). Social isolation and well-being. *Journal of Gerontology: Social Sciences, 44,* S169–S176.

Chou, K. L., & Chi, I. (1999). Determinants of life satisfaction in Hong Kong Chinese elderly: A longitudinal study. *Aging and Mental Health, 3,* 328–335.

Cobb, S. (1976). Social support as a moderator of life stress. *Psychosomatic Medicine, 38,* 300–314.

Cohen, S., Doyle, W. J., Skoner, D. P., Rabin, B. S., & Gwaltney, J. M. (1997). Social ties and susceptibility to the common cold. *Journal of the American Medical Association, 277,* 1940–1944.

Crohan, S. E., & Antonucci, T. C. (1989). Friends as a source of social support in old age. In R. Adams & R. Blieszner (Eds.), *Older adult friendship: Structure and process* (pp. 129–146). Beverly Hills, CA: Sage.

Cutrona, C., & Russell, D. (1986). Social support and adaptation to stress by the elderly. *Psychology of Aging, 1,* 47–54.

Dorfman, R. A., Lubben, J. E., Mayer-Oakes, A., Atchison, K. A., Schweitzer, S. O., Dejong, J., et al. (1995). Screening for depression among a well elderly population. *Social Work, 40,* 295–304.

Ell, K. (1984). Social networks, social support, and health status: A review. *Social Service Review, 58,* 133–149.

Ehrlich, P. (1979). *The mutual help model: Handbook for developing a neighborhood group program.* Washington, DC: Department of Health, Education, and Welfare, Administration on Aging.

Felton, B. J., & Berry, C. A. (1992). Do the sources of the urban elderly's social support determine its psychological consequences? *Psychology and Aging, 7,* 89–97.

Francis, D. (1991). Friends from the work place. In B. Hess & E. Markson (Eds.), *Growing old in America* (4th ed., pp. 465–480). New Brunswick, NJ: Transaction.

Gironda, M. W., Lubben, J. E., & Atchison, K. A. (1999). Social support networks of elders without children. *Journal of Gerontological Social Work, 27,* 63–84.

Glass, T. A., Mendes de Leon, C. F., Seeman, T. E., & Berkman, L. F. (1997). Beyond single indicators of social networks: A LISREL analysis of social ties among the elderly. *Social Science and Medicine, 44,* 1503–1507.

Heitzmann, C. A., & Kaplan, R. M. (1988). Assessment of methods for measuring social support. *Health Psychology, 7*(1), 75–109.

Henderson, S. (1977). The social network, support and neurosis: The function of attachment. *British Journal of Psychiatry, 131,* 85–91.

Hooyman, N. R., & Kiyak, H. A. (1988). *Social gerontology: A multidisciplinary perspective.* Needham Heights, MA: Allyn and Bacon.

House, J. S. (2001). Social isolation kills, but how and why? *Psychosomatic Medicine, 63,* 273–274.

House, J. S., Landis, K. R., & Umberson, D. (1988). Social relationships and health. *Science, 241,* 540–545.

Hurwicz, M. L., & Berkanovic, E. (1993). The stress process of rheumatoid arthritis. *Journal of Rheumatology, 20,* 1836–1844.

Johnson, D. P., & Mullins, L. C. (1989). Religiosity and loneliness among the elderly. *Journal of Applied Gerontology, 8,* 110–131.

Kaplan, G. A., Seeman, T. E., Cohen, R. D., Knudsen, L. P., & Guralnik, J. (1987). Mortality among the elderly in the Alameda County study: Behavioral and demographic risk factors. *American Journal of Public Health, 77*, 307–312.

Kaufman, A. V., & Adams, J. P. (1987). Interaction and loneliness: A dimensional analysis of the social isolation of a sample of older Southern adults. *Journal of Applied Gerontology, 6*, 389–404.

Kelsey, K., Earp, J. L., & Kirkley, B. G. (1997). Is social support beneficial for dietary change? A review of the literature. *Family and Community Health, 20*, 70–82.

Krause, N., Herzog, A. R., & Baker, E. (1992). Providing support to others and well-being in late life. *Journal of Gerontology: Psychological Sciences, 47B*, P300–P311.

Krause, N., & Jay, G. (1991). Stress, social support, and negative interaction in later life. *Research on Aging, 13*, 333–363.

Larson, R., Mannell, R., & Zuzanek, J. (1986). Daily well-being of older adults with friends and family. *Psychology and Aging, 1*, 117–126.

Levin, C. (2000). Social function. In R. L. Kane & R. A. Kane (Eds.), *Assessing older persons: Measures, meaning, and practical applications* (pp. 170–199). New York: Oxford University Press.

Lin, N., Ye, X., & Ensel, W. M. (1999). Social support and depressed mood: A structural analysis. *Journal of Health and Social Behavior, 40*, 344–359.

Litwak, E. (1985). *Helping the elderly: The complementary roles of informal networks and formal systems.* New York: Guilford Press.

Long, M. V., & Martin, P. (2000). Personality, relationship closeness, and loneliness of oldest old adults and their children. *Journal of Gerontology: Psychological Sciences, 55B*, P311–P319.

Lowenthal, M., & Haven, C. (1968). Interaction and adaptation: Intimacy as a critical variable. *American Sociological Review, 33*, 20–30.

Lubben, J. E. (1988). Assessing social networks among elderly populations. *Family Community Health, 11*, 42–52.

Lubben, J. E., & Gironda, M. W. (1996). Assessing social support networks among older people in the United States. In H. Litwin (Ed.), *The social networks of older people* (pp. 143–161). Westport, CT: Greenwood.

Lubben, J. E., & Gironda, M. W. (2000). Social support networks. In D. Osterweil, K. Brummel-Smith, & J. C. Beck (Eds.), *Comprehensive geriatric assessment* (pp. 121–137). New York: McGraw-Hill.

Lubben, J. E., Gironda, M. W., & Lee, A. (2002). Refinements to the Lubben Social Network Scale: The LSNS-R. *Behavioral Measurement Letter, 7*(2), 2–11.

Lubben, J. E., Weiler, P. G., & Chi, I. (1989). Health practices of the elderly poor. *American Journal of Public Health, 79*, 371–374.

Luggen, A. S., & Rini, A. G. (1995). Assessment of social networks and isolation in community-based elderly men and women. *Geriatric Nursing, 16*, 179–181.

Martire, L. M., Schulz, R., Mittelmark, M. B., & Newsom, J. T. (1999). Stability and change in older adults' social contact and social support: The Cardiovascular Health Study. *Journal of Gerontology: Social Sciences, 54B*, S302–S311.

Miller, P., & Ingham, J. (1976). Friends, confidants and symptoms. *Social Psychiatry, 11*, 51–57.

Mistry, R., Rosansky, J., McQuire, J., McDermott, C., & Jarvik, L. (2001). Social isolation predicts re-hospitalization in a group of older American veterans enrolled in the UPBEAT program. *International Journal of Geriatric Psychiatry, 16*, 950–959.

Mitchell, R., & Trickett, E. (1980). Social networks as mediators of social support: An analysis of the effects and determinants of social networks. *Community Mental Health Journal, 16*, 27–44.

Moon, A., Lubben, J. E., & Villa, V. M. (1998). Awareness and utilization of community long term care services by elderly Korean and non-Hispanic white Americans. *Gerontologist, 38*, 309–316.

Mor-Barak, M. E. (1997). Major determinants of social networks in frail elderly community residents. *Home Health Care Service Quarterly, 16*, 121–137.

Mor-Barak, M. E., & Miller, L. S. (1991). A longitudinal study of the causal relationship between social networks and health of the poor frail elderly. *Journal of Applied Gerontology, 10*, 293–310.

Mor-Barak, M. E., Miller, L. S., & Syme, L. S. (1991). Social networks, life events, and health of the poor, frail elderly: A longitudinal study of the buffering versus the direct effect. *Family Community Health, 14*, 1–13.

Mullins, L. C., Sheppard, H. L., & Anderson, L. (1991). Loneliness and social isolation in Sweden: Differences in age, sex, labor force status, self-rated health, and income adequacy. *Journal of Applied Gerontology, 10*, 455–468.

National Research Council. (2001). *New horizons in health: An integrative approach.* Washington, DC: National Academy Press.

Naughton, M. P., Henderson, A., Mirabelli, M. C., Kaiser, R., Wilhelm, J. L., Kieszak, S. M., et al. (2002). Heat-related mortality during a 1999 heat wave in Chicago. *American Journal of Preventative Medicine, 22*, 221–227.

Okwumabua, J. O., Baker, F. M., Wong, S. P., & Pilgrim, B. O. (1997). Characteristics of depressive symptoms in elderly urban and rural African Americans. *Journal of Gerontology: Medical Sciences, 52A*, M241–M246.

O'Reilly, P. (1988). Methodological issues in social support and social network research. *Social Science Medicine, 26*, 863–873.

Perlman, D. (1987). Further reflections on the present state of loneliness research. *Journal of Social Behavior and Personality, 2*, 17–26.

Peters, G. R., & Kaiser, M. A. (1985). The role of friends and neighbors in providing social support. In W. Sauer & R. Coward (Eds.), *Social support networks and the care of the elderly: Theory, research, practice, and policy* (pp. 123–158). New York: Springer.

Potts, M. K., Hurwicz, M. L., & Goldstein, M. S. (1992). Social support, health-promotive beliefs, and preventive health behaviors among the elderly. *Journal of Applied Gerontology, 11*, 425–440.

Pourat, N., Lubben, J., Wallace, S., & Moon, A. (1999). Predictors of use of traditional Korean healers among elderly Koreans in Los Angeles. *Gerontologist, 39*, 711–719.

Pourat, N., Lubben, J., Yu, H., & Wallace, S. (2000). Perceptions of health and use of ambulatory care: Differences between Korean and white elderly. *Journal of Aging and Health, 12*, 112–134.

Pyroos, J., Hade-Kaplan, B., & Fleisher, D. (1984). Intergenerational neighborhood networks: A basis for aiding the frail elderly. *Gerontologist, 24,* 233–237.

Regnier, V. (1980). *Community analysis techniques: Final report.* Los Angeles: University of Southern California, Andus Gerontology Center.

Rook, K. S. (1984). *Loneliness, social support and social isolation.* Prepared for the Office of Prevention, National Institute of Mental Health.

Rook, K. S. (1994). Assessing the health-related dimensions of older adults' social relationships. In M. P. Lawton & J. A. Teresi (Eds.), *Annual review of gerontology and geriatrics* (pp. 142–181). New York: Springer.

Rubenstein, L. Z., Aronow, H. U., Schloe, M., Steiner, A., Alessi, S. A., Yuhas, K. E., et al. (1994). A home-based geriatric assessment, follow-up and health promotion program: Design, methods, and baseline findings from a 3-year randomized clinical trial. *Aging (Milano) Clinical and Experimental Research, 6*(2), 105–120.

Rubinstein, R. L., Lubben, J. E., & Mintzer, J. E. (1994). Social isolation and social support: An applied perspective. *Journal of Applied Gerontology, 13,* 58–72.

Russell, D., Peplau, L. A., & Cutrona, C. E. (1980). The revised UCLA loneliness scale: Concurrent and discriminant validity evidence. *Journal of Personality and Social Psychology, 39,* 472–480.

Seeman, T. E., Singer, B. H., Ryff, C. D., Love, G. D., & Levy-Storms, L. (2002). Social relationships, gender, and allostatic load across two age cohorts. *Psychosomatic Medicine, 64,* 395–406.

Semenza, J. C., Rubin, C. H., Falter, K. H., Selanikio, J. D., Flanders, W. D., Howe, H. L., et al. (1996). Heat-related deaths during the July 1995 heat wave in Chicago. *New England Journal of Medicine, 335,* 84–90.

Sherbourne, C. D., & Stewart, A. L. (1991). The MOS Social Support Survey. *Social Science Medicine, 32,* 705–714.

Silverstein, M., Chen, X., & Heller, K. (1996). Too much of a good thing? Intergenerational social support and the psychological well-being of older parents. *Journal of Marriage and the Family, 58,* 970–982.

Solomon, D. H. (2000). Foreword. In D. Osterweil, K. Brummel-Smith, & J. C. Beck (Eds.), *Comprehensive geriatric assessment* (p. ix). New York: McGraw-Hill.

Steiner, A., Raube, K., Stuck, A. E., Aronow, H. U., Draper, D., Rubenstein, L. Z., et al. (1996). Measuring psychosocial aspects of well-being in older community residents: Performance of four short scales. *Gerontologist, 36,* 54–62.

Stone, R., Cafferata, G. L., & Sangl, J. (1987). Caregivers of the frail elderly: A national profile. *Gerontologist, 27,* 616–626.

Streiner, D. J., & Norman, G. R. (1995). *Health measurement scales: A practical guide to their development and use* (2nd ed.). New York: Oxford University Press.

Stuck, A. E., Walthert, J. M., Nikolaus, T., Bula, C. J., Hohmann, C., & Beck, J. C. (1999). Risk factors for the functional status decline in community-living elderly people: A systematic literature review. *Social Science and Medicine, 48,* 445–469.

Tremethick, M. J. (2001). Alone in a crowd. A study of social networks in home health and assisted living. *Journal of Gerontological Nursing, 27,* 4–5.

Thoits, P. A. (1982). Conceptual, methodological and theoretical problems in studying social support as a buffer against life stress. *Journal of Health and Social Behavior, 23,* 145–159.

Thoits, P. A. (1995). Stress, coping, and social support process: Where are we? What next? [Special Issue]. *Journal of Health and Social Behavior, 35,* 53–79.

Torres, C. C., McIntosh, W. A., & Kubena, K. S. (1992). Social network and social background characteristics of elderly who live and eat alone. *Journal of Aging and Health, 4,* 564–578.

Turner, R. J., & Marino, F. (1994). Social support and social structure: A descriptive epidemiology. *Journal of Health and Social Behavior, 35,* 193–212.

Vaux, A. (1988). *Social support: Theory, research and intervention.* New York: Praeger.

Wallsten, S. M., Tweed, D. L. K., Blazer, D. G., & George, L. K. (1999). Disability and depressive symptoms in the elderly: The effects of instrumental support and its subjective appraisal. *International Journal of Aging and Human Development, 48,* 145–159.

Weiss, R. S. (1973). *Loneliness: The experience of emotional and social isolation.* Cambridge, MA: MIT Press.

Wenger, G. C. (1996). Social isolation and loneliness in old age: Review and model refinement. *Aging and Society, 16,* 333–358.

Williams, A. W., Ware, J. E., & Donald, C. A. (1981). A model of mental health, life events, and social supports applicable to general populations. *Journal of Health and Social Behavior, 22,* 324–336.

Winemiller, D. R., Mitchell, M. E., Sutliff, J., & Cline, D. J. (1993). Measurement strategies in social support: A descriptive review of the literature. *Journal of Clinical Psychology, 49,* 638–648.

World Health Organization, Ageing and the Life Course Section. (2002). *Active ageing: A policy framework.* Geneva, Switzerland: Author.

Zuckerman, D. M., Kasl, S. V., & Ostfeld, A. M. (1984). Psychosocial predictors of mortality among the elderly poor: The role of religion, well-being and social contacts. *American Journal of Epidemiology, 119,* 410–423.

APPENDIX A
LUBBEN SOCIAL NETWORK SCALE—REVISED
LSNS-R

FAMILY: *Considering the people to whom you are related either by birth or marriage . . .*

1. How many relatives do you see or hear from at least once a month?
    0 = *none*   1 = *one*   2 = *two*   3 = *three or four*
    4 = *five thru eight*   5 = *nine or more*
2. How often do you see or hear from the relative with whom you have the most contact?
    0 = *less than monthly*   1 = *monthly*   2 = *few times a month*
    3 = *weekly*   4 = *few times a week*   5 = *daily*
3. How many relatives do you feel at ease with that you can talk about private matters?
    0 = *none*   1 = *one*   2 = *two*   3 = *three or four*
    4 = *five thru eight*   5 = *nine or more*
4. How many relatives do you feel close to such that you could call on them for help?
    0 = *none*   1 = *one*   2 = *two*   3 = *three or four*
    4 = *five thru eight*   5 = *nine or more*
5. When one of your relatives has an important decision to make, how often do they talk to you about it?
    0 = *never*   1 = *seldom*   2 = *sometimes*   3 = *often*
    4 = *very often*   5 = *always*
6. How often is one of your relatives available for you to talk to when you have an important decision to make?
    0 = *never*   1 = *seldom*   2 = *sometimes*   3 = *often*
    4 = *very often*   5 = *always*

FRIENDSHIPS: *Considering all of your friends including those who live in your neighborhood . . .*

7. How many of your friends do you see or hear from at least once a month?
    0 = *none*   1 = *one*   2 = *two*   3 = *three or four*
    4 = *five thru eight*   5 = *nine or more*

8. How often do you see or hear from the friend with whom you have the most contact?
   0 = *less than monthly*   1 = *monthly*   2 = *few times a month*
   3 = *weekly*   4 = *few times a week*   5 = *daily*

9. How many friends do you feel at ease with that you can talk about private matters?
   0 = *none*   1 = *one*   2 = *two*   3 = *three or four*
   4 = *five thru eight*   5 = *nine or more*

10. How many friends do you feel close to such that you could call on them for help?
    0 = *none*   1 = *one*   2 = *two*   3 = *three or four*
    4 = *five thru eight*   5 = *nine or more*

11. When one of your friends has an important decision to make, how often do they talk to you about it?
    0 = *never*   1 = *seldom*   2 = *sometimes*   3 = *often*
    4 = *very often*   5 = *always*

12. How often is one of your friends available for you to talk to when you have an important decision to make?
    0 = *never*   1 = *seldom*   2 = *sometimes*   3 = *often*
    4 = *very often*   5 = *always*

LSNS-R total score is an equally weighted sum of these twelve items. Scores range from 0 to 60.

APPENDIX B
LUBBEN SOCIAL NETWORK SCALE—ABBREVIATED LSNS-6

FAMILY: *Considering the people to whom you are related either by birth or marriage . . .*

1. How many relatives do you see or hear from at least once a month?
   0 = *none*   1 = *one*   2 = *two*   3 = *three or four*
   4 = *five thru eight*   5 = *nine or more*

2. How many relatives do you feel at ease with that you can talk about private matters?
   0 = *none*   1 = *one*   2 = *two*   3 = *three or four*
   4 = *five thru eight*   5 = *nine or more*

3. How many relatives do you feel close to such that you could call on them for help?
0 = *none*   1 = *one*   2 = *two*   3 = *three or four*
4 = *five thru eight*   5 = *nine or more*

FRIENDSHIPS: *Considering all of your friends including those who live in your neighborhood . . .*

4. How many of your friends do you see or hear from at least once a month?
0 = *none*   1 = *one*   2 = *two*   3 = *three or four*
4 = *five thru eight*   5 = *nine or more*

5. How many friends do you feel at ease with that you can talk about private matters?
0 = *none*   1 = *one*   2 = *two*   3 = *three or four*
4 = *five thru eight*   5 = *nine or more*

6. How many friends do you feel close to such that you could call on them for help?
0 = *none*   1 = *one*   2 = *two*   3 = *three or four*
4 = *five thru eight*   5 = *nine or more*

LSNS-6 total score is an equally weighted sum of these six items. Scores range from 0 to 30.

APPENDIX C
LUBBEN SOCIAL NETWORK SCALE—EXPANDED
LSNS-18

FAMILY: *Considering the people to whom you are related either by birth or marriage . . .*

(L1) 1. How many relatives do you see or hear from at least once a month?
0 = *none*   1 = *one*   2 = *two*   3 = *three or four*
4 = *five thru eight*   5 = *nine or more*

(L2) 2. How often do you see or hear from the relative with whom you have the most contact?
0 = *less than monthly*   1 = *monthly*   2 = *few times a month*
3 = *weekly*   4 = *few times a week*   5 = *daily*

(L3) 3. How many relatives do you feel at ease with that you can talk about private matters?
0 = *none*   1 = *one*   2 = *two*   3 = *three or four*
4 = *five thru eight*   5 = *nine or more*

(L4) 4. How many relatives do you feel close to such that you could call on them for help?
0 = *none*   1 = *one*   2 = *two*   3 = *three or four*
4 = *five thru eight*   5 = *nine or more*

(L5) 5. When one of your relatives has an important decision to make, how often do they talk to you about it?
0 = *never*   1 = *seldom*   2 = *sometimes*   3 = *often*
4 = *very often*   5 = *always*

(L6) 6. How often is one of your relatives available for you to talk to when you have an important decision to make?
0 = *never*   1 = *seldom*   2 = *sometimes*   3 = *often*
4 = *very often*   5 = *always*

NEIGHBORS: *Considering those people who live in your neighborhood . . .*

(L7N) 7. How many of your neighbors do you see or hear from at least once a month?
0 = *none*   1 = *one*   2 = *two*   3 = *three or four*
4 = *five thru eight*   5 = *nine or more*

(L8N) 8. How often do you see or hear from the neighbor with whom you have the most contact?
0 = *less than monthly*   1 = *monthly*   2 = *few times a month*
3 = *weekly*   4 = *few times a week*   5 = *daily*

(LN9) 9. How many neighbors do you feel at ease with that you can talk about private matters?
0 = *none*   1 = *one*   2 = *two*   3 = *three or four*
4 = *five thru eight*   5 = *nine or more*

(L10N) 10. How many neighbors do you feel close to such that you could call on them for help?
0 = *none*   1 = *one*   2 = *two*   3 = *three or four*
4 = *five thru eight*   5 = *nine or more*

(L11N) 11. When one of your neighbors has an important decision to make, how often do they talk to you about it?
0 = *never*   1 = *seldom*   2 = *sometimes*   3 = *often*
4 = *very often*   5 = *always*

(L12N)   12.   How often is one of your neighbors available for you to talk to when you have an important decision to make?
0 = *never*   1 = *seldom*   2 = *sometimes*   3 = *often*
4 = *very often*   5 = *always*

FRIENDSHIPS: *Considering your friends who do not live in your neighborhood . . .*

(L7F)   13.   How many of your friends do you see or hear from at least once a month?
0 = *none*   1 = *one*   2 = *two*   3 = *three or four*
4 = *five thru eight*   5 = *nine or more*

(L8F)   14.   How often do you see or hear from the friend with whom you have the most contact?
0 = *less than monthly*   1 = *monthly*   2 = *few times a month*
3 = *weekly*   4 = *few times a week*   5 = *daily*

(L9F)   15.   How many friends do you feel at ease with that you can talk about private matters?
0 = *none*   1 = *one*   2 = *two*   3 = *three or four*
4 = *five thru eight*   5 = *nine or more*

(L10F)   16.   How many friends do you feel close to such that you could call on them for help?
0 = *none*   1 = *one*   2 = *two*   3 = *three or four*
4 = *five thru eight*   5 = *nine or more*

(L11F)   17.   When one of your friends has an important decision to make, how often do they talk to you about it?
0 = *never*   1 = *seldom*   2 = *sometimes*   3 = *often*
4 = *very often*   5 = *always*

(L12F)   18.   How often is one of your friends available for you to talk to when you have an important decision to make?
0 = *never*   1 = *seldom*   2 = *sometimes*   3 = *often*
4 = *very often*   5 = *always*

LSNS-R total score is an equally weighted sum of these twelve items. Scores range from 0 to 90.

Note: (L*) codes refer to specific variable items as reported in Tables 14.2 and 14.3.

Chapter 15

HOME- AND COMMUNITY-BASED LONG-TERM CARE POLICIES AND PROGRAMS: THE CRUCIAL ROLE FOR SOCIAL WORK PRACTITIONERS AND RESEARCHERS IN EVALUATION

Stephanie A. Robert

Home- and community-based long-term care (HCLTC) programs and policies need to be improved and expanded to meet the needs and preferences of increasingly larger elderly and nonelderly populations who have long-term care needs in the United States. However, progress toward improving and expanding HCLTC programs and policies is hampered by the fact that policy makers and the general public have inadequate knowledge about the strengths and weaknesses of current HCLTC programs. This lack of knowledge is partly due to limitations in the types of program evaluations that have been conducted to date. Evaluations of HCLTC programs have generally focused on outcomes of cost-effectiveness, quality of health care, and health outcomes, to the exclusion of the quality-of-life outcomes that characterize many consumer goals for HCLTC. The contemporary emphasis on consumer-centered care in HCLTC policy, programs, and practice requires a similar emphasis on consumer-centered quality-of-life outcomes in HCLTC evaluation research. This chapter argues that social work practitioners and researchers can reshape public discourse on HCLTC program and policy issues by conducting or contributing to evaluation research that considers multiple perspectives, emphasizing consumer perspectives and outcomes.

SIGNIFICANCE TO GERONTOLOGY, HEALTH CARE, AND HEALTH PROFESSIONALS

Long-term care (LTC) services and supports are required by individuals who need assistance with daily activities due to chronic illness, long-term functional impairments, or both (Noelker & Harel, 2001). More than 12 million Americans need LTC supports. About 57% of them are older adults, aged 65 and older (National Academy on Aging, 1997). Projections suggest that by 2030, between 10.8 million and 14 million older adults will need LTC (Friedland & Summer, 1999). Of people with LTC needs, about 13% reside in nursing homes and the rest live at home or in various types of community residences. Almost two thirds of those with functional limitations who live in the community receive support exclusively from family, friends, and volunteers. Fewer than 10% of community residents with functional limitations rely exclusively on care and supports from formal, paid providers (U.S. Department of Health and Human Services, 1998).

Although most people with LTC needs reside in home or community settings, most public LTC expenditures go toward nursing home care. Medicaid, the primary public payer for LTC, is often criticized for its nursing home bias (Kane, Kane, & Ladd, 1998). States must cover nursing home care for those eligible for LTC services under Medicaid, but are not similarly required to cover LTC services and supports provided at home or in the community. In 1997, 56% of Medicaid LTC expenditures paid for nursing home care, 17% paid for intermediate care facilities for people with mental retardation, and only 24% paid for HCLTC (Citizens for Long Term Care, 2001).

Medicaid spends more on nursing home care than on HCLTC yet is the largest public payer of HCLTC services and supports. States are not required to cover HCLTC with Medicaid funds, but states can choose to provide optional Medicaid personal care services and can develop additional HCLTC services and programs by applying for Medicaid waivers. Under the Medicaid waiver programs, states can experiment with providing HCLTC services to different Medicaid target groups and can choose to limit services to certain geographic areas as well. In 1997, 77% of Medicaid home- and community-based waivers were for people with mental retardation or developmental disabilities, compared to 21% spent on older adults with disabilities (Harrington, Carillo, Wellin, Norwood, & Miller, 2000).

Need for Expansion in HCLTC

To prepare for the greater demand for LTC that is anticipated with a growing aging population, states are trying to find ways to increase and improve their ability to provide LTC services and supports in home and community settings rather than in nursing homes. Currently, about one in five adults with LTC needs who reside in the community reports an inability to receive necessary assistance (Feder, 2001). One survey of state Medicaid officials in 1998–1999 showed that 27 states had waiting lists for HCLTC waiver programs, and 42 states reported having an inadequate number of HCLTC waiver slots (Harrington, LeBlanc, Wood, Satten, & Tonner, 2000), reflecting a high consumer need and preference for HCLTC.

Murtaugh and colleagues (1999) conducted a survey of state units on aging and Medicaid departments in 1998 and found that the states' number one LTC priority was expanding HCLTC, followed by controlling nursing home expenditures and controlling expenditures on all LTC. The states reported particular interest in developing capitated or managed LTC programs and expanding assisted living or other supportive housing options. Indeed, the states have demonstrated their interest in expanding HCLTC services by (a) increasing expenditures for HCLTC services at a faster rate than increases in nursing home expenditures (Murtaugh et al., 1999); (b) asking the federal government to make HCLTC expansion easier by simplifying the Medicaid waiver application process; (c) spending state general revenues to pay for HCLTC (Kassner & Williams, 1997); (d) expanding access to Medicaid personal care services; and (e) designing, implementing, and testing pilot LTC programs (e.g., integrated acute and LTC programs, capitated LTC programs).

Many states are experimenting with new ways of financing, organizing, and delivering publicly funded HCLTC services. For example,

Wisconsin has multiple HCLTC programs, some that cover the whole state and others that are limited to certain counties. Wisconsin has multiple HCLTC Medicaid waiver programs for different target groups (e.g., frail elders, people with developmental disabilities); a Community Options Program funded entirely with state general funds; Medicaid personal care services; a Program of All-inclusive Care for the Elderly; and a Partnership program (combining Medicare and Medicaid funds to integrate and provide acute and LTC services to consumers in select counties). In addition, there is a new pilot HCLTC program in five counties, called Family Care, which is a capitated HCLTC model funded by combined federal, state, and county funds. Evaluations of each of these programs are necessary to determine which ones best serve which consumers, under what circumstances, at an acceptable cost.

Although states have generally been expanding HCLTC programs, there remains great variation between and within the states regarding the types of HCLTC programs available (Leutz, 1999). Spending on HCLTC waiver programs generally increased among all states in the 1990s, but the gap between low- and high-spending states increased significantly during this time as well (Murtaugh et al., 1999). Criteria vary greatly from state to state as to who is eligible to receive care, what services and how much service they are allowed to receive, and who is allowed to provide the paid services and supports. Even within a state, there is a surprising degree of variation, with residents in one county eligible for care that they might be ineligible for in the next county (Kane et al., 1998; Leutz, 1999). Despite the growing expansion of, and interest in, HCLTC services, states still devote only a modest share of their overall LTC expenditures on these services. In 1997, half the states spent less than 7.8% on HCLTC and three quarters spent less than 14.8%. Only five states spent more than 20% of their Medicaid LTC resources on HCLTC (Murtaugh et al., 1999).

Nationally, long-term care is not currently a hot policy topic, with most national efforts focused on providing modest funds to support caregivers, providing opportunities for individuals to purchase LTC insurance, and streamlining the Medicaid waiver process to support states' efforts to increase and improve HCLTC programs (Wiener, Estes, Goldenson, & Goldberg, 2001). The states' responsibility for providing HCLTC services, however, has been further encouraged as a result of the Supreme Court decision in *Olmstead v. L.C.* (1999). The Court held that states may be violating the Americans With Disabilities

Act of 1990 if they provide care to people with disabilities in institutional settings when those persons could be appropriately served in less restrictive home- or community-based settings. Although the full implications of *Olmstead v. L.C.* are not yet understood, most states have responded by preparing plans to expand HCLTC services (Rosenbaum, 2000).

Because of expectations of future LTC demands from the growing aging population, consumer demand and preference for HCLTC, high public costs of nursing home care, and pressure to deal more effectively with HCLTC as a result of *Olmstead v. L.C.* (1999), states are trying to implement and test old and new models of HCLTC services. Social workers should be advocates for increased access and improved equity in access to HCLTC options for people with LTC needs, but this requires that social workers help demonstrate which types of programs are most worth expanding. One of the crucial ways that social work practitioners and researchers can effectively increase knowledge about HCLTC is by improving the way HCLTC policies and programs are evaluated.

PRIOR RESEARCH

The types of knowledge systematically developed about HCLTC programs in the United States have been limited. Evaluations of HCLTC programs have overemphasized cost-effectiveness, quality of care, and health outcomes to the exclusion of quality-of-life outcomes and other consumer-centered and consumer-defined outcomes that are more consistent with the primary goals of HCLTC. As a result, the contemporary public and policy discourse around LTC issues has been hampered.

Overemphasis on Cost-Effectiveness

In the early 1980s, the Health Care Finance Administration (now known as Center for Medicaid and Medicare Services [CMS]) began funding Medicaid home- and community-based LTC waiver demonstration projects in some states. The Medicaid waiver option was developed in response to the criticism that Medicaid had a nursing home bias—that those needing publicly funded LTC services had no real choice but to enter nursing homes. In return for the ability to provide some HCLTC services to a limited group of people with LTC needs, states had to demonstrate that these HCLTC programs were budget neutral—that the cost of providing HCLTC services was no more than the cost of providing nursing home services. Therefore, right from the start, HCLTC waiver programs were justified by their potential cost-effectiveness, even if a primary impetus for implementing the HCLTC waiver program was the belief that providing such alternatives to nursing home care just seemed the right thing to do for community residents with LTC needs.

Federal policy that requires states to prove the budget neutrality of HCLTC programs, thereby emphasizing cost-effectiveness as a primary goal of HCLTC, has been detrimental to the knowledge base and to public discourse regarding LTC policy for two reasons. First, it established a very narrow definition of cost-effectiveness. The *public* costs of LTC are counted in such evaluations, but the *private* costs (in terms of social, psychological, health, and financial costs) to consumers and their families usually are not included in the cost-effectiveness equation. Moreover, even when limiting cost-effectiveness research to a narrow focus on public costs, there remains debate about how to measure cost-effectiveness.

Some research suggests that HCLTC programs are not cost-effective alternatives to nursing homes. HCLTC programs generally serve a less dependent population who have more numerous informal supports available; even if the per person cost of HCLTC is lower than the per person cost of nursing home care, the overall program costs are higher because many more people are being served (Weissert, Cready, & Pawelak, 1988; Weissert & Hedrick, 1999; Weissert, Lesnick, Musliner, & Foley, 1997). Others argue that some HCLTC programs are cost-effective because they have successfully targeted the most needy consumers (Alecxih, Lutsky, Corea, & Coleman, 1996; Nocks, Learner, Blackman, & Brown, 1986). However, these limited debates about whether HCLTC is cost-effective in the narrow sense of public costs diverts attention from the importance of examining cost-effectiveness in the broader sense of integrating private *and* public costs.

The second reason that the emphasis on cost-effectiveness has been detrimental to the public discourse regarding LTC policy is that it has shifted attention away from other important outcomes of HCLTC programs, such as quality-of-life. A true cost-effectiveness analysis would examine not only the money spent on HCLTC, but also whether HCLTC services are adding better value for the money spent (Harrington, Carillo, Wellin, Miller, & LeBlanc, 2000). This involves examining quality-of-care and quality-of-life outcomes in nursing homes, in HCLTC programs, and among people residing in the community with unmet needs, in order to compare the simultaneous costs and value of various arrangements to consumers, families, and society.

The federal government's requirement that Medicaid waiver programs demonstrate the cost-effectiveness of HCLTC programs has set up a self-fulfilling prophecy that ensures an overemphasis on this outcome in research and in public discourse. States developed complex systems to collect data on the HCLTC services provided and the costs of those services so that cost-effectiveness could be measured and demonstrated. Because it was not required, states were not motivated to put in place similar systems to collect data routinely that would measure the consumer-centered outcomes of HCLTC waiver programs. When researchers look to evaluate HCLTC programs, they find reasonable data available from the states regarding service use and cost, but not on quality-of-life outcomes. Therefore, published evaluations of HCLTC programs have consistently highlighted cost-effectiveness as an outcome. The overemphasis on cost-effectiveness in research on HCLTC programs then gets further perpetuated in public and policy discourse.

Overemphasis on Quality of Care

Research on the quality of health care in the United States has been conceptualized using Donabedian's (1966, 1980) differentiation among structures of care, processes of care, and outcomes of care. Quality issues in LTC have historically focused on nursing homes, where quality assurance has been attempted primarily through regulations (Kane et al., 1998; Wunderlich & Kohler, 2000). Nursing home quality regulations have focused on *structural variables* such as staffing adequacy and training, and on *process variables* related to how the services are actually provided. Process variables include what is done (appropriateness of care), when it is done (timeliness), and how well it is done (technical proficiency) (Noelker & Harel, 2001). Quality-of-care regulations and measurements have tended to focus on these structural and process measures of quality rather than on outcomes of care (Wunderlich & Kohler, 2000). This emphasis on structure and process factors in examining the quality of LTC diverts attention from the quality measures that ultimately matter most: quality-of-life outcomes for consumers. Emphasizing quality of care rather than quality of life permits professionals to focus on the structural and process determinants of quality of care rather than on the outcomes. Focusing on outcomes would ultimately necessitate examining more closely consumers' own perceptions of their quality of life, and the extent to which quality of life is maximized in LTC programs.

Overemphasis on Health-Condition Outcomes

When research has examined the actual outcomes of HCLTC for consumers, it often has emphasized outcomes related to physical health rather than quality of life (Kane et al., 1998; Noelker & Harel, 2001). Studies examine whether HCLTC services prevent hospitalizations, prevent negative acute-care health events (e.g., bedsores), or improve or maintain functional abilities. These are certainly important outcomes because many people with LTC needs also have or are at risk of having episodic acute-care needs. However, the overemphasis on these types of outcomes overlooks the fact that many of the important goals of LTC programs have to do with preserving quality of life in the face of chronic care and functional needs.

An emphasis on health outcomes hampers our understanding of HCLTC programs for a number of reasons. It limits our ability to examine the contribution of HCLTC programs to multiple aspects of the lives of consumers and their caregivers. Uniform data on quality of life, consumer satisfaction, and consumer-defined needs and preferences are not routinely or uniformly collected in HCLTC programs. When they are collected, they are not systematically documented and linked to other consumer records, precluding examination of which HCLTC service and support features led to positive outcomes for which consumers. A recent study by Chernew, Weissert, and Hirth (2001) examined the outcomes of a managed home-health-care program and demonstrated well the dilemma faced by researchers attempting to evaluate existing programs:

> Our analysis is limited to four outcomes, though the number that one could model is actually limited only by the availability of data. The outcomes we modeled were death, hospitalization, nursing home admission, and functional decline. . . . The most important omitted outcome is satisfaction of the client or caregiver, for which appropriate data are lacking. Others

omitted for similar reasons include patient locus of control, feelings of dignity, privacy, and self-determination, among others. (p. 1004)

Until quality-of-life outcomes are routinely collected in HCLTC programs, research will continue to judge the effectiveness of HCLTC programs by emphasizing the health outcomes that are more readily available. This results in an emphasis on health and patient safety, which is often accompanied by less emphasis on, and fewer expectations for, consumer autonomy, choice, and quality of life (Applebaum, Straker, & Geron, 2000; Kane, 2001; Kane et al., 1998). This emphasis perpetuates a medicalized model that is driven by professional perception of outcomes, making it harder to move toward and evaluate more consumer-centered and consumer-directed models of care.

In recent years, much attention has been paid to developing objective measures of health and functioning to use with consumers across different health-care settings. The preference for objective measures of health status stems from the belief that health status is most accurately determined by professionals who have specialized and objective knowledge about health conditions. This preference for objective, professional measures of health status in acute care settings has been transferred to LTC settings, although many of the outcomes of interest in LTC are not better determined by professionals than by consumers themselves (Applebaum et al., 2000; Benjamin, 2001; Benjamin, Matthias, & Franke, 2000; Geron et al., 2000). Even the recent development of multidimensional health-related quality-of-life measures does not go far enough in capturing aspects of individual preference for autonomy and choice that are necessary to characterize excellence in LTC settings (Capitman, Abrahams, & Ritter, 1997).

Finally, a focus on health outcome measures perpetuates the view that the best LTC programs can do is prevent or postpone negative health outcomes rather than promote positive outcomes. Instead, we should expect our LTC programs to produce positive outcomes for families and consumers (Caro, 2001; Kane et al., 1998). Research should evaluate the ways in which HCLTC can best achieve favorable consumer-centered quality-of-life outcomes.

FURTHER RESEARCH NEEDS

The research focus on HCLTC program cost-effectiveness, quality-of-care, and health outcomes has deterred progress in understanding how various HCLTC policies and programs contribute to quality of life for consumers. These quality-of-life outcomes are particularly salient in contemporary research on HCLTC because of the recent policy, program, and practice emphasis on consumer-centered care and on consumer-directed supports.

Consumer-centered care is responsive to consumers' needs and preferences rather than being determined and directed primarily by professionals. Consumer-directed supports are a particular way of implementing a consumer-centered HCLTC program. Consumer-directed supports involve consumers' choosing the degree to which they want to (a) determine how and by whom their needs should be met; (b) choose and supervise their care providers; and (c) monitor the quality of their care (Benjamin, 2001; DeJong, Batavia, & McKnew, 1992; Doty, Kasper, & Litvak, 1996; Kane et al., 1998; Wunderlich & Kohler, 2000). Consumer-directed supports are meant to provide consumers a full range of choice and control options, including, on one extreme, choosing to organize and manage their care themselves, or on the other extreme, choosing to have someone else make most decisions and plans. Over half of the states have introduced some form of consumer direction into their public HCLTC programs (Benjamin, 2001), and new consumer-directed models continue to proliferate.

Policy, program, and practice emphasis in consumer-centered care and consumer-directed supports in HCLTC programs requires that the professional perceptions of care should no longer drive measurement of HCLTC outcomes. Consumers should be viewed as the experts in evaluating their own outcomes. Ideally, this means that the ultimate outcomes of HCLTC programs are those selected and those reported by consumers themselves. At the very least, this means that many of the outcomes of interest in evaluating HCLTC policies must be those that are consistent with a consumer quality-of-life perspective.

The irony is that although the design of HCLTC programs increasingly focuses on consumer-centered care and on consumer-directed-supports models (Benjamin, 2001; Kane et al., 1998; Wunderlich & Kohler, 2000), research has not similarly moved toward consistently examining consumer-centered outcomes as the cornerstone of HCLTC program evaluation. Until research aligns with practice, discourse on LTC issues in policy and public arenas will remain similarly fragmented. Social work practitioners and researchers can play a pivotal role in aligning practice goals with the outcomes chosen, measured, and evaluated in HCLTC programs.

There is no single right way to measure outcomes of HCLTC programs. In fact, to promote productive discourse on the topic of LTC policies and programs, it is important to understand multiple perspectives on HCLTC issues, which requires that researchers and practitioners collect information that is consistent with the perspectives of different groups, including, but not limited to, the state (as financers of LTC), LTC professionals (e.g., case managers, social workers, nurses), service providers, consumers, and informal caregivers. Knowledge about HCLTC programs must include information about cost-effectiveness, quality-of-care, and health-condition outcomes. However, consumer perspectives on HCLTC quality-of-care outcomes and quality-of-life issues have been shockingly minimal in most evaluations of HCLTC policies and programs.

Because knowledge of multiple outcomes and multiple perspectives is necessary to further dialogue on LTC issues, social work practitioners and researchers can specifically improve knowledge of consumer perspectives by documenting consumer outcomes of HCLTC programs. The following discussion addresses some issues for social work practitioners and researchers to consider when deciding how to best contribute to improving knowledge about consumer perspectives and outcomes in HCLTC.

Examining Unmet Needs

Research on unmet needs or underuse of HCLTC services examines the assessment of an individual's need for assistance compared with the level of assistance actually received from informal or formal sources. Often, such research measures a person's need for assistance with activities of daily living (ADLs), such as toileting, bathing, transferring, eating, and dressing, or instrumental activities of daily living (IADLs), such as balancing a checkbook or preparing meals, and then measures whether or not assistance is being provided to meet those needs. Measures of unmet need have been important in helping to estimate the general extent of unmet need for LTC services in the community. However, these crude measures do not assess the extent of need, different types or domains of need, the extent of assistance, or the quality of assistance (Kane et al., 1998; Morrow-Howell, Proctor, & Dore, 1998; Wunderlich & Kohler, 2000).

Examining Adequacy of Care

Measuring adequacy of care goes a step beyond measuring unmet need by integrating quality of care considerations. As one example,

Morrow-Howell and colleagues (1998) examined adequacy of care by assessing need for assistance with 14 ADLs, assessing the degree to which those needs were met through informal and formal assistance, and assessing the quality of the care that was provided. Their approach produces a number of scores that indicate levels and types of unmet need, quality of formal help, quality of informal help, adequacy of quantity of help, and an overall measure of adequacy of care that takes into consideration quantity of care and quality of care. However, these measures focus primarily on quantity of care and quality of care with little attention to quality-of-life outcomes.

Examining Positive HCLTC Outcomes

Caro, Gottlieb, and Safran-Norton (2000) propose a quality of circumstances framework which, like the unmet need and adequacy-of-care models, incorporates content on ADLs and IADLs. In addition, it includes quality-of-life measures such as privacy, autonomy, and activity, emphasizing evidence for favorable outcomes of home care services. Caro (2001) suggests that "the home care field may be more successful in capturing public imagination and public resources when it presents evidence of 'improving lives' than when it demonstrates that it 'reduces unmet needs' " (p. 308).

Similarly, Kane and colleagues (1998) argue that a therapeutic approach to LTC should replace the prevailing compensatory approach to LTC. The compensatory care approach to LTC involves assessing a client's needs and developing a care plan to compensate for deficits. A successful intervention is often evaluated by whether the care plan was carried out and by the absence of negative events such as bedsores, hospitalizations, or client complaints. In contrast, a therapeutic approach emphasizes that good care should lead to positive outcomes rather than the absence of negative outcomes.

Examining Consumer-Centered Quality of Life

The policy and practice trend that emphasizes consumer-centered care, combined with the opportunity to highlight the underrecognized positive contributions of HCLTC policies and services to the lives of consumers, move us toward HCLTC research that emphasizes consumer-centered quality-of-life outcomes. Yet measuring quality-of-life outcomes in HCLTC programs is a difficult task. The components of quality of life vary across individuals and even vary over time and context for an individual (Brown, 2000). Moreover, which aspects of quality of life are likely to be most salient in an HCLTC setting? One reason some people want to avoid examining quality-of-life outcomes in LTC is that it is unrealistic to expect an HCLTC program to be responsible for a person's entire quality of life. Which aspects of quality of life are most likely to be affected, either positively or negatively, by an HCLTC program? Most of the factors contributing to an individual's quality of life, either positively or negatively, fall outside the purview of HCLTC programs.

However, social workers and other health professionals working in LTC recognize that a person's quality of life can become vulnerable when he or she needs LTC assistance. The degree to which and the way in which a person's LTC needs are met can, at the very least, contribute to the preservation of a consumer's quality of life. It is also clear, when listening to LTC consumers, that there are a number of quality-of-life themes that commonly arise, particularly when people are faced with health, functional, and cognitive impairments. Recent efforts to examine quality-of-life outcomes in LTC settings have been based on identifying these common quality-of-life domains expressed by consumers of LTC programs. For example, Kane and colleagues (Kane, 2001; Kane et al., 2000) have distinguished 11 domains of quality of life:

- sense of safety, security, and order
- physical comfort
- enjoyment
- meaningful activity
- relationships
- functional competence
- dignity
- privacy
- individuality
- autonomy and choice
- spiritual well-being

If these outcomes can be measured successfully, then researchers can examine how various HCLTC programs affect these outcomes (Kane, 2001). Each of the outcome domains can be measured in its positive or negative form. Emphasizing accentuating the positive form, Kane suggests that "absence of bedsores, absence of depression, absence of malnutrition—these are hardly evidence of a good quality of life or goals to inspire generations of care providers" (p. 297).

As another example, the Wisconsin Department of Health and Family Services is assessing the consumer outcomes of its pilot HCLTC program, called Family Care, by examining 14 personal outcomes and assessing the degree to which those outcomes are met in the Family Care program (Department of Health and Family Services [DHFS], 2002). The 14 outcomes are divided into three categories. In the category of self-determination and choice, the first seven outcomes include consumers' (a) being treated fairly, (b) having privacy, (c) having personal dignity and respect, (d) choosing their services, (e) choosing their daily routines, (f) achieving their employment objectives, and (g) being satisfied with services. In the category of community integration, three outcomes involve consumers' (a) choosing where and with whom they live, (b) participating in the life of the community, and (c) remaining connected to informal support networks. Regarding the health and safety category, four outcomes involve consumers' (a) being free from abuse and neglect, (b) having the best possible health, (c) being safe, and (d) experiencing continuity and security. These 14 personal outcomes were identified by a working group of consumers, providers, advocates, and staff of various divisions in the Wisconsin Department of Health and Family Services. The outcomes are meant to be global (applying to all people, old or young, with or without disabilities), holistic (covering quality-of-life aspects of community integration, self-determination, and choice, as well as health and safety), and flexible (designed to take into account each individual's attitudes, culture, etc.).

These are just two examples of the types of efforts being developed to examine quality-of-life outcomes in HCLTC settings. What is important to note is that there is no agreement yet on how best to measure consumer-centered quality-of-life outcomes. Until we develop better consumer-centered outcome-measurement strategies, it will be difficult to understand the impact of HCLTC programs on consumers' quality of life and even more difficult to compare the effectiveness of different programs.

Objective Versus Subjective Measures

One of the most important yet complicated decisions to make about measuring the outcomes of HCLTC programs is determining whether the measures should be objective or subjective. This decision is further complicated by the fact that objectivity and subjectivity can refer to two separate issues. Objectivity and subjectivity call into question who should report on the outcome measure (self-assessed, proxy, or professional assessment), as well as who should choose and define the outcome that is to be assessed in the first place.

Because outcome measurement in LTC has primarily focused on health outcomes and on quality-of-care structure and process variables, professional assessments of these outcomes have dominated LTC research. However, to the degree that a consumer's personal preferences and choices determine the quality of the outcome being measured, self-rating of the outcomes may be more appropriate than professional ratings in most HCLTC settings (Benjamin, 2001; Geron, 1998; Geron et al., 2000).

Research generally finds that self-reports of health, quality-of-care, and quality-of-life outcomes tend to be more positive than professional reports (Geron et al., 2000; Kane et al., 1998; Morrow-Howell et al., 1998; Wunderlich & Kohler, 2000). Most consumers report satisfaction with the services they receive and with the quality of their health and life, particularly when global or general measures are used. There are questions about whether a more positive self-report reflects a consumer's actual experience or instead reflects either (a) a consumer's reluctance to complain about his or her care or situation because of a desire to please or a fear of repercussions (fear of care providers or fear of being denied the ability to make choices); or (b) an unrealistic consumer assessment of his or her true situation.

Professionals are often chosen to evaluate HCLTC outcomes because of concerns that a consumer's positive self-report is due to one of the latter two explanations. Professionals are assumed to have objective standards that will lead to consistent measurement across consumers. Under this assumption, noted variations in consumer outcomes, as evaluated by professionals, will reflect true consumer differences. Although this consistency or objectivity is usually seen as an advantage, it can be a major flaw. Under consumer-centered models of care, researchers assume that consumers will differ in their preferences and choices, even under similar conditions. Therefore, researchers should also expect that consumers will differ in how they report experiences, based on their preferences. Under these assumptions, subjective reports of outcomes are not only preferred but are required in order to evaluate true quality of consumer-centered care (Geron, 1998; Geron et al., 2000; Kane, 2001).

There are concerns about whether people with severe physical or cognitive disabilities are able to evaluate their own condition and preferences. Proxy respondents (often informal care providers) are often used when consumers have cognitive impairments. Proxy respondents should be used only after serious consideration is given to whether it is truly necessary. There is evidence that consumers with mild to moderate cognitive impairments are able to consistently express their LTC preferences and choices (Brown, 2000; Feinberg & Whitlatch, 2001). There is also evidence that proxy respondents do not necessarily accurately represent either factual or preference information of consumers (Egan & Kadushin, 2000; Kane et al., 1998). Therefore, if an HCLTC evaluation is emphasizing consumer-centered outcomes, special attention should be given to facilitating consumer-reported outcomes as much as possible.

Although consumers are asked to report on their own outcomes in some HCLTC evaluations, and professional assessments of outcomes are gathered in other evaluations, a third option is the blended model. In this model, professionals (e.g., social workers, nurses) or trained interviewers conduct extensive interviews with consumers (and sometimes also with care providers and case managers) to elicit their responses about a number of quality-of-care and quality-of-life issues. The interviewer then completes the specific ratings of consumer quality-of-care and quality-of-life outcome measures, on the basis of comprehensive information gathered during the interviews. For example, Wisconsin's Family Care pilot LTC program is training interviewers in assessment techniques developed by the Council on Quality and Leadership. Assessments involve conducting interviews with consumers to determine a consumer's personal preferences related to outcomes, whether or not the outcomes are met, and how they are met. The process incorporates methods for ensuring interrater reliability, that is, making certain each interviewer conducts the interview process and the outcome survey in the same way. The process also involves flexibility based on the verbal skills of the consumer, on collecting complementary information from documents, and on collecting information from the lead professional on a consumer's care management team (DHFS, 2002).

The question of who should choose the appropriate outcomes to assess in HCLTC evaluations is even more complicated. In most HCLTC evaluations, consumers, proxy respondents, or professionals are asked predetermined, closed-ended questions about particular outcomes. The outcomes under study are usually chosen or defined by the researchers in advance. For example, in the unmet needs approach, ADL and IADL functional measures are used. In the adequacy-of-care approach, quality measures are added, although the choice of quality indicators is made by the researchers.

In a truly consumer-centered model of care, the goals and outcomes of a care plan are determined by the consumer. By definition, the goals of HCLTC services and supports will vary across consumers. Therefore, in order to understand the success of HCLTC programs, we ultimately need to understand each consumer's particular goals and then assess the extent to which those individual goals were met. Defining standardized measures of appropriate outcomes for HCLTC programs may, on average, map onto the goals and preferences of groups of consumers, but such measurement approaches will not measure the success of a program as defined by each consumer. However, conducting large-scale evaluations of HCLTC programs is difficult to do without developing standardized outcome measurements. There are advantages to developing reliable and valid measures of consumer outcomes in HCLTC, not the least of which is the ability to use these measures across different programs to compare the relative success of different types of programs. Successful evaluations of consumer-centered HCLTC programs will be those that are best able to match the measurement of consumer-centered goals with measurement of consumer-centered outcomes.

POLICY IMPLICATIONS

Expanding and improving HCLTC programs is not currently high on the national political agenda, leaving the states to face immediate dilemmas about how to do so. States recognize that the increasing need for formal LTC services and supports, the increasing demand for services to be available at home and in the community, the high costs of state-funded nursing home care, and the legal or moral challenges from *Olmstead v. L.C.* (1999) all require that HCLTC be made more accessible to consumers. Social work practitioners and researchers have a real opportunity and obligation to shape how HCLTC programs and policies develop and change to best meet the needs of consumers.

However, to take advantage of this opportunity, research is needed that can better inform us about what types of HCLTC programs work for whom, why, and in what circumstances. Previous HCLTC evaluation research has focused too heavily on cost-effectiveness, quality-of-care, and health-condition outcomes, to the exclusion of consumer-centered quality-of-life outcomes. Social work practitioners and researchers must help develop and conduct research that can better evaluate the quality-of-life outcomes that are most important to HCLTC consumers. At a time when a seemingly endless variety of pilot HCLTC programs are being implemented across the country, the successes and failures of different programs to maintain and improve consumer quality of life need to be examined and understood.

Moreover, a better understanding of the quality-of-life outcomes of HCLTC programs provides the information needed to inform policy and program debates regarding the potential trade-offs between different outcomes (such as quality-of-life, quality-of-care, and health-condition) and cost-effectiveness. Increasing and improving HCLTC programs will certainly require trade-offs. How much is society willing to pay for HCLTC services? What type of positive outcome is society willing to pay for? Until there is better information about the actual positive outcomes of model HCLTC programs for consumers, these discussions will continue to be incomplete and uninformed.

INTEGRATING KNOWLEDGE INTO THE CURRICULUM

As the demand for long-term supports and services grows, the need for social workers with interests and skills in this area is growing as well. Schools of social work should consider including a comprehensive advanced practice course on LTC from a generalist perspective. Consistent with developments in the field, this course would integrate students who have interests in serving older adults, people with developmental disabilities, and nonelderly adults with physical disabilities. It would emphasize cutting-edge practice on how to facilitate consumer-centered and consumer-directed supports in LTC. It would include content on how to conduct and evaluate research on LTC programs and policies. Moreover, it would also focus on how to use social work knowledge about LTC practice to inform changes in LTC programs and policies at local, state, and national levels.

All social workers are involved with people who are dealing either directly (as consumers) or indirectly (as family members or other informal supports) with LTC issues. Therefore, beyond advanced courses that focus specifically on LTC issues, some LTC content should be included throughout the social work curriculum. For example, foundation-year policy courses must include content on LTC policy and programs, describing the complex patchwork of institutional and community-based programs and policies that characterize LTC and discussing the implications of the *Olmstead v. L.C.* (1999) decision for the future of LTC policy. Moreover, because states are implementing a variety of different LTC pilot programs, comparing and contrasting these innovative programs can be used as a tool to explain general health policy concepts and terms such as capitation, cost-shifting, risk-adjustment, and devolution.

Social work courses or modules on ethical issues can use HCLTC issues to highlight many of the ethical dilemmas faced by social workers, such as issues around beneficence and safety versus autonomy. In particular, as social work in LTC moves more strongly toward consumer-centered care, social workers need to learn how to better address ethical issues related to the transition from professional-centered to consumer-centered care. In addition, because consumer-centered care is generally a strong value in social work, all students can benefit from learning how to facilitate consumer-centered care in an area where this is particularly challenging—long-term care.

Clearly, social work research courses need to include content on measuring consumer outcomes and on program evaluation. Long-term-care programs can be used as an excellent example to demonstrate topics such as the different methods of collecting data (e.g., survey, health records), dilemmas regarding whom information should be collected from (e.g., consumers, informal care providers, formal care providers, case managers), and measurement of outcomes (e.g., standardized outcomes, self-defined outcomes). Social workers also need to learn how to conduct research that integrates consumers as more than objects of study. Social workers need to integrate consumers in identifying important research questions and in defining research goals, processes, and outcomes.

Finally, and more generally, most schools of social work need to improve students' ability to translate social work knowledge into program and policy change at macro levels. This is not a skill that should be developed only by social work students who are majoring or concentrating in social policy. Improvements in LTC policy and other policy arenas will most effectively come about when social workers with frontline knowledge learn how to translate that knowledge into effective policy and program advocacy.

CONCLUSION

Many social workers in HCLTC settings know what works and what does not work in HCLTC. However, this social work knowledge and experience is not often reflected in the way research on LTC is conducted. Social workers may focus on maximizing quality-of-life outcomes among HCLTC consumers, yet research evaluations of HCLTC programs focus primarily or entirely on cost-effectiveness, quality-of-care, and health-condition outcomes rather than quality-of-life outcomes. What can social workers do to improve the way that HCLTC programs are evaluated? How can social work practitioners and researchers ensure that program evaluations examine the outcomes important to LTC consumers?

The Role of Social Work Practitioners in Improving HCLTC Research

Social work practitioner involvement can range from consulting on ongoing research efforts to conducting research oneself. Social work practitioners often hesitate to get involved in the research process even though they have crucial knowledge about the complexities of home care and understand the types of outcomes that can be expected for different types of consumers (Hughes, 1997). Social workers often take for granted their particular expertise, sometimes assuming that others share this knowledge as well. Researchers who are designing or conducting an HCLTC program evaluation may or may not have expertise regarding the full range of consumer outcomes that are important to consider in the HCLTC context. Thus, consumer quality-of-life outcomes are often overlooked or understudied. Social workers have expertise regarding the outcomes that may be appropriate to measure *and* the processes that would best facilitate the participation of consumers in developing appropriate outcome measures. At the very least, social workers should be involved as consultants on new and ongoing research projects and should ask to be involved if not already specifically invited to participate.

In addition, consistent with the consumer-centered care approach is the idea that consumers should be involved in designing research on the programs that impact their lives. Social workers can help advocate for consumer involvement when working with research professionals who may or may not have experience integrating consumers as participants in the research process. Social workers can also facilitate the participation of consumers by assisting with scheduling, transportation, functional assistance, and other support.

Social workers with little research expertise or no extra time can still initiate the research process in a number of ways. They can advocate with Medicaid and LTC program administrators in the state government to have the state conduct or fund HCLTC evaluation research. They can talk with researchers at a local university, gauging or stimulating other researchers' interest in collaborating. They can talk with local foundations or national foundations (such as the Robert Wood Johnson Foundation) that may have an interest in funding research on model HCLTC programs. In addition, some social workers themselves can conduct research on HCLTC programs. This is often unrealistic because most social workers in HCLTC settings are overworked and overcommitted already. However, if a social worker cannot or does not want to partner with researchers, there is a range of small-scale evaluation methods that could be used to improve knowledge about particular HCLTC programs, including focus groups, in-depth interviews, observation, diaries, and examination of documents, records, or case files (Applebaum et al., 2000).

Finally, social workers can elevate the ethical issues in HCLTC to the level of policy and public debate. Social workers in HCLTC settings deal with ethical issues all the time—balancing consumers' needs for safety with their need for autonomy, balancing cost and care priorities, or balancing the choices of consumers with the preferences of care providers (Clemens & Hayes, 1997; Clemens, Wetle, Feltes, Crabtree, & Dubitzky, 1994; Egan & Kadushin, 2000). Yet social workers deal with these ethical dilemmas privately in the practice setting rather than exposing and elevating these ethical dilemmas to public discourse. For example, instead of asking how a social worker should balance cost of care with quality of life for an individual consumer, policy makers should be addressing this dilemma at more macro levels. What is the balance between public HCLTC program costs and quality of life? What types of quality-of-life outcomes does society think are worth paying for? Social workers can provide policy makers and the public more knowledge about the ethical dilemmas inherent in HCLTC programs, particularly the ones created when consumer perspectives clash with organizational rules and perspectives. To do this effectively, the consumer perspectives and consumer outcomes so often neglected need to be well documented to submit to policy and public scrutiny.

The Role of Social Work Researchers in Improving HCLTC Research

Social work researchers can attend to each of the issues just described regarding involvement of practitioners in evaluation. In addition, social work researchers are urged to study aspects of HCLTC programs that have been understudied. Relatively few social work practitioners and researchers have been heavily involved in evaluating HCLTC programs (with some quite notable exceptions). In fact, Grenier and Gorey (2000) demonstrate that gerontological social work practitioners and researchers have not been heavily involved in evaluation of organizational or community programs more generally, and instead focus most gerontological intervention research on individuals, families, and small groups. When social workers do engage in research on HCLTC programs, the research often focuses on one component of the program such as case management or interdisciplinary teams. Although such research is valuable, social work researchers need to get more involved in evaluating the overall effectiveness of HCLTC programs, particularly those pilot programs that are testing new models of care that integrate several components such as capitated finances, interdisciplinary teams, flexible service plans, and consumer-directed supports.

One specific way that social work researchers can contribute to research on HCLTC programs is by expanding the definition and collection of consumer-centered quality-of-life outcomes. Limitations to program evaluation of HCLTC programs to date are best overcome by researchers who have an understanding of the goals and methods of consumer-centered care. An increasing focus on a consumer-centered approach to HCLTC requires new ways of thinking about and delivering care, determining success, and measuring outcomes. Because consumer-centered approaches are consistent with social work ideals and are taught in contemporary social work curricula, social work researchers are well suited to rise to the challenge of improving measurement of quality-of-life consumer outcomes in HCLTC programs.

There are other ways that social work researchers can also contribute to evaluation of new models of HCLTC programs. For example, with funding from the Hartford Geriatric Social Work Faculty Scholars Program and from the University of Wisconsin-Madison's Institute for Research on Poverty, I have been evaluating early phases of Wisconsin's new Family Care long-term care pilot initiative. I conducted phone interviews with care managers (nurses, social workers, and human service workers) during the first year of Family Care (Robert, 2001), and I am currently conducting follow-up interviews with care managers during the second year of the program. Most appropriately, consumer outcomes are not evaluated until a program is in full operation. However, conducting research on care managers' perceptions of the improvements and challenges of Family Care during its start-up phase provides early, valuable perspectives on the potentials and pitfalls of this new program. For example, the first wave of this study demonstrated that the goal of providing increased flexibility in HCLTC benefits to consumers through Family Care was somewhat hampered by the lack of people in the community who were willing and available to provide personal care services. Although the goals and the design of Family Care were meant to increase flexibility in the use of personal care services, external structural constraints of the workforce were preventing realization of program goals (Robert, 2001).

In addition, this research with care managers allows us to examine how the Family Care program goals of increasing consumer-centered and consumer-directed care are perceived and facilitated by care managers. To what degree do care managers focus on consumer-defined goals and outcomes? To what degree do care managers facilitate consumer-directed care rather than directing care themselves? Examining these process-oriented issues regarding consumer-centered and consumer-directed care provides valuable information in and of itself, but also these process measures can eventually be linked to the consumer outcomes that result.

I am also using research on Family Care to begin documenting the diverse values and beliefs that people hold regarding LTC issues more generally. I asked care managers to rate their level of agreement or disagreement with a series of value statements about LTC, such as "People owe it to their parents to care for them in their old age" or "People should be willing to spend their own savings on their long-term-care needs before the government pays for such care." I intend eventually to collect information on this series of value statements from other interest groups as well, such as from LTC consumers, caregivers, the general public, and state legislators. By directly examining values that surround LTC issues, and demonstrating differences within and between interest groups in these values, I hope to encourage more open debate and discussion about the LTC program and policy issues our society must face.

REFERENCES

Alecxih, L. M. B., Lutsky, L., Corea, J., & Coleman, B. (1996). *Estimated cost savings from the use of home and community-based alternatives to nursing facility care in three states.* Washington, DC: American Association of Retired Persons.

Applebaum, R. A., Straker, J. K., & Geron, S. M. (2000). *Assessing satisfaction in health and long-term care.* New York: Springer.

Benjamin, A. E. (2001). Consumer-directed services at home: A new model for persons with disabilities. *Health Affairs, 20*(6), 80–95.

Benjamin, A. E., Matthias, R. E., & Franke, T. M. (2000, April). Comparing consumer-directed and agency models for providing supportive services at home. *Health Services Research,* 351–366.

Brown, R. I. (2000). Learning from quality-of-life models. In M. P. Janicki & E. F. Ansello (Eds.), *Community supports for aging adults with lifelong disabilities.* Baltimore: Paul H. Brookes.

Capitman, J., Abrahams, R., & Ritter, G. (1997). Measuring the adequacy of home care for frail elders. *Gerontologist, 37,* 303–313.

Caro, F. G. (2001). Asking the right questions: The key to discovering what works in home care. *Gerontologist, 41,* 307–308.

Caro, F., Gottlieb, A., & Safran-Norton, C. (2000). Performance based home care for the elderly: The quality of circumstance protocol. *Home Health Care Services Quarterly, 18*(4), 1–48.

Chernew, M. E., Weissert, W. G., & Hirth, R. A. (2001). Heterogeneity of risk in a managed home health care population. *Medical Care, 39,* 1002–1013.

Citizens for Long Term Care. (2001). *Defining common ground: Long term care financing reform in 2001.* Washington, DC: Author.

Clemens, E. L., & Hayes, H. E. (1997). Assessing and balancing elder risk, safety, and autonomy: Decision-making practices of health care professionals. *Home Health Care Quarterly, 16,* 3–20.

Clemens, E., Wetle, T., Feltes, M., Crabtree, B., & Dubitzky, D. (1994). Contradictions in case management: Client-centered theory and directive practice with frail elderly. *Journal of Aging and Health, 6,* 70–88.

DeJong, G., Batavia, A. I., & McKnew, L. B. (1992, Winter). The independent living model of personal assistance in national long-term care policy. *Generations,* 89–95.

Department of Health and Family Services. (2002). *Family care quality, CMO member outcomes: The 2001 assessment.* Madison, WI: Author.

Donabedian, A. (1966). Evaluating the quality of medical care. *Milbank Memorial Fund Quarterly, 44,* 166–206.

Donabedian, A. (1980). *Explorations in quality assessment and monitoring: Vol. 1.* Ann Arbor, MI: Health Administration Press.

Doty, P., Kasper, J., & Litvak, S. (1996). Consumer-directed models of personal care: Lessons from Medicaid. *Milbank Quarterly, 74,* 377–409.

Egan, M., & Kadushin, G. (2000). The social worker in the emerging field of home care: Professional activities and ethical concerns. In S. M. Keigher, A. E. Fortune, & S. L. Witkin (Eds.), *Aging and social work* (pp. 373–388). Washington, DC: NASW Press.

Feder, J. (2001). Long-term care: A public responsibility. *Health Affairs, 20*(6), 112–113.

Feinberg, L. F., & Whitlatch, C. J. (2001). Are persons with cognitive impairment able to state consistent choices? *Gerontologist, 41,* 374–382.

Friedland, R., & Summer, L. (1999). *Demography is not destiny.* Washington, DC: National Academy on an Aging Society.

Geron, S. M. (1998). Assessing the satisfaction of older adults with long-term care services: Measurement and design challenges for social work. *Research on Social Work Practice, 8,* 103–119.

Geron, S. M., Smith, K., Tennstedt, S., Jette, A., Chassler, D., & Kasten, L. (2000). The home care satisfaction measure: A client-centered approach to assessing the satisfaction of frail older adults with home care services. *Journal of Gerontology: Social Sciences, 55B,* S259–S270.

Grenier, A. M., & Gorey, K. M. (2000). The effectiveness of social work with older people and their families: A meta-analysis of conference presentations. In S. M. Keigher, A. E. Fortune, & S. L. Witkin (Eds.), *Aging and social work* (pp. 227–234). Washington, DC: NASW Press.

Harrington, C., Carillo, H., Wellin, V., Miller, N., & LeBlanc, A. (2000). Predicting state Medicaid home- and community-based waiver participants and expenditures, 1992–1997. *Gerontologist, 40,* 673–686.

Harrington, C., Carrillo, H., Wellin, V., Norwood, F., & Miller, N. (2000). *1915(c) Medicaid HCBS waiver participants, services, and expenditures, 1992–1997.* San Francisco: University of California, Department of Social and Behavioral Sciences.

Harrington, C., LeBlanc, A., Wood, J., Satten, N., & Tonner, M. C. (2000). *Medicaid home and community based services in the states: Policy issues and future directions.* Unpublished manuscript, University of California, San Francisco.

Hughes, S. L. (1997). Impact of expanded home care models. *Social Work Research, 21,* 165–172.

Kane, R. A. (2001). Long-term care and a good quality of life: Bringing them closer together. *Gerontologist, 41,* 293–304.

Kane, R. A., Kane, R. L., Giles, K., Lawton, M. P., Bershadsky, B., Kling, K., et al. (2000). *First findings from Wave 1 data collection: Measures, indicators, and improvement of quality of life in nursing homes.* Minneapolis: University of Minnesota, Division of Health Services Research, Policy, and Administration, School of Public Health. Submitted to the Health Care Financing Administration.

Kane, R. A., Kane, R. L., & Ladd, R. C. (1998). *The heart of long-term care.* New York: Oxford University Press.

Kassner, E., & Williams, L. (1997). *Taking care of their own: State-funded home and community-based care programs for older persons.* Washington, DC: AARP PPI.

Leutz, W. (1999). Policy choices for Medicaid and Medicare waivers. *Gerontologist, 39,* 86–93.

Morrow-Howell, N., Proctor, E. K., & Dore, P. (1998). Adequacy of care: The concept and its measurement. *Research on Social Work Practice, 8,* 86–102.

Murtaugh, C. M., Sparer, M. S., Feldman, P. H., Lee, J. S., Basch, A., Sherlock, A., et al. (1999). *State strategies for allocating resources to home and community-based care.* New York: Center for Home Care Policy and Research.

National Academy on Aging. (1997). *Facts on long-term care.* Washington, DC: Author.

Nocks, B. C., Learner, M., Blackman, D., & Brown, T. E. (1986). The effects of a community based long-term care program on nursing home utilization. *Gerontologist, 26,* 150–157.

Noelker, L. S., & Harel, Z. (2001). Humanizing long-term care: Forging a link between quality of care and quality of life. In L. S. Noelker & Z. Harel (Eds.), *Linking quality of long-term care and quality of life* (pp. 3–26). New York: Springer.

Olmstead v. L.C., (98-536) 138 F.3d 893 (1993).

Robert, S. A. (2001). *Early evidence from Wisconsin's Family Care Long-Term Care Pilot Program: Continuity and change in the provision of formal services* (Special Report No. 80). Madison: University of Wisconsin-Madison, Institute for Research on Poverty.

Rosenbaum, S. (2000). The *Olmstead* decision: Implications for state health policy. *Health Affairs, 19*(5), 228–232.

U.S. Department of Health and Human Services. (1998). *Informal caregiving: Compassion in action.* Washington, DC: Author.

Weissert, W. G., Cready, C. M., & Pawelak, J. E. (1988). The past and future of home and community-based long-term care. *Milbank Memorial Fund Quarterly, 66,* 309–388.

Weissert, W. G., & Hedrick, S. C. (1999). Outcomes and costs of home and community-based long-term care: Implications for research-based practice. In E. Calkins, C. Boult, E. H. Wagner, & J. T. Pacala (Eds.), *New ways to care for older people* (pp. 143–157). New York: Springer.

Weissert, W. G., Lesnick, T., Musliner, M., & Foley, K. A. (1997). Cost savings from home and community-based services: Arizona's capitated Medicaid long-term care program. *Journal of Health, Politics, Policy, and Law, 22,* 1329–1349.

Wiener, J. M., Estes, C. L., Goldenson, S. M., & Goldberg, S. C. (2001). What happened to long-term care in the health reform debate of 1993–1994? Lessons for the future. *The Milbank Quarterly, 79,* 207–252.

Wunderlich, G. S., & Kohler, P. (Eds.). (2000). *Improving the quality of long-term care.* Washington, DC: National Academy Press.

Chapter 16

MEETING THE CHALLENGES OF SOCIAL WORK PRACTICE IN HEALTH CARE AND AGING IN THE 21ST CENTURY

Daniel S. Gardner and Bradley D. Zodikoff

This book explores the fundamental populations, settings, and challenges relevant to social work practice in health care with older adults and their families. In an endeavor to integrate the domains of gerontology and health care into social work education, policy, practice, and research, each author has examined a particular problem or area of social work practice in aging within the context of a changing health-care world. Dramatic shifts in population growth and transformations in the delivery of health care services have had enormous impacts on the lives of older adults and their families. With age, adults are increasingly vulnerable to physical and mental conditions that can affect their independent functioning and quality of life. Radical changes in the financing and distribution of health care, fragmentation in the delivery of social and medical services, and movements toward community-based and consumer-directed care have shaped the ways in which older adults access and utilize health care. Families, which have themselves undergone dramatic changes in recent generations, have taken on expanded roles and functions in the support and care of their kin in later life.

Based on our experiences as health care social workers and as gerontological researchers, the authors of this chapter review significant trends affecting the health and mental health of older adults and their caregivers, in the context of transformations in health care. We explore the implications of these demographic, social, economic, and political trends for effective social work practice, and identify the knowledge and skills critical to enhancing the health and well-being of older adults and their families. Finally, we briefly describe projected interrelated trends in aging and health and suggest directions for future gerontological social work practice in health care.

What are the major trends affecting the health and well-being of older adults and their families?

An Aging Population

Technological and biological advances in medicine and public health in the last century have significantly extended the lives of current generations in the West. As the baby boom generation (the largest birth cohort in our history) reaches the age of 65, the proportion of older adults relative to the rest of the population is expected to mushroom. Census projections suggest that the number of individuals aged 65 or older in the United States will double in the next 30 years to approximately 70 million, representing 20% of the total population (Federal Interagency Forum on Aging Statistics [FIFAS], 2000).

The older adult population is increasingly diverse in terms of age, race, ethnicity, gender, and socioeconomic status. In the next 50 years, for example, the proportion of Hispanic individuals aged 65 or older is expected to triple, representing an estimated 16% of the population. The age gap between the young-old and the oldest-old is widening as well, with the oldest-old representing the fastest growing sector of the population (FIFAS, 2000). Such differences are associated with greater disparities in health and access to care in later life. Chadiha and Adams (chapter 7) suggest, for example, that older women of color are uniquely vulnerable to chronic conditions such as heart disease, diabetes mellitus, and hypertension, and they experience more comorbid conditions than do White women. Gender plays a central role in the experience of aging. Demographically, women live longer and live alone longer than do men. Women of all races are more likely to have more chronic illnesses and functional limitations and to live in poverty (Hooyman & Kiyak, 2002; Sharlach, Damon-Rodriguez, Robinson, & Feldman, 2000).

Increasing Prevalence of Chronic Illness and Disability

Aging itself is associated with increased vulnerability to a variety of chronic physical and mental health conditions (Berkman, 1996; Burnette & Kang, chapter 6). Chronic illnesses and conditions such as diabetes, heart disease, and cancer are enduring and episodic in nature and often require monitoring and management for extended periods. In older adults, chronic illnesses contribute to declines in functioning and quality of life as well as increases in mortality and health care costs (Adamek, chapter 2; Burnette & Kang, chapter 6). Mental health concerns such as late-life depression (see Adamek, chapter 2), dementia (see Semke, chapter 3), and developmental disabilities (see McCallion & Kolomer, chapter 9) may present additional risks due to the associated stigma. In addition, there are significant gaps in knowledge about geriatric mental health among formal and informal caregivers.

Physical and mental conditions that diminish one's capacity to function independently often lead to a need for long-term care in community or residential settings. Dementia, for example, is one of the primary precursers to the need for long-term care among older adults (Semke, chapter 3). Despite recent declines in nursing home residence, in 1997 an estimated 1.5 million individuals aged 65 or older (4% of the older population) resided in nursing homes (FIFAS, 2000). Nursing home residents were more likely to be women (75% of all residents) and to have serious functional limitations (e.g., incontinence and problems with feeding or mobility) that limit their ability to live on their own.

The Intergenerational Context of Aging

Because of declining mortality and extended life expectancy, families have evolved to include multiple generations and a diversity of kinship relationships. Older adults spend an increasing amount of time occupying a variety of intergenerational roles, and many rely more on their spouses and other family members for instrumental and emotional support (Hooyman & Kiyak, 2002; Scharlach et al., 2000). The family is by far the primary source of support for older adults with serious illnesses or disabilities and those requiring long-term care (National Alliance for Caregiving/American Association of Retired Persons [NAC/AARP], 1997; Penrod, Kane, Kane, & Finch, 1995). Although most older adults live and function within the context of multigenerational families, health care and social service systems continue to focus on the individual as the unit of care (Golden & Corely Saltz, 1997).

Many older adults are themselves caregivers. More than 12% of caregivers of older adults are aged 65 years or older (NAC/AARP, 1997). Caregiving most often involves a reciprocal relationship with an ill partner, spouse, or parent. In addition, a growing number of older women have assumed the role of custodial grandparents, due most often to the biological parent's substance abuse, incarceration, physical disability, or death (Kropf & Wilks, chapter 8). These intergenerational family relationships often carry both "strains and gains" (Poindexter & Boyer, chapter 10). Although custodial grandparents often derive emotional rewards (e.g., companionship, pride, a sense of mastery) from their caregiving roles, assuming parenting responsibilities in later life is developmentally dissonant and can negatively affect one's psychosocial and physical health (Kropf & Wilks; Poindexter & Boyer).

One risk associated with the increased burden of family caregiving is the problem of elder mistreatment. Paveza and VandeWeerd (chapter 11) point out that although most social workers are aware of the individual and societal costs of elder mistreatment, little is known about the incidence, the precipitating factors, the consequences, and effective treatment. As with other types of family violence, elder abuse is believed to be underreported and underdiagnosed, due to a lack of thorough assessment and knowledge of the problem among health care professionals. There remains a serious need for empirical research, comprehensive planning, and policy to address this multifaceted public health concern.

Cost Containment and Focus on Outcomes

The rising cost of health care in the second half of the last century has led to radical changes in the public and private financing of health care. Efforts to contain the costs of care have resulted in the implementation of a variety of managed care and prospective payment systems in physical and mental health care (Berkman, 1996; Naleppa, chapter 5; Robert, chapter 15). The increased use of the primary care physician as gatekeeper and of precertification requirements has served to complicate an already complex system and to limit older adults' access to health care (Berkman, 1996).

This transformation of health care to a more market-driven economy is associated with a greater emphasis on producing effective outcomes with the least possible investment of resources. Third-party and public insurers are much more actively involved in specifying and directing treatment protocols through their selective financing of activities that produce cost-effective outcomes. This trend affects older adults because the drive to save health care costs may overshadow concerns about the needs of consumers (Robert, chapter 15).

Decentralization and Fragmentation in Health Care

Efforts at cost containment, paired with the development of diagnostic and treatment technologies that can be delivered more cost-effectively in ambulatory settings, have led to the rapid decentralization and deinstitutionalization of hospital-based care. Hospital admissions and lengths of stay have declined dramatically, and most medical procedures are now performed in community-based ambulatory-care settings (Berkman, 1996; Shortell, Gilles, & Devers, 1995).

With decentralization, physical and behavioral health-care settings that deliver acute, rehabilitative, and long-term-care services have proliferated. Health care has grown increasingly fragmented, requiring consumers to interact with a growing number of health care professionals in a complex array of settings in order to obtain care (Volland, 1996). Older adults, who often cope with multiple illnesses that involve several medical disciplines, are perhaps most affected by the increasing fragmentation in health care (Berkman & Harootyan, chapter 1). Navigating among these often disjointed services demands a working knowledge of health care systems and resources that is daunting to many older adults and their caregivers.

Community-based options have also emerged for long-term care (Lee & Gutheil, chapter 4; Robert, chapter 15). Alternatives to nursing home care such as community residential care and home health care have grown in use during the past 15 years. Valuing the philosophy of "aging in place," such services offer more individualized care in less institutionalized settings (Semke, chapter 3; Lee & Gutheil, chapter 4). Despite individual and family preferences for alternatives to nursing homes, community residential care is still in its infancy; there is little consistency in the design, regulation, or financing of such services across the United States (Semke, chapter 3). There remains a lack of affordable long-term-care alternatives for middle and lower income individuals, reflecting a structural lag in the development of services to meet the changing needs of older adults and their families.

Consumer-Centered and Consumer-Directed Care

Another trend associated with the aging of the baby boom generation is that more individuals are seeking active participation in their own care. Accordingly, the philosophies of consumer-centered care and consumer direction have grown increasingly popular in health and long-term-care services. Representing a continuum of approaches based on levels of consumer involvement in designing and implementing their own care, " 'consumer-direction' has become part of the lexicon among state and some federal policy makers" (Stone, 2000, p. 8). Consumer-centered services specifically prioritize the needs of clients over the needs of professionals. Consumer-directed supports empower older adults and their families with increased choice and control over their own care (Naleppa, chapter 5; Robert, chapter 15). This growing emphasis on consumer-centered care and consumer direction has led to the implementation of public demonstration projects in home and community long-term care (Robert, chapter 15) and of standardized measures to assess consumer satisfaction with home care services (Geron & Little, chapter 12).

What knowledge and skills do social work practitioners need in order to respond to the needs of older adults and their families?

The contributors to this volume have identified a broad range of knowledge and areas of expertise that are essential to effective social work practice in aging, in rapidly changing social, political, and health care environments.

Knowledge About Health and the Emerging Health Care World

Social workers in aging must build continuously upon their knowledge of basic mechanisms of health promotion, illness prevention, and the impact of illnesses and treatment on individuals and families. As diagnosis and treatment become increasingly specialized and older persons interact with a greater variety of medical disciplines, social workers in aging are faced with the challenge of knowing about disease-specific medical and psychosocial issues across virtually the entire range of medical specialty areas (e.g., cardiology, oncology, neurology, psychiatry, endocrinology, rheumatology). Therefore, it is increasingly essential to apply a holistic biopsychosocial approach to understanding physical and mental health, that takes into account older persons' *complete* medical and psychiatric presentation in addition to their coping capacities and social support resources (Berkman, 1996; Netting & Williams, 1998).

Knowledge of mental health and illness, specifically regarding manifestations of psychopathology and symptomatology in later life, is an essential piece of understanding that has clearly been missing in some geriatric settings. For example, as Adamek (chapter 2) points out, depression among older persons in long-term-care settings is underdiagnosed and undertreated. Raising awareness among social workers and other health professionals of the indicators and treatment of geriatric mental-health concerns (including depression, dementia, and developmental disabilities) can make significant differences in their contributions in clinical settings.

In addition, it is critical to understand the workings of health care systems and their financial structures and processes (including prospective payment and managed care systems), as well the availability of public and private resources that support health maintenance and rehabilitation (Berkman, 1996). Social workers must be familiar with eligibility requirements for these resources and know how to disseminate the information effectively among older individuals and their caregivers.

Practice Skills in Health and Aging

Given the transformations in the biological, psychological, social, and political contexts for health care described throughout this book (see

Berkman & Harootyan, chapter 1), health care practitioners in aging must strengthen their foundation skills as well as develop new skills in order to keep pace with the velocity of societal change. Many of these skills are familiar to social work practitioners, in that they have and will continue to form the core skill base of the field. In some areas, social work practitioners will find new ways to accomplish familiar tasks. Social workers will adapt to new modes of information technology and integrate their knowledge of rapidly developing scientific advances in the treatment of disease in order to enhance their abilities to address the psychosocial implications of these discoveries for older patients and their families. Additionally, as evidence-based knowledge on psychosocial interventions is disseminated more rapidly in our information-intensive environment, it is likely social workers will be required to modify and adapt their practice skills and intervention techniques at a rate of change much faster than previously experienced.

In other areas of practice, social workers in aging will be pressed to build upon current competencies and to develop new skills as they are thrust into roles that demand increased preparation and training. The contributors to this book have delineated several core areas in which practitioners must broaden their capacities and skills. These areas—biopsychosocial assessment, counseling and case management over the continuum of care, family practice and advocacy for the needs of individuals and their families—will remain the essential practice skills of all social workers in health care in the twenty-first century.

Cultural Competency Skills

Several contributors to this volume have highlighted the rich heterogeneity of the aging population of the United States. Current and projected cohorts of older persons are increasingly racially, ethnically, and culturally diverse. Gerontological social workers must remain sensitive to the interactions of health and age, race, ethnicity, gender, and socioeconomic status, and they must practice competently and creatively with individuals from a variety of cultural backgrounds. Maramaldi and Guevera (chapter 13) discuss the importance of developing culturally sensitive health services that focus greater attention on the social and cultural contexts of health and illness. They specifically highlight the critical role social workers can play in assessing the culturally influenced health beliefs and health-related quality of life of older adults and their families. By virtue of their biopsychosocial perspective and training, social workers are strategically well-positioned on interdisciplinary teams to assess the impact of health care recipients' and health care providers' cultures on the effective delivery of health care services. It is also essential to facilitate communication among patients, families, and health care providers about culturally related perceptions of wellness, illness, and treatment.

Burnette and Kang (chapter 6) explore the role of self-care among African American elders and add to our understanding of the complex cultural and symptom-specific processes involved in management of chronic conditions. Chadiha and Adams (chapter 7) examine some of the complex associations between poverty and health that put older Black women at risk for developing chronic medical conditions, and suggest the use of empowerment techniques in social work practice with older Black women. Self-awareness, cultural competence, and sensitivity to the influences of culture are essential for promoting health and preventing illness among older adults of all cultural backgrounds.

Case Management Skills and Standardized Assessment

In the midst of dramatic changes in health care, social workers in aging must be able to define their roles and unique contributions to other health care professionals and funders (Netting & Williams, 1998). Berkman (1996) suggests that social workers are uniquely qualified to perform two basic, overlapping roles in health care settings. *Clinical specialists* teach older adults about health and health promotion; counsel and advocate for individuals and families to help them better manage health conditions and treatment; and collaborate with multidisciplinary health-care teams around psychosocial issues, patient and family management, treatment adherence, and ethical issues. *Clinical case managers* engage in education, counseling, and social brokerage designed to guide older individuals and their families through the health care system and gain access to essential resources. In an increasingly fragmented service environment, geriatric social-work case management ensures integration and promotes "seamless service" across the continuum of care (Berkman, 1996; Naleppa, chapter 5).

Effective case management with older adults and their families requires the use of a variety of interrelated skills. Perhaps most fundamental is the use of comprehensive, biopsychosocial geriatric assessment, long the principal tool with which a social worker develops an "appropriate and effective" response to the needs of older individuals and families (Geron & Little, chapter 12). Standardized measures that cover physical, psychological, and social functioning are used for preventive screening and early identification of individual and family needs, to demonstrate the need for social work involvement, to monitor the effectiveness of interventions, and to ensure accountability (Berkman, 1996; Robert, chapter 15). According to Geron and Little (chapter 12), the assessment tools that best support the clinical and policy practice aims of social work practitioners are comprehensive in scope, functional in design, and uniform across users. They also incorporate established measures, balance psychometric precision with practicality, support objective and multiple sources of information, are easy to read and administer, and are culturally sensitive.

As Lubben and Gironda point out (chapter 14), social relations are an essential component of physical and mental functioning in later life. Assessment of the extent and strength of social supports is therefore an important element of the assessment of an older person's health and well-being (Lubben, 1988). Older adults often lack the social ties and related resources that promote emotional and psychological adaptation to illness (Lubben & Gironda, chapter 14). Lubben and Gironda suggest that further research is needed in developing measurement tools, identifying risk factors for social isolation, and developing interventions that integrate the importance of supportive social ties to quality of life in older adults and their families.

Intergenerational Family Practice Skills

The chapters in this volume attest to the importance of multigenerational relationships across the continuum of social and health problems for older adults. The family has long been a core concern of social work assessment and intervention (Germain & Gitterman, 1996; Woods & Hollis, 2000). It is essential, however, to broaden social workers' understandings of health promotion, illness prevention, and treatment in order to incorporate an intergenerational family systems context. Practice with family caregivers and with custodial grandparents, for example, is enhanced by the use of family therapy to help clarify boundaries, roles, and functions (Kropf & Wilks, chapter 8). Social workers must also promote "family practice" in health settings, by communicating familial concerns and advocating that the health care team view and treat families as the primary unit of care (Berkman, 1996; Volland, 1996).

Research Skills and Evidence-Based Practice

Social workers must demonstrate the benefits of assessment, case management, and clinical intervention by focusing on research outcomes in their case planning and by utilizing evidence-based interventions (Vourlekis, Ell, & Padgett, 2001). The application of best practices and developing "critical-path treatment models" are preferred methods to monitor and improve practice with older adults and to demonstrate the effectiveness of social work interventions (Berkman & Harootyan, chapter 1). Research is also an essential component of advocacy for increased funding and policy making to enhance the lives of older adults and their families.

In discussing research on elder mistreatment, Paveza and Vande-Weerd (chapter 11) delineate several areas of necessary research that can be generalized to other areas in gerontological health. Research is needed on the incidence and prevalence of social and health conditions or concerns, and on the etiology of these concerns. Empirical evaluations of practice modalities and approaches are also increasingly important in this outcomes-oriented health care environment. In addition, it is essential that researchers explore and develop the theoretical underpinnings of inquiries into such areas as self-care among older adults (Burnette & Kang, chapter 6) and elder abuse (Paveza & Vande-Weerd, chapter 11).

Advocacy and Empowerment Skills

Social workers must continue to intervene actively on multiple levels to ensure the development and delivery of "a just and quality" system of care for older adults and their families (Lee & Gutheil, chapter 4). Practitioners in aging are ideally positioned to advocate within health care systems to balance the desire for cost efficiency and successful outcomes with services that best meet the needs of older adults and their families. In today's constantly changing health care environment, practitioners must feel comfortable shifting between and integrating

their roles and skills in micro-level, meso-level, and macro-level interventions. Chadiha and Adams (chapter 7), for example, suggest that
empowerment strategies are best implemented with older Black
women through collaboration and teamwork with a variety of health
care providers, across various levels of practice.

Skills for Ethical Practice

Given current trends, it is probable that social workers will increasingly be called upon to serve as family therapists, mediators, consultants, and advocates in addressing ethical dimensions of medical
decision-making, particularly in the arena of end-of-life care. Ethical
issues involving the decision to continue or withhold life-sustaining
interventions at the end of life are particularly prominent in the current
health care environment, especially in hospitals where the majority
of deaths of older persons occur. Social workers will also need to
address ethical issues surrounding the expectations and responsibilities placed on family caregivers who must assume longer term and
more technologically advanced care tasks with minimal training and
support from an overburdened health care system (Levine & Zuckerman, 1999). Mediating between the individual needs, perspectives,
values, and quality of life of *all* members of a family system demands
a high skill level of ethical practice.

*How can social workers best prepare for the future of health care
practice with older adults?*

Many of the demographic, social, economic, and political trends described earlier in this chapter are expected to continue well into the
future. It is clear that the aging of society will continue for most of
the twenty-first century, as will evolutions in health care and the
practice of health care social work. The expansion and diversification
of the older adult population will most probably generate increasing
demand for home health care and long-term care services (Cornman &
Kingson, 1996). As society grows older and a greater proportion of
adults experience chronic illnesses and conditions, our expectations
of later life will change dramatically with respect to employment,
housing, social relationships, independent functioning, and quality of
life. In fact, the notion of what constitutes "productive" aging is an

evolving construct in the research literature as reflected by these changes in society at large (Morrow-Howell, Hinterlong, & Sherraden, 2001).

Given the present descriptors of the older baby-boom cohort, Silverstone (1996) predicts that older adults of tomorrow will be more confident, will remain in the workforce longer, and will take active roles in advocating for themselves in terms of health care policies and health resources. It is likely that the demand for consumer-directed care in physical, mental, and long-term-care settings will increase, and a variety of individual options will emerge in the near future. The ability of older adults to take control over their care will need to be balanced, however, with the cost-effectiveness of services and the needs of the larger population. Cornman and Kingson (1996) suggest that diminishing economic resources and competing needs among an increasingly diverse population might lead to a decline in public financing of health care (including Social Security) for older adults. In turn, aging families will continue to absorb a growing share of the care and support of older adults, and a larger proportion of families will include multiple intergenerational care arrangements.

In the face of increasing diversity, fragmentation of services, and dwindling public funding for health care, the use of social brokerage and advocacy skills for the needs of vulnerable older populations and social workers' skills in cultural competency will grow in importance. Gerontological social workers of the future will need to be flexible, knowledgeable, and independent in their practice. Research will become an increasingly vital part of developing, implementing, and evaluating effective and efficient services. And social work practitioners, researchers, and educators in aging and health care will need to define their roles further and to collaborate with other health care professionals in a continually evolving health care world.

CONCLUDING THOUGHTS

The John A. Hartford Foundation launched the Geriatric Social Work Initiative in 1999 to build the capacity of the social work profession to improve the health and well-being of older adults and their families. This book represents the scholarship of a few of the many gerontological social work researchers, practitioners, and educators who are a part of the Hartford Initiative. What has been learned about the practice of gerontological social work in health care from the work presented here? Several themes have emerged that run through each of the chapters in this book.

First, social work practice in aging is inextricably linked with social work practice in health care. Effective gerontological social workers are active and essential participants of the evolving health-care world, and they practice creatively and independently across a continuum of services in order to enhance the health and well-being of older adults and their families. Social work fulfills an important role in developing and delivering health care services and, through the process of case management, in helping older adults and their families gain access to the appropriate services for their unique situations (Naleppa, chapter 5). Given what we know about disparities in health and in access to health care, it is essential that the profession continue to advocate for equitable distribution of resources and to attend to issues of gender, race, ethnicity, and class (Chadiha & Adams, chapter 7).

Second, it is increasingly clear that it is no longer possible to view aging as solely the purview of gerontological social workers (Berkman & Harootyan, chapter 1). In light of current and future demographic shifts, the profession as a whole will be at a costly disadvantage if it continues to ignore the needs of older adults and their families. Social work practitioners, educators, researchers, and policy makers must "fully embrace gerontological practice" (Scharlach et al., 2000, p. 525) and develop, implement, and evaluate intergenerational approaches to meet the evolving needs of this population. The shortage of trained, competent practitioners and educators in aging needs to be addressed as does the infusion of gerontological content throughout social work curricula in bachelor's and master's-level programs (Scharlach et al., 2000; Volland, 1996). Moreover, there is a need to address the negative attitudes and myths about work in aging that may prevent social workers from participating in this emerging and rewarding field of practice.

Third, the future of social work in geriatric health care relies on social work's ability to generate meaningful research into the epidemiology and theoretical bases of health-related psychosocial problems and to develop and evaluate effective interventions for addressing these concerns. The authors in this book, for example, suggest the need for further research that tests existing methods of assessment and develops new ones (Lubben & Gironda, chapter 14); evaluates outcomes in case management (Naleppa, chapter 5) and long-term-care models (Robert, chapter 15); and explores the impact of staff attitudes toward mental illness on the care of older long-term-care residents (Adamek, chapter 2). Professional social-work programs must integrate evidence-based research into their curricula and teach students to use empirically derived intervention approaches and "critical-path treatment models" in gerontological practice (Berkman & Harootyan, chapter 1). Social work research in gerontology needs to be practice-based and must incorporate theoretical, ethical, social, and political contexts of physical and mental health and health care.

Finally, aging occurs primarily within a familial context. An individual's experience of physical and mental illness profoundly influences and is influenced by his or her reciprocal relationships (or lack of relationships) with family members. In addition, a great many older adults provide care for physically or mentally ill or disabled family members (see, for example Semke, chapter 3; McCallion & Kolomer, chapter 9). Gerontological social workers, trained in a biopsychosocial perspective that views an individual in the context of person-in-environment, know the importance of family and intergenerational social relationships in later life. In a health care system that views the individual as the unit of care, social workers must identify and address the psychosocial needs of family members, as well as communicate their concerns to other health care professionals. Social workers must also work to support and advocate for families' efforts to care adequately for the health and long-term-care needs of their elder kin.

Aging is an inexorable feature of living, an experience that has great potential to enhance an individual's quality of life and development while at the same time posing genuine threats to health and independence. Social work practitioners in health and aging are fortunate to work in a field of practice that provides abundant challenges and opportunities to have positive impacts on people's lives. In an era characterized by dramatic changes in population and health care, gerontological social workers are rising to these challenges by working in a variety of ways to enhance the health and well-being of older adults and their families.

REFERENCES

Berkman, B. (1996). The emerging health care world: Implications for social work practice and education. *Social Work, 41*, 541–553.

Cornman, J., & Kingson, E. (1996). Trends, issues, perspectives and values for the aging of baby boom cohorts. *Gerontologist, 36,* 15–26.

Federal Interagency Forum on Aging Statistics. (2000). *Older Americans 2000: Key indicators of well-being.* Washington, DC: U.S. Government Printing Office.

Germain, C., & Gitterman, A. (1996). *The life model of social work practice* (2nd ed.). New York: Columbia University Press.

Golden, R., & Corley Saltz, C. (1997). The aging family. *Journal of Gerontological Social Work, 27*(3), 55–64.

Hooyman, N., & Kiyak, H. (2002). *Social gerontology: A multidisciplinary perspective* (6th ed.). Boston: Allyn and Bacon.

Levine, C., & Zuckerman, C. (1999). The trouble with families: Toward an ethic of accommodation. *Annals of Internal Medicine, 130,* 148–152.

Lubben, J. (1988). Assessing social networks among elderly populations. *Family Community Health, 11,* 42–52.

Morrow-Howell, N., Hinterlong, J., & Sherraden, M. (2001). *Productive aging: Concepts and challenges.* Baltimore: Johns Hopkins University Press.

National Alliance for Caregiving/American Association of Retired Persons. (1997). *Family caregiving in the U.S.: Findings from a national study.* Washington, DC: National Alliance for Caregiving.

Netting, F. E., & Williams, F. (1998). Can we prepare geriatric social workers to collaborate in primary care practices? *Journal of Social Work Education, 34*(2), 195–210.

Penrod, J., Kane, R., Kane, R., & Finch, M. (1995). Who cares? The size, scope and composition of the caregiver support system. *Gerontologist, 35,* 489–497.

Scharlach, A., Damron-Rodriguez, Robinson, B., & Feldman, R. (2000). Educating social workers for an aging society: A vision for the 21st century. *Journal of Social Work Education, 36*(3), 521–538.

Shortell, S., Gilles, R., & Devers, K. (1995). Reinventing the American hospital. *Milbank Quarterly, 73*(2), 131–159.

Silverstone, B. (1996). Older people of tomorrow: A psychosocial profile. *Gerontologist, 36,* 27–32.

Stone, R. (2000). Consumer direction in long-term care. *Generations, 24*(3), 4–9.

Volland, P. (1996). Social work practice in health care: Looking into the future with a different lens. *Social Work in Health Care, 24*(1/2), 35–51.

Vourlekis, B., Ell, K., & Padgett, D. (2001). Educating social workers for health care's brave new world. *Journal of Social Work Education, 37*(1), 177–191.

Woods, M., & Hollis, F. (2000). *Casework: A psychosocial therapy* (5th ed.). New York: McGraw-Hill.

Appendix

SELECTED BOOK RESOURCE LIST

Aronson, M. K. (Ed). (1994). *Reshaping dementia care: Practice and policy in long-term care*. CA: Sage Publications.

Bandura, A. (1986). *Social foundation of thought and action: A social cognitive theory*. Englewood Cliffs, NJ: Prentice-Hall.

Barnouw, V. (1985). *Culture and personality*. Belmont, CA: Wadsworth Publishing Co.

Beaulieu, E. M. (2001). *A guide for nursing home social workers*. New York: Springer Publishing Co.

Blazer, D. (2001). *Depression in later life* (3rd edition). New York: Springer Publishing Co.

Burbank, P. M., & Riebe, D. (Eds.). (2001). *Promoting exercise and behavior change in older adults: Interventions with the transtheoretical model*. New York: Springer Publishing Co.

Coon, D. W., Gallagher-Thompson, D., & Thompson, L. W. (Eds.). (2002). *Innovative interventions to reduce dementia caregiver distress: A clinical guide*. New York: Springer Publishing Co.

Dreher, B. B. (2001). *Communication skills for working with elders* (2nd edition). New York: Springer Publishing Co.

Dziegielewski, S. F. (2003). *The changing face of health care social work: Professional practice in managed behavioral health care* (2nd edition). New York: Springer Publishing Co.

Emlet, C. A., Crabtree, J. L., Condon, V. A., & Treml, L. A. (1996). *In-home assessment of older adults: An interdisciplinary approach*. Gaithersburg, MD: Aspen.

Estes, C. L. (2001). *Social policy and aging: A critical perspective*. Thousand Oaks, CA: Sage Publications.

Gallo, J. J., Fulmer, T., Paveza, G. J., & Reichel, W. (2000). *Handbook of geriatric assessment* (3rd ed.). Gaithersburg, MD: Aspen Publishers.

Geertz, C. (1973). *The interpretation of cultures: Selected essays*. New York: Basic Books.

Gelfand, D. E. (1998). *The aging network: Programs and services* (5th ed.). New York: Springer Publishing Co.

Greene, R. R. (2000). *Social work with the aged and their families* (2nd edition). New York: Aldine de Gruyter.

Gudykunst, W. B., & Kim, Y. Y. (1992). *Communicating with strangers: An approach to intercultural communication*. New York: McGraw-Hill, Inc.

Hofstede, G. (1991). *Cultures and organizations: Software of the mind*. London: McGraw-Hill Book Co.

Hooyman, N. R., & Kiyak, H. A. (2002). *Social gerontology: A multidisciplinary perspective* (6th edition). Boston: Allyn & Bacon.

393

Hummert, M. L., Wiemann, J. M., & Nussbaum, J. L. (Eds.) (1994). *Interpersonal communication in older adulthood: Interdisciplinary theory and research.* Thousand Oaks, CA: Sage.

Janicki, M. P., & Ansello, E. F. (Eds.). (2000). *Community supports for aging adults with lifelong disabilities.* Baltimore: Paul H. Brookes Publishing Co.

Kane, R., & Kane, R. (2000). *Assessing older persons: Measures, meaning, and practical applications.* Oxford: Oxford University Press.

Kane, R. A., Kane, R. L., & Ladd, R. C. (1998). *The heart of long-term care.* New York: Oxford University Press.

Kane, R. A., & Kane, R. L. (1987). *Long-term care: Principles, programs, and policies.* New York: Springer Publishing Company.

Keigher, S. M., Fortune, A. E., & Witkin, S. L. (Eds.). (2000). *Aging and social work: The changing landscapes.* Washington, DC: NASW Press.

Kleinman, A. (1988). *Rethinking psychiatry: From cultural category to personal experience.* New York: Free Press.

Kramer, B. J., & Thompson, Jr., E. H. (Eds.). (2001). *Men as caregivers: Theory, research, and service implications.* New York: Springer Publishing Co.

Lee, E. (Ed.). (1997). *Working with Asian Americans: A guide for clinicians.* New York: The Guilford Press.

Leutz, W., Greenlick, M. R., & Nonnenkamp, L. (2002). *Linking medical care and community services: Practical models for bridging the gap.* New York: Springer Publishing Co.

Lichtenberg, P. A. (Ed.). (2000). *Handbook of assessment in clinical gerontology.* New York: John Wiley.

McInnis-Dittrich, K. (2001). *Social work with elders: A biopsychosocial approach to assessment and intervention.* Boston: Allyn & Bacon, Inc.

Mezey, M. D., et al. (Eds.). (2000). *The encyclopedia of elder care: A comprehensive resource on geriatric and social care.* New York: Springer Publishing Co.

Minkler, M., & Estes, C. L. (Eds.). (1999). *Critical gerontology: Perspectives from political and moral economy.* Amityville, NY: Baywood Publishing Company, Inc.

Misra, D. (Ed.). (2001). *Women's health data book: A profile of women's health in the United States* (3rd ed.). Washington, DC: Jacobs Institute of Women's Health and the Henry J. Kaiser Foundation.

Nathanson, I., & Tirrito, T. (1998). *Gerontological social work: Theory into practice.* New York: Springer Publishing Co.

Noelker, L. S., & Harel, Z. (Eds.). (2001). *Linking quality of long-term care and quality of life.* New York: Springer Publishing Co.

Obeyesekere, G. (1990). *The work of culture: Symbolic transformation in psychoanalysis and anthropology.* Chicago: University of Chicago Press.

Olson, L. K. (Ed.). (2001). *Age through ethnic lenses: Caring for the elderly in a multicultural society.* Lanham, MD: Rowman & Littlefield Publishers.

Ory, M. G., & DeFriese, G. H. (Eds.). (1998). *Self-care in later life.* New York: Springer Publishing Co.

Osterweil, D., Brummel-Smith, K., & Beck, J. (Eds.) (2000). *Comprehensive geriatric assessment.* New York: McGraw-Hill, Inc.

Pynoos, J., & Liebig, P. S. (1995). *Housing frail elders: International policies, perspectives, and prospects*. Baltimore: The Johns Hopkins University Press.

Richardson, V. E. (1993). *Retirement counseling: A handbook for gerontology practitioners*. New York: Springer Publishing Co.

Scherer, M. (2002). *Assistive technology: Matching device and consumer for successful rehabilitation*. Washington, DC: American Psychological Association.

Schneider, R. L., Kropf, N. P., & Kisor, A. J. (Eds.). (2000). *Gerontological social work: Knowledge, service settings, and special populations* (2nd edition). Belmont, CA: Brooks/Cole.

Shweder, R. A. (1991). *Thinking through cultures: Expeditions in cultural psychology*. Cambridge, MA: Harvard University Press.

Spilker, B. (Ed.). (1996). *Quality of life and pharmacoeconomics in clinical trials*. Philadelphia: Lippincott-Raven Publishers.

Swanson, E. A., Tripp-Reimer, T., & Buckwalter, K. C. (2001). *Health promotion and disease prevention in the older adult: Interventions and recommendations*. New York: Springer Publishing Co.

Teresi, J. A., Lawton, M. P., Holmes, D., & Ory, M. (Eds.) (1997). *Measurement in elderly chronic care populations*. New York: Springer Publishing Co.

Toseland, R. W., & McCallion, P. (1998). *Maintaining communication with persons with dementia*. New York: Springer Publishing Co.

Triandis, H. C., & Berry, J. W. (Eds.). (1980). *Handbook of cross-cultural psychology*. Boston: Allyn & Bacon, Inc.

Trotman, F. K., & Brody, C. M. (Eds.). (2001). *Psychotherapy and counseling with older women: Cross-cultural, family, and end-of-life issues*. New York: Springer Publishing Co.

Wacker, R. R., Roberto, K. A., & Piper, L. E. (1997). *Community resources for older adults: Programs and services in an era of change*. Thousand Oaks, CA: Pine Forge.

Zarit, S. H., Pearlin, L. I., & Schaie, K. W. (Eds.). (2002). *Personal control in social and life course contexts*. New York: Springer Publishing Co.

INDEX

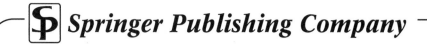

Springer Publishing Company

Innovative Interventions to Reduce Dementia Caregiver Distress

A Clinical Guide

David W. Coon, PhD,
Dolores Gallagher-Thompson, PhD, ABPP,
and Larry W. Thompson, PhD, Editors

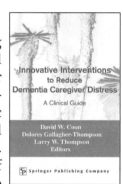

This volume provides an overview of emerging themes in dementia caregiving research and presents a broad array of practical strategies for reducing caregiver distress, including interventions for specific populations such as ethnic minority caregivers, male caregivers, and caregivers with diverse sexual orientations. Innovative approaches include the value of partnering with primary care physicians to improve quality of life for both patient and caregiver and the use of technological advances to help distressed caregivers.

Partial Contents:

Part I: Background Issues • Family Caregivers, *D.W. Coon, M.G. Ory, and R. Schulz* • Monitoring and Evaluating Interventions, *B.H. Gottlieb, et al.*

Part II: Practical Interventions for the Reduction of Caregiver Distress: Experience from the Field • Specific Stressors of Spousal Caregivers: Difficult Behaviors, Loss of Sexual Intimacy, and Incontinence, *M. Mittelman, A. Zeiss, H. Davies, et al.*

Part III: Case Examples of Interventions Tailored to Specific Caregiving Groups • Ethnic Minority Caregivers, *E. Edgerly, L. Montes, E. Yau, et al.*

2003   328pp   0-8261-4801-8   hardcover

536 Broadway, New York, NY 10012 • Fax: 212-941-7842
Order Toll-Free: 877-687-7476 • Order On-line: www.springerpub.com